STRESS, COPING, AND DEVELOPMENT IN CHILDREN

STRESS, COPING, AND DEVELOPMENT IN CHILDREN

Norman Garmezy, Ph.D.
Michael Rutter, M.D.
Editors

THE JOHNS HOPKINS UNIVERSITY PRESS
BALTIMORE

This volume is dedicated to
The Center for Advanced Study in the Behavioral Sciences—its conception and its staff

Originally published in a hardcover edition in July 1983 by the McGraw-Hill Book Company. The Johns Hopkins Paperbacks edition is published by arrangement with the McGraw-Hill Book Company.

Johns Hopkins Paperbacks edition, 1988

The Johns Hopkins University Press, 701 West 40th Street,
Baltimore, Maryland 21211

Library of Congress Cataloging-in-Publication Data

Stress, coping, and development in children.

Reprint. Originally published: New York:
McGraw-Hill, c1983.
Includes bibliographies and index.
1. Stress in children. I. Garmezy, Norman.
II. Rutter, Michael.
BF723.S75S77 1988 155.4'18 87-46302
ISBN 0-8018-3651-4

CONTENTS

EDITORS' PREFACE

THIS VOLUME GROWS OUT of a seminar that was held at the Center for Advanced Study in the Behavioral Sciences during the academic year, 1979–1980. During that period seven Fellows, then in residence, joined together to discuss two constructs of uncertain definition—*stress* and *coping* in children. That theme, until recently, has been an area of research neglected by those interested in the study of normal and abnormal developmental processes as well as by practitioners in child psychiatry and child clinical psychology.

The seven who agreed to participate were Garmezy, Kagan, Lipsitt, Patterson, Rutter, Segal, and Wallerstein. Diversity of interest and varying degrees of research commitment to the study of stress and coping characterized the group. Two (Garmezy and Rutter) had research programs already under way on risk factors and stress-resistance in children. Kagan and Lipsitt, developmental psychologists, had a broad expertise in research with infants and young children and strong ongoing research programs with these age groups. Patterson brought to the seminar a long-term research commitment to the study of antisocial children and of related coercive family practices; his work provided a continuing effort to generate intervention techniques for this highly refractory disorder. Segal and Wallerstein shared backgrounds of experience with two of the most powerful stressors of childhood—loss and separation. Wallerstein's research on children of divorce had drawn the nation's attention to a growing psychosocial trauma implicating millions of children. Segal had been asked repeatedly by the federal government to assist in problems concerning returning POWs, the stress of wartime separation in military families, and the repatriation of displaced Vietnamese refugee children and their families. In his role as Director of the Division of Scientific and Public Information for the National Institute of Mental Health, Segal bore a major responsibility for the dissemination of accurate mental health information to the public. Rutter contributed a broad knowledge of the etiology and epidemiology of many forms of childhood psychopathology. Garmezy had been very active in research with children at risk for schizophrenia and other forms of psychopathology and in the emergent area of research with stress-resistant children.

At mid-year Leiderman joined the group, bringing his knowledge of both adult and child psychiatry together with a normative and cross-cultural perspective in research on infant development, the nature of attachment and bonding, and a growing interest in the adaptation of families with infants born with severe congenital physical handicaps.

The seminar met 29 times over a span of nine months. Eighteen of the sessions were given over to individual research presentations by seminar members together with discussions of the implications of the methods and findings for the study of stress and coping. Eleven other sessions were used for colloquia presentations by invited speakers. The authors acknowledge their appreciation to the following guests: Thomas Almy, Paul Baltes, Deena Flowers, Norma Haan, Herbert Haynes, Mardi Horowitz, Seymour Kety, Joseph Kriss, Richard Lazarus, Seymour Levine, Clark Slayde, and Emmy Werner.

From February to April 1980 a series of sessions was devoted to discussions by the group as participants outlined the structure and content of the chapters they intended to write for a projected volume. Group discussions that followed led to a consensus that the volume would be one that emphasized the different authors' perspectives on stress and coping in children using their research interests as a frame for the contents of the chapters.

It was evident to the group, as the outline of the volume took shape, that several important broad perspectives would be missing unless other researchers were invited to participate. In particular, a major orientation that was absent from our group was a biological perspective on stress. To remedy this shortcoming, invitations were extended to Roland Ciaranello and Seymour Levine of the Department of Psychiatry, Stanford University, to contribute individual chapters. Their acceptance of the invitation has provided a better balanced and more representative volume that reflects more adequately the interdisciplinary nature of stress research. Two other chapters were also invited, again in the interest of balance. Social and emotional development is a fundamental key to an understanding of coping, particularly with older children, but it was not reflected in the composition of our group. Eleanor Maccoby agreed to fill this gap and provided an important chapter. Sociology, which has contributed greatly to stress research, also remained unrepresented, and Lee Robins' acceptance of our invitation to contribute a chapter not only brought sociology into the fold but did so by contributing a much needed methodological critique of relevance to all researchers studying stress factors and behavioral responsiveness.

As a result of these additions, twelve investigators have examined the problems of stress in children from a multiplicity of viewpoints. The book's organization encompasses five areas.

1. The first two chapters serve as an introduction to the chapters that follow. Rutter has contributed his views on the central issues and perspectives from which to consider the three concepts that dominate the volume: stress, coping, and development. Garmezy has followed with a discussion of the literature of two stressor categories, both implicating loss and separation for children: the first concerns the interpersonal trauma of a child's loss of a significant caregiver, the other looks at war and its effects on children as a trauma that brings in its aftermath profound familial and social dislocations and instability. The chapter concludes with a brief overview of various types of research that reaffirm the resilience of children even in dire circumstances.

2. The next two chapters, by Ciaranello and Levine, emphasize neurochemical and physiological contributions to stress research. Ciaranello presents the nature of neurochemical systems, indicating how they respond to stress; also, he provides necessary technical details on the nature of such processes. His emphasis is on the need to recognize the significance of model building that is designed to integrate these processes into a higher-order conceptual framework of behavior. Levine summarizes the role of the pituitary-adrenocortical system in stress, reaffirming the critical importance of a psychobiological perspective. He has illustrated this orientation with findings from his laboratory's primate research. This research demonstrates the central importance given by Levine to the organism's exercise of control over the traumatic situation, with the attendant feedback that follows. The control factor is seen as responsible for effective coping across species—reaching its greatest power among primates. Levine's observations on attachment and the effect of maternal deprivation on the adaptation of the infant monkey provide important parallels to human behavior. Experimental interventions to ameliorate social deficits in the infant caused by separation are more than mere analogues. Primate research has added to our understanding of the stressful effects of separation and their reduction through peer participation, substitute mothering ("aunting"), and surrogate mother rearing. Similarly, his examination of the role of the mother's presence on arousal of the infant, the effects of reunion on cortisol response, the impact of separation on the mother-infant dyad, all these have relevance for the human mother-infant interaction before and after separation.

3. The third part of the volume comprises four chapters devoted to a developmental-psychological perspective. These are provided in sequence by Leiderman (the newborn), Lipsitt (infancy), Kagan (early childhood), and Maccoby (middle-childhood and beyond). In these transitions from newborn status to middle childhood each of our four contributors has examined significant stressors of the age period they have focused upon. Leiderman begins his chapter with an evaluation of the three major perspectives on stress in the adult—biological, psychological, and social—and then turns to their applicability to children. He emphasizes the impact of the rapidity of biological and psychological growth in children on the internal and external perturbations to which children are subjected. The interaction of child and environment during these formative years calls for a meticulous description of the environment in which the child must function. Leiderman moves from these general statements to a specific environment he has come to understand as a researcher. He has selected prematurity and the environment of the stressed premature infant—the newborn nursery—as a central theme. In this setting a highly stressed dyad—mother and infant—must cope with the temporally earliest separation. Leiderman's discussion of bonding and the facilitative environment that has now become the hallmark of many nurseries housing premature infants is the focus of the latter portion of his chapter. In the context of factors that facilitate the coping process, these environmental changes can be thought of as another manifestation of the redemptive power of an external support system. In the case of prematurity it helps mother and child, to some extent, to reduce the stress to which each has been subjected.

Lipsitt focuses on the universals of certain developmental tasks in infancy, which he links in a speculative fashion to a little understood disorder of infancy—sudden infant death syndrome (SIDS). He places the origins of coping behavior in the earliest days of life, pointing to the defensive behaviors of infants as they seek to promote physiological integrity. Defensive behaviors in the face of aversive stimuli represent early prototypes of the coping behaviors to come, with initial biological defensiveness the precursor to the psychological defenses that will follow.

Kagan's perspective is also a universalistic one, in which he demonstrates (with cross-cultural replications) distress evocation in two-year-olds facing the challenge of a specific task that calls for imitation of an adult model in which the child's appraisal leads to an anticipation of failure to perform effectively. For Kagan, distress engendered in this way reflects a critical transition in the life of the young child, a growth of awareness of self and one's limitations, during a period in which a profound interaction comes to exist between temperamental qualities, parental practice, and the behavior of two- and three-year-olds.

Maccoby has provided a review of social-emotional responsiveness in middle childhood and beyond in which she presents a set of developmental principles linking increasing age, transitional stressor events, children's vulnerabilities, and emerging coping patterns in the move from childhood to adolescence. Her examples of these developmental principles provide content that reveals the child's world of stress as seen in two ecologies: the real world and the laboratory.

4. The fourth area relates to the ecology of the family as the stress agent and is represented by chapters written by Patterson and by Wallerstein. These investigators are concerned with children at risk. In Patterson's research, the focus is on antisocial behavior. In Wallerstein's work, divorce is the antecedent for a variety of children's ills including depression, "acting-out" behavior, and potential neurotic conflicts in seeking close relationships with others. Patterson searches for the mechanisms and processes implicated in antisocial behavior in children in the hope that their discovery will provide a rationale for relevant interventions with such children. His locus is the family and the pattern of escalating coercive regulatory interactions between aggressive child and mother, which seems amenable to behavioral change in some families, not in others. Where such shifts away from coercive practices can be obtained, a diminution in antisocial behavior in the child is also evident. Patterson's complex methods of interaction analysis serve as an exciting example of a transposition from laboratory procedures to their utilization in the therapeutic management of children at risk for antisocial behavior.

Wallerstein also provides a view of process-oriented research engaged in by a very sensitive and sophisticated clinician. Hers is a long-term longitudinal prospective study of children's efforts to cope with divorce. She points to important developmental tasks for children of divorce—tasks that must be met and constructively realized for the child's ultimate freedom from the trauma induced by divorcing parents. She traverses a broad age range for children caught up in such a stressful experience, providing many clinical examples of the emotional impact of the divorce experience on a cohort she has seen in treatment at the Center for the Family in Transition, which she directs.

5. The fifth segment of the volume focuses on two important issues for stress researchers: 1) the dissemination of scientific findings and 2) methodological issues that raise questions about presumed causal relationships in studies of stress.

Segal's theme is a provocative one. There are massive mental health problems that extend beyond the treatment room and are evident in a substantial portion of the population. At what point and in what manner can we provide this large group with scientific information that may help to create a better, less stressful life for them and for their children? What level of confidence in the data of our sciences and in their reliability is needed before release is permitted of such information to the media for distribution to the citizenry? Segal's answer is one of caution. The inconclusiveness of research findings and the cautionary notations of investigators tend to be bypassed by media—not out of maliciousness but out of a felt need to simplify the findings of researchers. At what point, then, does information, often partial and incomplete, become the basis for advocacy? What does one do with the mass of oversimplified self-help books that fill the bookstores and that can damage as well as elevate? These are the essential concerns of Segal, whose life work has been concerned with the transmission of helpful mental health data to millions of America's citizens.

The last chapter in the volume is provided by a distinguished sociologist, Lee Robins. Her chapter is a methodological one in which she, too, provides a cautionary note with regard to two stress themes elaborated elsewhere in the volume—divorce and its effects on children, and antisocial behavior. Drawing on her own research Robins presents a series of caveats and a planned program of epidemiological research aimed at stress prevention in children. She describes the need for baseline measures and the creation, now under way, of instruments that will help to secure measures of children's behavioral status as a basis for learning about the efficacy of different modes of intervention.

These are some of the contents of this volume. Do they provide a coherent answer to the complex problems of the effects of stress and the quality of different patterns of coping in childhood? The conservative and appropriate answer must be no. We now stand at the starting point for studying stress and its vicissitudes in children. Perhaps this volume will contribute one solid step into that future. That is the only compensation we can offer for those whose expectation was to gain a sense of closure into a complex and fascinating area.

The completion of this volume has been facilitated by many persons and agencies. Collectively our dedication represents our acknowledgment to the Center and staff that supported our stay there. To our colleagues in the venture go our heartfelt thanks not only for their contributions to the volume but to the deep friendships that emerged from our year together. Special words of appreciation from individual authors to foundations, federal agencies, and support figures who were responsible for facilitating their stay at the Center and their writing of individual chapters appear in the acknowledgments.

We all join in an expression of gratitude to Dr. Robert Haggerty, President of the William T. Grant Foundation, for his foreword to this volume and to the Foundation for the support that enabled the authors to meet together at the Center in March 1981, to review draft chapters of the volume and to participate in a conference sponsored by the Foundation on stress and coping in children following that editorial review.

The authors express their collective thanks to Mr. Tom Quinn, McGraw-Hill's Editor-in-Chief of Social Sciences, for his strong support of this volume from its inception to its publication.

In Minneapolis, we wish to acknowledge the role of Janis Abraham in bringing this volume to fruition. In London, we express our gratitude to Joy Maxwell for assaying a similar role.

NORMAN GARMEZY
MICHAEL RUTTER

FOREWORD

STRESS IS AN INTERESTING WORD. Most laypersons have no difficulty saying when they are under stress, and attributing all manner of problems to stress. Researchers, on the other hand, have considerable difficulty defining stress. They have tended to avoid the concept as too global, although, in recent years, there has been a modest amount of research on the physiological and psychological consequences of environmental stimuli perceived to be stressful. Most of this work on stress has been limited to adults. The work reported by the authors of this volume is unique for it focuses on stress in the developing organism—the child. The group of pioneers who report their work in this volume have examined the developmental aspects of stress, its definition, its effects upon children, and the ways in which children cope and adapt to stress.

We have found it useful at the William T. Grant Foundation to use the concept of stress and coping as an umbrella term, fairly easily understood by the public, to cover the area on which we focus our support—research on problems of adjustment in the school age and adolescent period. As the scientists whose work is reported in this volume emphasize, the definition of the concept of stress needs considerably greater precision before it can be used for research. But it has withstood the rigors of careful scrutiny by this group and has still emerged as a useful concept. Part of its usefulness lies in the fact that it brings several diverse problem areas and external events together—problems such as school failure, school-age pregnancy, and drug and alcohol abuse; and environmental stressful events as different as divorce, a death in the family, or the upset caused by a chronic physical disease. All of these may have a common theme if one relates them to stress. It is the nature of science to proceed by reduction, which usually leads to workers having difficulty communicating across disciplines or across problem areas. Rarely do workers on these problems or life events coordinate their work or collaborate. The term stress counters this reductionism with an integrated theme and brings together possible common causes of diverse outcomes.

Stress combines, in one term, the external stimulus, such as death of a relative, divorce, or a move, and the host or individual's response to the stimulus, such as anxiety or depression. There is still an argument among research workers as to whether the stimulus must be aversive or not to be stressful, or whether any life change is in itself stressful, even if it leads to beneficial results for the individual and his family. We recognize that stress is a part of all life, and that learning how to cope successfully with stress is an important aspect of children's development. Our goal in sponsoring research on stress in children is not to lead to elimination of stress, but to discover how children learn to cope with stress in ways which do not lead to disease or maladaptation. We believe that with this information we will be better able to develop programs that will help children learn, during critical phases of their development, how to cope with the inevitable stresses that will occur during their later life.

The William T. Grant Foundation is very pleased to have been able to assist some members of the group, whose work is published in this volume, during their stay at the Center for Advanced Study of the Behavioral Sciences at Stanford, and also to sponsor the conference which brought together additional research workers to consider the issues and opportunities in the field of stress, coping, and development in children. We are especially grateful to the participants and to their leaders, Dr. Norman Garmezy and Dr. Michael Rutter. Together these research workers have defined the state of the field and outlined the research needs for the future in this important area. Their work should lead ultimately to better health for children.

ROBERT J. HAGGERTY, M.D.
President, William T. Grant Foundation

CHAPTER 1

STRESS, COPING, AND DEVELOPMENT: Some Issues and Some Questions

MICHAEL RUTTER, M.D.
PROFESSOR OF CHILD PSYCHIATRY AND HONORARY DIRECTOR
M.R.C. CHILD PSYCHIATRY UNIT
INSTITUTE OF PSYCHIATRY, LONDON

INTRODUCTION

"The single most remarkable historical fact concerning the term 'stress' is its persistent, widespread usage in biology and medicine in spite of almost chaotic disagreement over its definition" (Mason, 1975). It is a concept which is familiar to both layperson and professional alike, and hence it is understood by all, so long as it is used in a sufficiently vague and *general* context (Cox, 1978). On the other hand, because "stress" lacks any agreed upon definition, it is understood by very few, and even by those few in totally contradictory ways, whenever a precise account is required. This confusion over the meaning of "stress" is not new. As the *Oxford English Dictionary* makes clear, the use of the term goes back to at least the early fourteenth century, at which time the word had already acquired several rather different meanings. Thus, stress seems to apply equally to a form of stimulus (or stressor), a force requiring change of adaptation (strain), a mental state (distress), and a form of bodily reaction or response (that is, Selye's general adaptation syndrome of stress).

In view of this all-too-evident chaos, confusion, and controversy, why has the concept of stress proved to be so enduring? After all, as Miller (1960)

A slightly modified version of this chapter has appeared in the *Journal of Child Psychology and Psychiatry*, vol. 22, 1981.

put it, the discipline of the philosophy of science "craves wary walking in the thicket of ill-defined concepts," and there is no doubt that stress constitutes just such a thicket, with an unusually rich growth of tangled thoughts and thorny assumptions. The answer lies in the fact that, for all its overinclusiveness, the concept of stress draws attention to some interesting and important phenomena. Moreover, in the absence of a good understanding of the mechanisms involved, it has been impossible to agree on which term or terms should replace it.

The two other concepts in the title are at least as diffuse and unsatisfactory as that of stress, but, nevertheless, they too refer to issues of great consequence in developmental psychopathology. The first issue, which perhaps may be thought to involve the notion of "coping," is that of individual differences in children's responses to all manner of stressful events, happenings, and circumstances. As part of this general topic, there has grown an increasing interest in the phenomenon of resilience, as shown by the young people who "do well," in some sense in spite of having experienced a form of stress which in the population as a whole is known to carry a substantial risk of an adverse outcome (Anthony, 1974; Antonovsky, 1979; Coelho, Hamburg, & Adams, 1974; Garmezy, 1976, 1981; Lazarus, 1966; Moos, 1976; Murphy & Moriarty, 1976; Rutter, 1978, 1979; Vaillant, 1977; Werner & Smith, 1982).

The second issue focuses on the further specific questions which arise whenever a developing organism is concerned. That is, not only do we have to ask whether the processes involved in stress and coping differ according to the child's stage of development, but more particularly we need to determine whether adverse experiences or happenings in early life alter the course of subsequent development or influence the ways in which an individual responds to much later stress events.

The question of how far early experiences have long-term effects extending into later childhood or even adult life has proved remarkably difficult to answer (Rutter, 1980a). However, it is clear that the links between infancy and adulthood are complex, indirect, and uncertain.

STRESS

Association between Life-Event Stress and Psychiatric Disorder

In considering the topic of stress it is appropriate to begin with the basic question of whether there is an association at all between stressful life events of any type and the development of some kind of psychiatric disorder. There are numerous methodological problems involved in this seemingly straightforward question. Not the least of them concerns the definition and measurement of life events and of psychiatric disorder. However, there is also the more troublesome point of the meaning of any correlations found. Do stressful events *cause* psychiatric disorder or, conversely, does the presence of disorder (or its precursors in the form of personality or lifestyle variables) increase the likelihood of *having* stressful experiences? Or, alternatively, are both stress and disorder due to some third set of variables with the intercorrelation between the first two purely artifactual? These difficulties are by no means entirely resolved (Dohrenwend & Dohrenwend, 1974, 1980) but, even so, there is reasonably strong evidence that, *in adults*, stressful life events play a significant role in provoking the onset of suicide, depressive conditions, neurotic disorders and, to a lesser extent, schizophrenia (Andrews & Tennant, 1978; Brown & Harris, 1978a; Lloyd, 1980b; Paykel, 1978). Evidence is mounting, too, that such events serve to precipitate and to maintain physical illnesses (Cohen, 1979).

The main research strategy has been some kind of case-control comparison, in which psychiatric patients (or individuals identified as having a disorder on the basis of an epidemiological survey) are contrasted with members of the general population found to be free of psychiatric disorder. A typical finding is that some three-fifths of patients have experienced a "severe" life event in the weeks prior to the onset of a disorder compared with about one-fifth of controls (Brown & Harris, 1978a). The main grounds for supposing that the stresses may have truly provoked the psychiatric disorder are: (1) that the differences still apply when life events are rigorously defined and when information is obtained through similarly searching, standardized interviews in both groups, ensuring that there is no contamination between the measurements of events and of disorder; (2) that the differences are much more marked in the period immediately preceding the onset than during any earlier period prior to the onset; and (3) that the differences are maintained even when events are restricted to those which appear independent and outside the control of the person (such as bereavement, or discovering a burglary, or learning of a father's serious illness).

Pooling data of this type, Paykel (1978) estimated that life events involving threat led to a sixfold increase in the risk of suicide during the subsequent six months, to a two- to five-fold increase in the risk of depression, and to a two- to three-fold increase in the risk of schizophrenia. It should be added that most of the events preceding psychiatric illness are not major crises such as bereavement, life-threatening illness, or financial ruin, but rather more everyday disturbances such as marital disruptions, difficulties at work, or personal rebuffs and rejections. As Paykel concluded, the findings indicate effects of some importance, but, equally, it remains true that many major threatening life events are *not* followed by psychiatric disorder and, conversely, that many disorders are not preceded by life events of any severity. Marked individual differences in response to stressors have been striking in all studies.

Many questions remain in connection with the role of stress events in adult disorders, but there is a substantial mass of studies providing empirical evidence in support of such a relationship. In sharp contrast, there is a great paucity of evidence on the possible importance of stressful life events in the genesis of psychiatric disorders in *childhood*.

Of course, under the rather broad and general heading of "maternal deprivation," there have been many studies showing that adverse experiences of various kinds may substantially increase the risk of psychiatric disorder in childhood (see Rutter, 1981a). But most of these refer to rather chronic and long-lasting adversities such as those involved in prolonged family discord and disharmony, parental rejection and neglect, or an institutional upbringing; however, less is known about the effects of relatively acute stressful life events such as those investigated in adults.

However, there are some relevant findings which come from several different sources. One of the most important early studies was that by Meyer and Haggerty (1962), in which for one year they followed prospectively 100 children in 16 families, undertaking throat cultures for streptococci every two weeks, and having the family keep a diary of "upsetting" events which occurred to family members and a record of illnesses. They found in the two weeks prior to documented streptococcal infections there was a marked increase in upsetting events as well as clinically recognizable upper respiratory infections. Although only about a quarter of streptococcal infections were preceded by such stressors, the risk of infections increased several fold after a stressful event. In the eighteen years since that pioneering study there have been only a handful of other investigations into the links between extrinsic stressors and physical disease in childhood. These vary in rigor and, in view of their methodological limitations, they provide no more than somewhat equivocal modest support for the notion that there may be a link (Haggerty, 1980; Heisel, Ream, Raitz, Rappaport, & Coddington, 1973).

There have been equally few attempts to study the psychiatric sequelae of acute stresses in childhood, but there are a few scattered investigations that point to their possible importance. For example, Hudgens (1974) noted a relationship between severe personal stressors and depression, in a group of adolescents with medical disorders; Douglas (1973) found that a high number of stress events in the first four years of life was associated with an increased likelihood of later enuresis; and Heisel et al. (1973) found that a high number of stresses were more common in children with psychiatric disorder than in general population controls. None of these studies made differentiations according to the type of stress event and none was able to examine the effects of independent events which were not also associated with chronic adversity.

Perhaps a better test is provided by the study of isolated specific events. Three rather different events—*hospital admission*, *birth of a sibling*, and *parental divorce*—may serve as examples of this style of approach. So far as hospital admission is concerned, there are numerous studies which show that many, but not all, preschool children exhibit emotional disturbance at the time (see Rutter, 1981a; Vernon, Foley, Sipowicz, & Schulman, 1965). Such disturbance may persist for some months after the child returns home. However, one hospital admission of less than a week is *not* associated with any significantly increased risk of long-term disorder some years later (Douglas, 1975; Quinton & Rutter, 1976). We may conclude that a single hospital admission constitutes a precipitant of short-term distress and disorder in young children but that longer-lasting sequelae are unusual.

Less is known about children's reactions to the birth of a sibling, but Moore's (1975) small scale longitudinal study of London children showed that some 15% developed difficulties—most often in the form of "problem" behavior or a disturbed mother-child relationship. The recent longitudinal study by Dunn and her colleagues (1981) provides more detailed findings. They found that more than half of the 40 two- to three-year-old children studied became more tearful after the birth of a sibling, one-fourth developed sleeping difficulties, and nearly half showed new toileting problems. The study design did not include a control group so that we do not know what proportion of children would have shown these changes even without the birth of a sibling. Nevertheless, the magnitude and timing of the changes make it highly likely that, at least in large part, the changes in behavior were indeed precipitated by the events surrounding the addition to the family of a brother or sister.

Little is known regarding the long-term effects. However, there is some indication that eldest children, but not only children, may have a slightly increased risk of emotional disturbance later in childhood (see Rutter, Tizard, & Whitmore, 1970). Both share the experience of being first born (which has implications for patterns of parent-child interaction—see Rutter, 1982) but only eldest children experience the birth of a sibling. The evidence is fragmentary and inconclusive and, even if the association proves valid, it is open to more than one interpretation. Nevertheless, one possibility is that sibling rivalry plays some part in the process, although whether such rivalry, when it occurs, stems from events in the period immediately following the birth of a sibling has yet to be determined.

The third example, parental divorce, differs from the other two in that the stress event, namely the separation of the parents, generally takes place following a rather prolonged period of discord and disharmony. Numerous studies indicate that much of the disturbance in the children stems from such discord, rather than from the separation per se (Rutter, 1971, 1982). Nevertheless, the recent longitudinal studies by Hetherington and her colleagues (1978, 1979a, 1979b) and by Wallerstein and Kelly (1980) clearly show that, in many children, emotional disturbance tends to worsen immediately following a divorce. It would appear that the circumstances associated with the divorce do constitute an additional stressor which may aggravate or precipitate emotional difficulties.

While the evidence is not as strong as one would wish, we may conclude that stress events in childhood, as in adult life, may serve to provoke at least short-term disturbance. Up to this point stress events have been considered in a rather general way, taking a commonsense view on the sorts of happenings which might prove upsetting to people. However, if the concept of stress is to take us beyond the banal conclusion that bad experiences may have bad effects, we need to undertake a more searching analysis that would implicate three factors: (1) which features of life events may predispose to (2) which types of disorder (3) by which underlying processes or mechanisms.

Physiological Responses to Stressors

In this connection, the first striking point is that the kinds of stressors studied by psychophysiologists bear little relationship to those studied by social scientists (Mason, 1975). Selye (1950, 1956) conceptualized stress as a nonspecific physiological pattern consisting of hypertrophy of the adrenal cortex, atrophy of the thymus, and gastric ulceration. In his early work, the stressors involved noxious physical stimuli such as mechanical trauma or the injection of foreign substances which constituted a physiological challenge to the organism. However, more recent experimental studies with animals have extended the range of stressors to include events that cause arousal as a result of novelty, uncertainty, or unpleasantness, but not necessarily as a result of physiological threat or challenge (Hennessy & Levine, 1979). Similarly, human studies with adults have dealt with a variety of life events such as examinations, parachute jumping, admission to the hospital, wartime combat, and various fear-evoking stimuli (Cox, 1978; Rose, 1980).

The results of these biological studies are reasonably consistent in showing a fairly predictable and similar endocrine response to most important changes in the environment. Initially, there is an increase in cortisol, in catecholamine secretion, in growth hormone, and in prolactin, but a fall in testosterone (Rose, 1980; Ursin, Baade & Levine, 1978). However, there is a rather rapid adaptation to repetition of the stress stimuli, particularly with respect to the cortisol response. Moreover, the nature and timing of the endocrine response alters with further exposure to the stressor, so that the main reaction takes place during the anticipation phase rather than in the period following the event. On the other hand, heart rate and epinephrine secretion tend to increase afresh with each new encounter even in individuals well-habituated to that particular stressor—indicating that there are different components of the physiological response which function in disparate ways. However, these group findings convey a misleading picture of consistency since numerous investigations have affirmed very marked individual differences in the response to potentially stressful events (Rose, 1980). For example, studies of the parents of children dying of leukemia (Wolff, Friedman, Hofer, & Mason, 1964), of women undergoing breast biopsy for possible malignancy (Katz, Weiner, Gallagher, & Hellman, 1970), and of children admitted to the hospital for tonsillectomy (Knight, Atkins, Eagle, Evans, Finkelstein, Fukushima, Katz, & Weiner, 1979) have all found that some people fail to exhibit the expected increase in cortisol secretion. On the whole, it seems that these differences in endocrine response are linked to variations in how people perceive the event and how they respond emotionally to the situation.

Crucial questions remain regarding the implications of these findings for psychopathology, four of which may be singled out as fundamental. First, the endocrine response appears to be one that applies to a very wide range of stimuli, many of which have no known association with disease or disorder of any kind. Indeed, increases in catecholamine excretion have been found following both tennis and sexual intercourse (see Rose, 1980), which many regard as pleasurable activities that facilitate coping with daily stresses. Whether cortisol secretion also increases with pleasant forms of activation is not known at this time.

Second, little is known about endocrine responses to chronic stress. On the whole, it seems that there are rather few changes.[1] For example, Rose, Jenkins, and Hurst (1978) found no consistent relationship between cortisol response and work load in air traffic controllers. Of course, it could be suggested that in actuality the work did not constitute a chronic stressor. However, this does not seem to constitute a sufficient explanation in that, as a group, air traffic controllers *were* found to have a substantially increased rate of hypertension which was thought to have arisen as a result of work stress. The matter must remain open in the absence of data on endocrine

[1] As expected, there are autonomic changes in relation to recurrent life events known to act as stressors. Thus, Tarrier, Vaughn, Lader, & Leff (1979) found skin conductance and heart rate changes in the home (but not in the laboratory) in schizophrenic patients following life events. However, endocrine responses were not assessed, and it is not known whether the autonomic changes predicted relapse.

responses to chronic stress situations known to carry a much increased risk of psychiatric disorder.

Third, there is a paucity of data on the links or lack of links between the endocrine response to stressors and the development of psychiatric disorder. Very few of the studies have examined any kind of disease or disorder as an outcome variable, and those that have done so have produced rather inconclusive findings. Thus, for example, in the air traffic controllers study cited above, those with a high rate of physical illness tended to have *lower* cortisol levels and *less* variability in blood pressure readings; those who developed hypertension had an *increased* blood pressure response on high workload days; and those who developed psychiatric disorder did not differ in blood pressure level but had a slightly above average level of cortisol (Rose et al., 1978). Cortisol responsivity, however, was more strongly associated with the concurrent *presence* of psychiatric disorder than with a predisposition to develop disorder later. In the Ursin et al. (1978) study of parachute jumpers, endocrine responsiveness did not clearly differentiate the seven men who quit after the first jump, although in those men there was a strong association between norepinephrine and expressed fear that was not evident in the group as a whole. It remains quite possible that the physiological response to stressors *may* ultimately prove to be linked with the development of psychopathology, but such a link has yet to be demonstrated.

The fourth point concerns the variety of sequelae which may follow stressful life events—ranging from anxiety states and depression to schizophrenia in the behavioral domain, and from streptococcal infections to hypertension in the field of physical disease. Does this type of physiological response to the life event predict the type of outcome? Currently very little is known on this point, but it is a question that warrants further study.

Types of Life-Event Stress on Adults

In the stress events studies by social scientists we encounter rather a different range of stressors. Instead of the very brief physically noxious stimuli unconnected with chronic psychosocial adversity favored by psychophysiologists, we have sets of events which tend to occur as part of a broader network of chronic problems (such as divorce or a marital quarrel); or which necessarily involve lasting or permanent life changes (such as bereavement or becoming unemployed); or which may stem in part from the person's own behavior (such as losing a friend, or being arrested, or having an abortion). Accordingly, we need to ask: Is there any evidence as to the types of events which are and which are not liable to provoke psychiatric disorder?

In attempting to answer that question we immediately run into twin problems: (1) how should types of events be categorized; and (2) how far should the personal meaning of an event to each individual be taken into account? Is bereavement automatically regarded as an unpleasant experience or may it be considered pleasurable or at least neutral in its capacity for emotional arousal if it involves release from an intolerable relationship? How should immigration be judged when it may be perceived as a splendid challenge and opportunity with the chance of a fresh start, but also may be seen as an oppressive burden, the breaking of old ties, and a frightening threat involving all the uncertainties of the unknown? It is all too apparent that there is no easy answer to these questions. On the one hand, it seems obvious that stress responses must be viewed in terms of a transaction between the individual and the environment with the meaning and appraisal of the event intrinsic to its definition (Lazarus & Launier, 1978). On the other hand, this carries the danger of becoming a tautology in that the people who see a change as a threat rather than an opportunity may have that perception just because they have responded to the event with a depressed mood.

These constitute difficult methodological issues. Nevertheless, the distinctions are real enough, and, moreover, observers agree well on ratings of meaningfulness, such as the "contextual threat" of an event (Tennant, Smith, Bebbington, & Hurry, 1979). The first distinction we need to consider is that between pleasant and unpleasant life changes. Much of the early work, based on the Holmes and Rahe scale (Holmes & Rahe, 1967), utilized an approach in which events were rated in terms of the *degree* of life change involved, regardless of whether the change was for better or worse. However, more recent research has been reasonably consistent in showing that the associations with psychiatric disorder are largely confined to unpleasant or undesirable events (Gersten, Langner, Eisenberg, & Orzek, 1974; Paykel, 1974; Tennant & Andrews, 1978; Vinokur & Selzer, 1975). Even major changes such as engagement, marriage, or promotion at work, do not seem to provoke disorder if they are predominantly pleasurable in quality.[2]

Paykel (1974) also drew a somewhat different distinction—that between "entrances" and "exits," with the former including items such as the birth of a child or the addition of a new person to the home, and the latter including such items as a child marrying or leaving home. He found that "exits" were most strongly associated with psychiatric disorder, with "entrances" linked with attempted suicide but not depression. The suggestion is that the loss of

---

[2] This statement must be qualified by adding that in certain predisposed individuals even pleasurable events may act as stressors because of the threat implicit in the degree of change (as in the cases of engagement neurosis described by Davies, 1956, in which the magnitude of the decision constituted the stress, which was then relieved by the act of marriage which resolved the uncertainty), or because of the physiological upheaval (as in the psychiatric disorders arising in the puerperium—Kendall, Wainwright, Hailey, & Shannon, 1976). Moreover, there are some events which involve major adaptations but which are neither clearly pleasurable nor unpleasant in quality—for example, starting to attend school for the first time.

an important relationship is more likely to provoke disorder than the gaining of a new one. However, presumably much depends on the particular meaning of specific entrances and exits and, so far as children are concerned, it should be noted that the entrance event of the birth of a sibling does seem to constitute a significant stressor. Of course, that may well be because the arrival of the sibling results in an alteration of the parent-child relationship, but that only serves to emphasize the importance of considering the meaning of the event as well as the crude fact of whether a person has been added to or lost from the family (or social) circle.

Yet another differentiation is that between events within the control of the person (such as marriage) and those (such as serious illness in a family member) which are outside his control (Paykel, 1974). Both types of event seem to be linked with psychiatric disorder, but Paykel (1974) found that the link was substantially stronger in the case of "uncontrolled" events.

Brown and Harris (1978a) compared events according to the duration of threat in terms of the social context. In essence, short-term threat events referred to those which were anxiety-provoking or unpleasant at the time, but which involved no long-term consequences. They give as examples witnessing a serious accident or having to deliver a neighbor's baby in the middle of the night. In contrast, events with a long-term threat were those with necessary sequelae of some kind such as the loss of a relationship, the threat of death implicit in a very serious illness, or the change in lifestyle which follows the loss of a job. It was found that it was only events with a *long-term* threat which provoked depressive disorders. A more detailed analysis of the events showed that the great majority involved loss or disappointment of some kind. Brown and Harris (1978a) suggest that this is indeed the key feature of those stressors which predispose to psychiatric disorder in adult life.

Stress Events in Childhood

There are no comparable studies of children in which the effects of different types of stress are contrasted systematically. However, we may utilize the adult findings as a guide in considering which might be the crucial aspects of life events that make them liable to provoke psychiatric disorder in children.

With respect to hospitalization, the most obvious feature is the child's age at the time. Distress is most marked in those aged between about 6 months and 4 years (Illingworth & Holt, 1955; Prugh, Staub, Sands, Kirschbaum, & Lenihan, 1953; Schaffer & Callender, 1959). As this is the age when selective attachments are first forming and yet when children are only just beginning to be able to maintain relationships during a period of separation, the implication is that the interference with attachment implicit in a hospital admission may constitute one of the features which make it stressful. Two other findings tend to support this suggestion. First, young children's distress is much reduced by either daily visits or the presence of a familiar person such as a parent or a sibling. Second, individualized family care during a period of separation from the family reduces young children's distress (Robertson & Robertson, 1971), and a supportive relationship with a consistently present nurse reduces emotional disturbance during hospital admission (Visintainer & Wolfer, 1975). It seems that the immediate disturbance during hospital admission is due in part to the child's separation from all people to whom he is attached, together with a lack of opportunity to form new attachments.

But, is that all that makes going into a hospital stressful? It seems not, in that quite a variety of measures *not* involving attachment—including reading preparatory booklets about hospital procedures, a preadmission home contact, and a peer modeling film—have all been found to lower significantly the incidence of emotional disturbance during and immediately after admission (Ferguson, 1979; Wolfer & Visintainer, 1979). It is clear that a hospital is anxiety-provoking for reasons intrinsic to hospital care and to medical or surgical treatment, quite apart from the stress of separation. It should be added that these same studies which have evaluated different means of preparing children for hospitalization also suggest that, to a considerable extent, the benefits to the children stem from the effects of the measures in allaying *parental* anxiety. Children may be affected as much by their parent's attitudes and mental state as by any hospital procedures that apply to them as individuals.

We may conclude, then, that part of the immediate distress caused by hospital admission stems from the combination of a strange and frightening environment and parental anxiety. Measures designed to reduce either are likely to reduce the child's distress in the hospital. However, reducing immediate distress and reducing the effect of admission in provoking psychiatric disorder are not necessarily the same thing at all. Thus, hospital admission rarely provokes disorder in older school-age children, although they may find the experience unpleasant (see Rutter, 1981a). Indeed, Ferguson (1979) found that the experience of hospital admission tended to *reduce* fears of hospital in school-age children, but not in preschoolers. Moreover, Brown, Chadwick, Shaffer, Rutter, and Traub (1981), in a study of children admitted to the hospital for orthopedic injuries, found *no* increase in the rate of psychiatric disorder four months after the accident. It seems that, except occasionally, a single hospital admission does not constitute a significant factor in the evocation of psychiatric disorder in older children.

In younger children, emotional distress lasting some months after admission is appreciably more frequent. The question is whether the *after* effects of admission are purely explicable in terms of distress experienced during admission. Unfortunately, good data are lacking on this crucial point. Nevertheless, there are indicators to suggest that other factors concerned with experiences after reunion with the family are operative. First, it seems that persisting disturbance is more likely if the child comes from a deprived or disturbed family, or if the previous parent-child relationship was poor (Douglas, 1975; Quinton & Rutter, 1976; Stacey, Dearden, Pill, & Robinson, 1970). Second, primate studies indicate that an infant's disturbance after separation is strongly connected with the quality of the mother-infant relationship (Hinde & McGinnis, 1977). The implication is that the nature of the parent's response to a child's difficult and clinging behavior on return home from the hospital may help determine whether the emotional distress is rapidly alleviated, or instead goes on to constitute a more persistent psychiatric disorder. The issue calls for systematic study.

Similar issues arise with respect to children's responses to the birth of a sibling. Dunn and Kendrick (1980b) found that, following the birth of a second child, mothers tended to engage in less playful interaction with the first child, and also evidenced more prohibitions, confrontations, and negative verbal interactions. The development of emotional and behavioral problems in the firstborn was linked in part to temperamental variables and with the mother's mental state (children of depressed mothers were more likely to exhibit signs of withdrawal) as well as with changes in the mother-child relationship (Dunn, Kendrick, & MacNamee, 1981). As Dunn and her colleagues conclude, the relationship between a mother and her 2- to 3-year-old is often a difficult one, and it seems that the constellation of changes involved when a sibling is born is enough to heighten these difficulties, even when the second child is born at home so that there is no separation of the mother and firstborn. In the case of the birth of a sibling, the stress to the elder child seems to lie largely in the effects that this has on the patterns of family interaction.

The third childhood stressor considered above was parental divorce. Sometimes there has been a tendency to view divorce as if it were only a positive solution to destructive family functioning. For the child, according to that view, the resolution of the family conflict should be generally beneficial, with the loss of one parent from the household as the only likely stressor in the situation. Recent research, especially that by Hetherington and her colleagues (Hetherington, Cox, & Cox, 1978, 1979a, 1979b; Hetherington, 1980), by Wallerstein and Kelly (1980), and by Hess and Camara (1979), has clearly shown that those assumptions are wrong. It is true that, in the long-term, a conflict-ridden intact family is more deleterious than a stable home situation in which the parents are divorced. It also appears that an inaccessible, rejecting, or hostile parent is more detrimental to the development of a child than is the absence of a parent (Hetherington, 1980). On the other hand, the assumption that divorce necessarily brings conflict to an end is mistaken, and certainly it is not the case that the absence of one parent is the only potential stressor for the child. In the immediate aftermath of divorce, both parents tend to be inconsistent, less affectionate, and lacking in control over their children (see Wallerstein's chapter). In many divorcing families, there is a period during the first year following divorce when mothers become depressed, self-involved, erratic, less supportive, and ineffectually authoritarian with their children. Fathers often begin by being unduly indulgent and permissive, but then increase in restrictiveness and in the use of negative sanctions. The postdivorce family relationships—between the parents and between each parent and the child—play a major role in determining the consequences of divorce for the children.

Differential Effects of Different Types of Stressor

At least so far as hospital admission, birth of a sibling, and parental divorce are concerned, it seems that much of the stressful quality of the event lies in its effects on patterns of family interaction and relationships. This is an important observation, but the particular effects on interaction and relationships are not necessarily the same in all three cases; nor can it be assumed that they will be the same with all other varieties of apparently stressful life events. Accordingly, we need to ask whether different types of events lead to different types of outcome.

The evidence on this point is decidedly limited for children and not much greater for adults, but the suggestion is that there may be different effects with different stressors. Thus, for example with adults, Jacobs, Prusoff, and Paykel (1974) found that the recent life events associated with depression tended to be particularly those which involved disturbed interpersonal relationships, whereas those associated with schizophrenia were less specific in type; Brown and Harris (1978a) found that long-term threat was crucial in evoking depression but not schizophrenia; and Leff and Vaughn (1980) found that the interaction between expressed emotion in the family and life events was quite different in the cases of schizophrenia and depression. The onset or relapse of schizophrenia was associated with *either* highly expressed emotion *or* an independent life event, whereas for depression it was the *conjunction* of a relative prone to be critical and a life event which proved to be provocative. Brown and Harris (1978a) also tentatively suggested that loss events tended to be particularly associated with depression whereas *non*-loss events involving uncertainty were more likely to lead to anxiety. In the somatic arena, it is striking (and puzzling) that "Type A" personalities (i.e., hard-driving, competitive, impatient, aggressive people) tend to have an increased risk of coronary artery disease (Glass, 1977; Marmot, 1980; Rosenman, Brand, Sholtz, & Friedman, 1976) but apparently a *decreased* risk of hypertension; the latter tends to be associated instead with "Type B" personalities (Rose et al., 1978), characterized by a more calm and relaxed approach and a tendency to seek goals in a less pressured, less intense manner.

The findings with children are rather sparse but they, too, suggest differential outcomes. Thus, Felner, Stolberg, and Cowen (1975), in a study of primary school children in Rochester, compared the behavioral patterns associated with parental death and with parental divorce or separation. They found that the bereaved children tended to manifest heightened shyness, timidity, and withdrawal; whereas those from divorced or separated families were more likely to show aggressive antisocial problems.

Concepts of Psychosocial Stress

The utility of the concept of psychosocial stress needs to be considered with this rather meagre and scattered array of empirical findings in mind. Does the use of the term "stress" in any way add to our understanding of the processes involved or clarify our thinking about underlying mechanisms? Its use ought to suggest that the experiences included under its umbrella have some essential quality in common, or have similar consequences, or are comparable in terms of their provocation to disorder. But is this the case?

In attempting to answer that question, perhaps reference should be first made to research on neuroendocrine processes. As we have seen, a very wide range of stimuli have been found to give rise to a rather similar endocrine response, leading Hennessy and Levine (1979) to suggest that the terms "psychological stress" and "arousal" are essentially synonymous. Ursin, Baade, and Levine (1978), indeed, view stress in terms of neuroendocrine activation and actually define successful coping with stress in terms of a response decrement in the physiological activation processes accompanying the response to threat. Similarly, Rose (1980) and Levine (1982) both point out that endocrine findings may show a marked stress response when this is not evident in behavior or self-reports.

Should we then adopt a neuro-endocrine definition when considering psychosocial stress? I suggest not, for four rather separate reasons. First, just as it is possible to show a neuro-endocrine response without observable behavioral change, so too is the converse true. For example, Curtis, Buxton, Lippman, Nesse, and Wright (1976), in a study of seven phobic patients undergoing "flooding in vivo" treatment, found that whereas confrontation with the feared object led to a very marked upsurge in anxiety and obvious emotional distress, it was *not* accompanied by any changes in plasma cortisol. Second, the events leading to neuro-endocrine activation include many that reveal *no* tendency to provoke disaster. Third, physiological measures have been found to be rather poor predictors of the likelihood of developing psychiatric disorder (see, e.g., Rose et al., 1978). Fourth, an absence of a neuro-endocrine response to a psychosocial stressor may mean that the individual has not been affectively aroused by the situation, but it does not mean that he has coped with it successfully in any other sense. For example, Katz, Weiner, Gallagher, and Hellman (1970) found that women with breast tumors who responded by denying the risk of malignancy had low cortisol levels; from a neuro-endocrine viewpoint they had coped successfully but only at the cost of waiting a dangerously long period before seeking medical attention. Similarly, in terms of the psychosocial tasks involved in coping successfully with a threatening situation, a degree of activation (or neuro-endocrine stress) may be helpful (see, e.g., Hofer, Wolff, Friedman, & Mason, 1972).

If, on these grounds, neuro-endocrine definition for psychosocial stress is abandoned, what do we put in its place? It appears that most of the stressors which provoke psychiatric disorder involve some form of loss or disappointment on the one hand or disturbed interpersonal relationshps on the other. It seems generally unhelpful to lump these all together under the broad rubric of stress. Rather it would be better, I suggest, to differentiate the several various types of life events according to their psychological meaning and consequences. It is true that we do not yet know exactly how such events are best classified, but it seems likely that progress will come through further attempts to do so by using differences in empirically identified processes or consequences as the validating criteria rather than by aggregating various heterogeneous happenings. Leads as to how to proceed are available from prior research, based primarily on adults rather than children, but it remains to be seen whether the variables studied so far will prove ultimately to be the most effective differentiators.

Does this approach mean that we have to reject the notion that short-lived events which involve no loss or disappointment and no disturbance of interpersonal relationships, but which do lead to physiological arousal and activation, are of no psychiatric consequence? These events might include such well-known stressors as the taking of examinations, being involved in an accident, experiencing a robbery, being taken hostage, undergoing shelling or a bomb attack, or being bitten by a dog. It would be foolhardy to suppose that these are without effect. Indeed, it is obvious that they may be accompanied by considerable short-term anxiety and also that they may lead to conditioned fear reactions which affect later behavior, especially when subsequent similar situations are encountered. However, it does seem that, on the whole, frightening events without personal connotations in terms of loss, discord, and the like, are probably less likely to provoke psychiatric disorder than those with persisting consequences in terms of altered personal relationships or negative self-appraisal. Whether "pure" fear-provoking events may be relatively more important in the genesis of particular types of psychopathological reaction (such as anxiety states) remains to be determined. The matter warrants study and the term "stress events" is worth retaining for this group of happenings. In that connection, it is necessary to take into account the sheer number of such events per unit time. It could be that single fear-provoking events are of very limited consequence but that many experienced over a short period of time are more likely to be damaging.

Other considerations are also required. In lay parlance, annoying or unpleasant events are often said to be stressful, even though they do not involve fear. Irritating and intrusive noises such as aircraft flying overhead for those people living under flight paths near an airport, or the constant yapping of noisy dogs in a neighbor's garden, or the blaring of pop music through the wall of the adjoining house, all fall into that category. Regrettably, we know surprisingly little about the effect of such unwanted stimuli. However, Tarnopolsky, Barker, Wiggins, and McLean (1978) and Tarnopolsky, Watkins, and Hand (1980) did examine the effects of aircraft noise on adults. They confirmed that most people found high levels of aircraft noise very annoying, but, overall, there was no difference in rates of psychiatric disorder according to whether people lived in a high or low aircraft noise area. In general, it seemed that noise was not a very important factor in the precipitation of psychiatric disorder, but, on the other hand, there was some suggestion that there might be more of an effect on certain subgroups. No information was obtained of the effects on children.

Most of the findings discussed so far have applied to major events or circumstances of some kind, but it is not self-evident that it is these that matter most. Lazarus (1978) quotes Charles Bukowski in making this point poetically: "It's not the large things that send a man to the madhouse. . . . No, it's the continuing series of small tragedies that send a man to the madhouse . . . not the death of his love but a shoelace that snaps with no time left. . . ." In his own work, Lazarus (1978) has therefore focused on daily "hassles" and positive events as well as major changes. There are immense methodological problems in this approach, if only because so many of the minor hassles and pleasures of the day are brought about, at least in part, by persons themselves as a consequence of the way they are feeling. The person who travels to work with a smile is more likely to have a pleasurable encounter and less likely to have an irritating and unpleasant interchange than a colleague who pushes through the crowd with a scowl. Nevertheless, it is not an unreasonable suggestion that the balance between pleasant and unpleasant events might be important in predisposing to mental health or ill-health (Lazarus, Cohen, Folkman, Kanner, & Schaefer, 1980).[3] Indeed, Norman Cousins (1976), in describing his own unexpected recovery from a serious collagen disease, argued that if negative emotions produce harmful chemical changes in the body then perhaps positive emotions should have a therapeutic value. He attributed much of his own beneficial outcome to his self-generated program which included "laughter therapy," consisting of watching old *Candid Camera* vignettes and being read selections from humorous books.

It is clear that it is still too early to bury completely the concept of stress. Nevertheless, it does seem that it has little use (and indeed is obfuscating) in its more general form. Like the somewhat comparable global term "maternal deprivation" (Rutter, 1981a), it has served a purpose in drawing our attention to important phenomena, but now it is time to undertake a more discriminating analysis of the different effects that are likely produced by the various contrasting types of life events sometimes considered "stressful."

COPING

In doing so, it will also be necessary to consider the different ways in which people *respond to* or *cope with* stressful events or situations. Most forms of psychosocial stress do not constitute a short-term single stimulus but rather a complex set of changing conditions that have a past history and a future one (Mechanic, 1978). Hence, adaptation or coping need to be considered as a process extending over time. In recent years this process has come to be seen as the key to an understanding of stress reactions. Thus, Lazarus and Launier (1978) suggest that "the ways people cope with stress [may be] even more important to overall morale, social functioning and health/illness than the frequency and severity of episodes of stress themselves," (p. 308). By coping, they mean "efforts, both action-oriented and intrapsychic to manage (i.e., master, tolerate, reduce, minimize) environmental and internal demands, and conflicts among them, which tax or exceed a person's resources" (p. 311). The steps a person takes to deal actively with stress may well be important, but that topic needs to be considered as part of the broader issue of individual differences. Clearly, it would be wrong

---

[3] There is some preliminary evidence from studies of adults that satisfaction and well-being are indeed correlated with the presence of positive life experiences as well as the lack of negative ones. However, the data do not adequately test the hypothesis that it is the balance between them that matters with respect to deviant outcomes of any kind (Kanner, Kafry, & Pines, 1978).

to assume that the only source of differences in the outcome following stress events concerns strategies or tactics for dealing with the challenges or threats implicit in the events.

Individual Characteristics

The personal qualities and characteristics that an individual brings to the stress interaction are likely to be important; relevant variables of this type include age, sex, genetic factors, temperament, intelligence, and other problem-solving skills.

Age

The effects of age have already been noted with respect to hospital admission. With that particular stress event the age period of greatest risk has proved to be about 6 months to 4 years. Circumstantial evidence suggests that this is a consequence of two rather different factors. Children below the age of 6 or 7 months are relatively immune because they have not yet developed selective attachments and therefore are not able to experience separation anxiety. Children above the age of 4 years or so, on the other hand, are less vulnerable, probably because they have the cognitive skills needed to appreciate that separation does not necessarily mean abandonment or loss of a relationship and to understand better what is involved in hospitalization and the necessity of unpleasant medical or surgical procedures.

With the birth of a sibling, age is perhaps less critical, but both Dunn et al. (1981) and Moore (1975) found that younger children were those most likely to show at least some forms of disturbed behavior—particularly increased clinging. The reasons for this age-effect are not well understood, but it might be suggested that older children are less at risk because the greater age gap means that the new baby is less likely to be felt as a rival, or because it is easier to give an older child a role of responsibility with the baby (so that the sibling serves to enhance the firstborn's feeling of self-esteem and importance), or because mothers are less likely to alter their pattern of interaction with an older child, or because an older child is less dependent on mother for play activities. Whatever the explanation, it seems likely that the factors are not identical to those that apply to hospital admission.

The *form* of children's responses to parental divorce, naturally, is modified by their age and level of development (Wallerstein & Kelly, 1980; Wallerstein, this volume), but it does not seem that there are marked age differences in the general threshold of vulnerability to the effects of divorce. Children of different ages tend to react to rather different aspects of the divorce, and their patterns of coping, too, are not the same. However, it does not seem that vulnerability is markedly increased or decreased in any specific age period.

Bereavement, perhaps, is worth particular mention because it brings out an additional point—namely that age may influence the short-term and long-term effects in rather different ways. Adequate systematic data on representative samples are lacking, but the findings suggest that immediate grief reactions are both milder and of shorter duration in young children compared with those in adolescents or adults (see Bowlby, 1980; Kliman, 1968; Rutter, 1966). The reasons for the age difference probably lie in the child's cognitive level and in the consequent variations in the ability to conceptualize both the past and the meanings of death. On the other hand, although the *immediate* grief reactions seem to be more short-lived in younger children, the *delayed* consequences in terms of psychiatric disorder may well be greater (Rutter, 1966). These long-term effects are probably a result of factors consequent upon the death, as much as the death itself. These include hazards such as the breakup of the home, frequent changes of caregiver, changes in family roles, financial and material disadvantage, the effects of bereavement on the surviving parent, and the arrival of a stepparent (Furman, 1974; Rutter, 1966). It is clear that with bereavement—as with many other supposedly acute stresses—the event as defined may be brief in duration but the consequences are both chronic and complicated.

But age may be important, too, for reasons separate from age-specific vulnerabilities. Thus, in part, the meaning and impact of events may be influenced by whether or not they occur at what are usually regarded as the "appropriate" times in the life cycle (Hultsch & Plemons, 1979). For example, Bourque and Back (1977) suggest that events in adult life, such as the departure of children or retirement, are felt to be more disruptive if they occur at a "nonnormative" age.

Age, then, is an important variable for some types of stress events, but even in those for which it is important, the effects and the mode of operation vary according to the category of the event.

Sex

In contrast, at least with prepubertal children, sex differences in response to most kinds of stress events seem to operate in the same direction. That is to say, boys appear to be more vulnerable (Rutter, 1970, 1982). The evidence is least striking with respect to the effects of hospital admission, but with this event too, there has been some tendency for more males to show adverse effects (Rutter, 1981a). With the birth of a sibling, Dunn et al. (1981) found that boys were more likely than girls to show an increase in withdrawal behavior (sex differences for other forms of behavioral change were not statistically significant). With divorce, both Hetherington (1980) and Wallerstein and Kelly (1980) found that disturbance tended to be more severe and more prolonged in boys. Similarly, there has been a tendency for boys to show more behavioral change in response to day-care (Rutter, 1981b) and more aggressive behavior in relation to parental discord and disharmony (Rutter, 1982).

The reasons for this general sex difference in children's reactions to stress events or indeed to changed situations of any type remain unclear. Various suggestions have been put forward. These include the possibility that parents are less supportive of boys in their attempts to cope with the changing life circumstances or are more likely to respond negatively to their distress reactions (Elder, 1979; Hetherington, 1980); that the patterns of interaction are affected by temperamental differences associated with sex (Eme, 1979); that the salience of the stress events may sometimes be greater for boys (Block, Block, & Morrison, 1981); and that there may be a biologically determined increased male vulnerability to physical hazards (Rutter, 1970). We lack evidence on which to base a choice between these (and other) alternatives and it is not at all certain whether the explanation for the sex difference will prove to be the same or different for different types of stressors.[4]

Genetic Factors

It is, of course, well recognized that genetic factors play a significant part in determining individual differences in both development and in susceptibility to disorder. However, it is perhaps less generally appreciated that hereditary influences may affect either the *extent* to which individuals respond to environmental variables (ordinal interaction) or indeed sometimes the *direction* of their responses (disordinal interaction) (Shields, 1980). For example, studies of both Crowe (1974) and Hutchings and Mednick (1974) suggest that the genetic variables associated with criminality may operate in this way, at least in part. It seems from their data that the presence of a genetic predisposition to criminality may render children more vulnerable to adverse environmental influences—influences which have little impact on children who are not susceptible (see Rutter, 1978). The finding in both studies is based on quite small numbers, and replication is needed before firm conclusions are drawn. Nevertheless, their observations open up a potentially important area for future research—the relevance of individual differences in response to stress events.

---

[4] Sex differences also may not be the same for immediate and for enduring effects. For example, Hennessy and Levine (1979) found that female mice were more likely than male mice to show a sensitization effect to repeated electric shock stimulation.

Temperament

There is now considerable evidence that infants and young children show wide individual differences in behavioral *styles*, that is, in the "how" of their behavioral responses to differing situations (Dunn, 1980; Keogh & Pullis, 1980). In part these temperamental differences are genetically determined (Torgersen & Kringlen, 1978). The observation that children may vary in their temperamental features as they grow older, and also may behave differently in different situations, led some commentators to dismiss the importance of individual characteristics of this kind. However, this dismissal is misconceived for two separate reasons. First, there is some evidence that the nature of this individual variability across situations and across ages is itself genetically determined to a significant extent (Matheny & Dolan, 1975). Second, even though individual temperamental features change as children grow older (as indeed they do change), nevertheless, such features may still play an important part in determining individual-environment interactions at any one time (Rutter, 1977).

It must be added that there is very limited direct evidence on either the extent or the nature of the contribution of temperament in modifying children's reactions to stress events. Nevertheless, in spite of continuing problems with both the concepts and the measures (Bates, 1980), significant associations have been found between temperamental features and psychiatric disorder, and between temperament and other people's responses to the child (see Rutter, 1977; Dunn, 1980; Keogh & Pullis, 1980). What are largely lacking are studies of the role of temperament in reactions to stress events. The study of children's responses to the birth of a sibling by Dunn et al. (1981) constitutes one of the very few exceptions. They found not only that the child's temperament [using interview measures shown to agree well with direct observations (Dunn & Kendrick, 1980a)] significantly predicted changes in behavior after the birth of a sibling, but also that there were significant interactions with the mother's emotional state and with the pattern of mother-child interaction. The implication is that the child's temperamental features increased the liability to behavioral changes after the birth of a sibling, but that this increased liability was due in part to the effect of temperamental features in modifying children's responses to altered parental behavior. It may also be that children of differing temperament *elicit* different parental behaviors. For example, in our own work with the families of mentally ill patients, we found that children with adverse temperamental characteristics were twice as likely as other children to be the target of parental criticism (Rutter, 1978). It seemed that, to an appreciable extent, a child's temperament protected him or put him at risk by virtue of its effect on parent-child interaction.

Intelligence and Other Skills

There is a slight but consistent tendency for children of above average intelligence to have rather low rates of psychiatric disorder (Rutter, Tizard, & Whitmore, 1970) and of sociobehavioral deviance generally. There is also some evidence that good intelligence and good scholastic attainment may exert a protective effect in the presence of chronic psychosocial adversity (Rutter, 1979). Little is known of the mechanisms involved, and even less as to whether intelligence is also important with respect to children's responses to acute stressors. However, the possibility warrants study. Such an hypothesized effect could operate through the protective influence of high self-esteem and a sense of achievement; or it could reflect greater problem-solving skills (Shure & Spivack, 1979); or it could be just that, for other reasons, intellectually able children are constitutionally more resilient.

It is evident that there is much still to be learned about the effects of individual characteristics such as these, and even more to be discovered about how they operate in increasing or decreasing vulnerability to various stressors. But it is already clear that their role is likely to be an important one.

Chronic Psychosocial Adversity

Although the stressors considered refer to acute events of one type or another, many of them often occur against the background of more chronic psychosocial adversity. The question, therefore, arises as to whether the presence or absence of chronic adversity influences the child's responses to acute life events. The matter has been minimally investigated up to now, but there is some suggestion that it does. For example, in our own epidemiological studies (Quinton & Rutter, 1976), we found that the effect of repeated hospital admissions in provoking emotional disturbance was greater in conjunction with high psychosocial adversity than it was in more favored family circumstances (Rutter, 1979). It was not just that the adverse effects summated but rather that they *potentiated* one another so that the combined effects of the two together was greater than the sum of the two considered separately. This potentiating interactive effect was also found for a combination of chronic stressors. Whether it similarly applies to a combination of acute stressors is not known. It also remains to be determined how far this multiplicative effect is a general occurrence.

Vulnerability and Protective Factors

In the combination of chronic and acute stressor, we are dealing with the effects of two variables, both of which, even in isolation, predispose towards disorder. However, interactive effects may also occur when one of the variables has *no* effect on its own. The notion here, then, is of factors which are largely inert on their own but which serve as *catalysts* when combined with acute stressors of some type—to use a chemical analogy. If the catalytic variables tend to *increase* the effect of stressors, they may be called "vulnerability" variables (as in Brown and Harris's 1978a work); when they tend to *reduce* the effect of stressors, they are usually termed "protective" factors (as those considered by Rutter, 1979). Such factors may be of various different types, but, in relation to the growing interest in theories of attachment in recent years (see Bowlby, 1969, 1973, 1980; Rutter, 1980b), researchers have increasingly focused on the possible importance of social networks and close personal relationships.

Social Networks and Close Personal Relationships

This is evident, for example, in Brown and Harris's (1978a) studies of origins of depression in women.[5] They identified three contemporaneous items as vulnerability factors—employment outside the home, a confiding relationship, and the presence of three or more children less than 14 years old. The findings may be illustrated by considering the presence of children. Of the women *without* any stressor, 2% of those without young children developed depression as against 0% of those with young children—clearly showing that the presence of children on its own did not predispose towards depression (if anything, the contrary). However, in the women *subjected to* a stressor, the presence of young children increased the risk of depression 2½ fold (from 17% to 43%). Broadly similar findings applied to the two other contemporaneous vulnerability factors. We may conclude, with Brown and Harris, that their data do show the kind of catalytic or potentiating effect of otherwise natural variables which they postulated.

However, the real test of the notion is not the application of statistics to one set of data but rather whether the findings can be independently replicated. Other investigations have used somewhat different sets of measures, but comparable interaction effects have been found in several studies. Examples include: Paykel, Emms, Fletcher, and Rassaby's (1980) study of life events and social support in the puerperium; Nuckolls, Cassel, and Kaplan's

---

[5] There has been a rather pointless controversy over the statistical models implicit in their concept of vulnerability (see Bebbington, 1980; Brown & Harris, 1978a, 1978b, 1980; Everitt & Smith, 1979; Tennant & Bebbington, 1978). The controversy lacks point because the crux of the issue does not lie in the particular sort of statistical interaction found, but rather in the much simpler notion that there are vulnerability variables which have a negligible effect in the absence of stressors and a significant effect in the presence of stressors—an effect, that is, which exceeds both the effect of the stressor on its own and also the sum of the separate effects of the vulnerability factor and the stressors when they occur in isolation. The chief limitation of the multivariate statistics usually employed to test for this interactive effect is that they use as their starting point the assessment of whether the vulnerability factor shows a significant main effect. Unfortunately, this is *not* the same as determining whether the variable has an effect in the absence of the stressor—the one datum crucial to the hypothesis (see Brown & Harris, 1978b; Rutter, 1979). As a result, the usual multivariate statistics are inappropriate for testing for this particular sort of vulnerability or protective effect.

(1972) study of psychosocial assets, life crises, and complications of pregnancy; Theorell's (1976) study of life crisis, discord, and illness; Eaton's (1978) analysis of life crisis, social supports, and psychiatric symptoms in the New Haven study; Gore's (1978) study of social support in moderating the health consequences of unemployment; Jenkins's (1979) analyses of psychosocial modifiers of response to stress in air traffic controllers; and Lin, Simeone, Ensel, and Kuo's (1979) study of the effects of social support and stressful life events on psychiatric symptoms in a Chinese-American sample. These studies vary in rigor, in the quality of statistical analysis, and in sample size, but the general pattern of findings is supportive of the suggestion that good personal relationships and social supports may mitigate the effects of stressful life events, and that a lack of such intimate relationships increases the adverse effects of stressors.

However, it should be added that protective factors need not necessarily involve features which appear intrinsically beneficial (Hultsch & Plemons, 1979). For example, Hinkle (1974), in commenting on his long series of life-change studies, noted that the people who seemed most immune to stress had an almost "sociopathic" flavor to their personality, in that they seemed to have a shallow attachment to people, goals, or groups; and they readily shifted to other relationships when established relationships were disrupted. Many of these people had an accurate awareness of their own needs and limitations and avoided situations that made demands on them that they did not want or felt that they could not meet. Similarly, Lieberman (1975) noted that the elderly people who best survived crises were often aggressive, narcissistic, and demanding. Jenkins (1979), too, in the air traffic controllers study, found that persons who rated high on "anomie" (meaning a feeling of alienation from other people), as a group had a higher rate of problems in impulse control, but, conversely, that the anomic group were *less* likely to develop such problems in high life-stress situations. These findings are interestingly provocative in their implications, but, obviously, replication is required before they can be accepted as valid.

These data all apply to adults, and, once again, less is known about comparable effects in childhood. However, in his study of children reared during the economic depression between the two world wars, Elder (1979) found that supportive relationships between the parents much reduced the likelihood of a helpless, passive, "failure" response. We, too, in our studies of the families of psychiatric patients, looked at the possible protective effect on the child having a good relationship with at least one parent (Rutter, 1971, 1979). In families without discord, the presence of one good relationship made little difference, although it provided a substantial protective effect. Of the children in discordant homes with one good relationship, only a quarter showed a conduct disorder, compared with three-quarters of those lacking such a relationship. The findings are based on very small numbers, the stressor concerned was chronic rather than acute, and there is conceptual overlap between the protective factor and stressor. For all these reasons, caution is needed in the interpretation of the effects shown. Nevertheless, if nothing more, the observation suggests the utility of looking for the possible effects of vulnerability and protective factors in childhood, as in adult life.

The Social Group and the Social Context

The protective effect of personal relationships, in the studies just mentioned, was considered in individual terms. However, the possible protective effect of the social context must also be considered in group terms. This is most obvious, perhaps, in some of the wartime studies. For example, Bourne, Rose, and Mason (1967) found that helicopter ambulance medics showed neither behavioral signs of stress nor changes in urinary 17-hydroxycorticosteroids (17-OHCS) when flying combat missions under enemy fire. Interview data suggested that the job prestige and gratification led to a sense of high morale which counteracted the real threat of death or mutilation. Similarly, another study by the same investigators (1968) of Special Forces troops in Vietnam showed a drop (rather than an increase) in 17-OHCS on the day when attack by the Vietcong was expected. The increased morale associated with the relief from boredom and the flurry of productive activities countered the potential stress of possible death. In contrast, however, the captain and radio operator, who remained rather apart from the group, in that they spent most of the time in communication with headquarters, showed sharp increases in 17-OHCS levels—indicating that the situation was indeed stressful in the absence of group support. Perhaps the Israeli finding (Ziv & Israeli, 1973) that anxiety levels were higher among children from kibbutzim undergoing frequent shelling than among those from nonbombarded kibbutzim reflects a similar social group cohesion effect.

There is evidence that social organizational factors influence behavior in childhood. This is shown, for example, by the studies looking at school influences (Rutter, Maughan, Mortimore, Ouston, & Smith, 1979). Schools have been found to vary markedly in rates of disruptive behavior and absenteeism, and it has been shown that these variations are systematically related to the characteristics of the schools themselves, with their general ethos or social climate as one important feature. The findings suggest that schools can act as a force for good (or bad) even with children living under conditions of psychosocial disadvantage. Nevertheless, that is not the same as saying that the effect of the social group modifies children's response to stress events. That remains a plausible hypothesis, but one that has yet to be tested systematically.

But, quite apart from the possible modifying effect of the social group in altering people's perceptions of and reactions to stress events, school influences might operate in two other ways. First, just as good personal relationships in the family seem to be protective, perhaps good relationships with peers or with other adults outside the family may also serve to mitigate the effects of stress. Second, it is generally thought that people function better if they have a high self-esteem and an appropriate positive sense of their own worth. Does the experience of personal success at school or in the peer group aid the development of this confident feeling of being a worthwhile and competent person, and if it does, then does such positive self-esteem modify a child's response to acute stress events?

Cognitive Appraisal of the Stress Event

Although some of the early work on psychosocial stressors seemed to assume that life events could be studied without reference to their meaning to the individual, this view is no longer held by most investigators. Empirical findings suggest that a person's cognitive appraisal of life events strongly influences his response (Lazarus & Launier, 1978).[6] The same event may be perceived by different individuals as irrelevant, benign, and positive, or threatening and harmful. Hinkle (1974) cites the example of the Hungarian refugees at the time of their flight during their revolution in the mid-fifties. Regardless of the physical dislocation and the social, emotional, and psychological changes they had to undergo, it is claimed that most felt pleasurable excitement and anticipation, and experienced improved health and well-being during that time. At a more everyday level, people are likely to vary in whether a change of school or a move to another residence is seen as providing much-wanted opportunities or just additional burdens and problems. Hence, although little considered in children, it is highly likely that a person's primary cognitive appraisal of the positive or negative meaning of particular life events will determine whether they are experienced as stressful.

However, this is not the only form of appraisal which is important. Lazarus and Launier (1978) use the term "secondary appraisal" to deal with a person's conceptualization of the implications of the event in terms of coping resources and options. Seligman and his colleagues (Abramson, Seligman, & Teasdale, 1978; Seligman, 1975, 1978), in putting forward the concept of "learned helplessness," postulate a learned cognitive attribution style which varies on the dimensions (1) of the extent to which people anticipate positive outcomes; (2) of the extent to which they perceive the outcomes as within or outside their control; and (3) of the extent to which failure is attributed to

[6] Nevertheless, there is the major methodological problem that the use of subjective reactions and reports involves contamination of the event with the reaction to it (Mechanic, 1978).

unalterable faults in themselves, rather than either to behaviors which they can modify or to external factors which may change. Brown and Harris (1978a), too, utilize a somewhat similar cognitive model. They suggest that their "vulnerability" factors operate by creating feelings of low self-esteem and lack of mastery. This feeling of hopelessness, of being unable to do anything about their fate, in turn makes them less able to deal with stressful life events which persons without such a negative cognitive set may confidently take in their stride.

There is a good deal of evidence in favor of the *general* proposition that an individual's attributional style influences how he responds to life events, although data are lacking on the specific link in terms of the hypothesized mediating influence on the outcome with respect to stressors. Little of the research in this area has been undertaken with children, but that which has is interesting in its implications. Dweck and her colleagues (Dweck & Bush, 1976; Dweck, Davidson, Nelson, & Enna, 1978) have shown that whereas boys tend to respond with *greater* efforts when they receive feedback from adults that they are failing, girls tend to give up and attribute their failing to their own lack of ability. One of the reasons for girls being more likely to give up seems to lie in the sex-differentiated pattern of feedback from adults. The pattern seems to be one likely to increase girls' tendency to feel that they cannot succeed whatever they do, whereas boys are given the message that their failure is a consequence of their misbehaving or not trying hard enough and hence that they *could* cope if they chose to do so. It has been suggested that the increasing experience of feedback from adults during the school years may make girls more likely to adopt an attributional style of "learned helplessness," which could perhaps explain, in part, why depression is more prevalent in women (Rutter, 1980c). The suggestion, of course, remains highly speculative but the role of cognitive sets and attributional styles in determining how children react to stress events seems to be worth empirical investigation.

Coping Processes

That reaction, of course, includes the coping process itself—i.e., what the person does about the stress situation. Coping mechanisms include individuals' attempts directly to alter the threatening conditions themselves, and the attempts to change only their appraisal of them so that they need not feel threatened.[7] That is, coping must have the dual function of problem-solving

---

[7] Coping has usually been discussed and studied in terms of the behavior of *individuals*, but, particularly so far as children are concerned, it may be at least as important to consider the coping process in terms of family *styles* and strategies—i.e., in terms of a group response which may not necessarily correspond to just the sum of the behaviors of the individuals in that group (see, e.g., Hansen & Johnson, 1979).

and of a regulation of emotional distress. Similarly, the means of meeting these objectives may involve both manipulation of the environment and intrapsychic processes.

Various attempts have been made to classify the different types of coping mechanisms. Some writers, such as Haan (1963, 1977), have made a differentiation between coping mechanisms (which are seen as healthy, reality-oriented, and conscious), defense mechanisms (which are regarded as rigid, distorting, and involving unconscious elements), and fragmentary processes (which are repetitive, unresponsive to requirements, and determined by affect needs). However, although the Haan (1977) model has some limited empirical support, these distinctions have not proved particularly helpful so far, and they seem to be based on a host of unwarranted assumptions (with respect to the use of terms, the grouping of attributes, and the concept of their constituting a personality dimension). Lazarus and his colleagues (Lazarus & Launier, 1978; Roskies & Lazarus, 1980) have proposed a classification based first on whether the function is to alter the troubled person-environment transaction, or to regulate emotion (i.e., problem-solving or palliation); and based second on the coping mode used. The coping modes are subdivided into information-seeking, direct action (either on the self or the environment), inhibition of action, and various intrapsychic modes. These categories are, of course, rather broad, and it remains quite uncertain whether they reflect dimensions which relate in any way to outcome. It should be added that coping can be anticipatory (i.e., initiated before an expected stressful encounter) or consequent upon the event (Lazarus, 1975). Thus, in anticipation, people may take on only those tasks they feel they can handle, they may insulate themselves against failure, or they may plan ahead and rehearse various solutions (Mechanic, 1978).

It is evident that some coping processes may *increase* the risk of maladaptation or disorder, while others may improve adaptation and reduce the risks of a deviant outcome (Lazarus et al., 1980). Hence, a further essential dimension is between effective and ineffective coping. The dilemma here is how to conceptualize, let alone measure, effectiveness. Obviously, the criterion of efficacy cannot be the avoidance of disorder, as that simply forces the tautology of successful coping being the "explanation" of resilience in the face of stress situations. "Solving" the problem cannot be used as the criterion either, as some problems do not admit of a solution. Discovering that you have an incurable cancer is, of course, extremely stressful, but whether that stress leads to depression need not depend on a new medical discovery which brings cure. Resolution of conflict, too, cannot be employed as a criterion as, in some circumstances, conflict may be resolved in ways which are profoundly damaging to health or to social functioning. The issues are summarized in the Alcoholics Anonymous prayer: "God grant me the serenity to accept the things I cannot change, courage to change the things I can, and the wisdom to know the difference."

It is clear that there can be no one (or even several) most successful coping strategy—the mode which is most effective is likely to vary with the type of stress and with the circumstances. But it may also be the case that some strategies are better suited to one person, whereas others are more appropriate to another person. Or, within a very broad range, does it not matter very much which coping mechanism is used so long as the obviously maladaptive and damaging ones are avoided? Or is it that the important thing is to do something, to make a decision, and act accordingly? Or, in the longer term, does successful coping depend on flexibility, adaptability, and an adequate range of strategies and tactics? Perhaps, as Pearlin and Schooler (1978) put it, "having a particular weapon in one's arsenal is less important than having a variety of weapons. . . . The single coping response, regardless of efficacy, may be less effective than bringing to bear a range of responses to life strains."

Intuitively, it seems that the coping process ought to play a role in determining the outcome following stress events. But, up to the present, both the concepts and the measures have proved elusive, and there is a lack of evidence that the particular coping mechanism adopted in fact matters at all in terms of the risk for psychiatric disorder (in adults or in children). But it may matter and the possibility should be studied.

DEVELOPMENT

Prior experiences remain the one major factor not so far mentioned which might influence the outcome of a stress encounter. Various developmental issues have been touched on already, for example with respect to age specificities in children's reactions to particular stressors. But the central issue has yet to be discussed—namely, the effect of stress events on the developmental process, and on subsequent functioning more generally. Of all the topics considered here, probably this is the one most difficult to investigate rigorously, if only because of the problems of separating the effects of early events from those of later events (see Rutter, 1980a). Not unexpectedly, the two tend to be linked.

There are, perhaps, five main ways in which early experiences might be linked with disorder some years later. First, early events might lead to disorder at the time, which then persists for reasons which are largely independent of the initial causation or provocation. The National Survey findings provide what may constitute an example of this kind. Douglas and Mann (1979) found that family adversities in childhood (such as the death of a sibling or parental divorce) were statistically associated with psychiatric problems in early adult life. However, a more detailed analysis of their data showed that this link was almost entirely a function of the prior associations between adversities in childhood and disorder in childhood. The link was with disorders provoked in childhood which then persisted into adult life. Another example of this kind would be the persistence of a conditioned fear response in the form of a phobia initially provoked by some acute stress event.

Second, the early events may lead to bodily changes which in turn influence later functioning. For example, a quarter of a century ago, Levine, Chevalier, and Korchin (1956) found that rat pups subjected to electric shock showed an enhanced resistance to later stress. Subsequent research has repeatedly confirmed the finding and has shown that it applied to a wide range of aversive experiences in infancy (Thompson & Grusec, 1970; Hunt, 1979). The explanation in this case seems to lie in changes in the neuroendocrine system which generates a more adaptive response to later stress (Hennessy & Levine, 1979).

Third, the early events may lead directly to altered patterns of behavior which, although changed at the time of the event, take the form of an overt disorder only some years later. No well-established example of this kind can be cited, but it may be that the social abnormalities which sometimes follow an institutional upbringing with frequently changing caretakers (see Rutter, 1980a) constitute a case in point.

Fourth, early events may lead to changed family conditions which, in turn, later predispose to disorder. In some circumstances the death of a parent may function in this way, with disorder developing some years later, not so much because of the death as such, but rather because of the chain of psychosocial adversities which followed (Rutter, 1966).

Fifth, however, early events may operate through their action in altering sensitivities to stress or in modifying styles of coping which then protect from, or predispose towards, disorder in later life only in the presence of later stress events.

Attention is focused on this last possibility, not because it is necessarily more important than the others, but rather because it is central to the overall theme of stress, coping, and development. Several points need to be made before turning to a few of the empirical findings. The most obvious and important is that the long-term effects of early stress events may be either beneficial or harmful (or, of course, they may be entirely without long-term consequences). There may be *sensitization* to the effects of later stressors, but also there are *steeling* effects involved in overcoming stress and adversity. Nor should it be assumed that the effects of stress are usually harmful. Many examples of adaptive consequences are well documented. The neuroendocrine studies on the effects of early stimulation, already mentioned, are a case in point. The effects of repeated acute stressful events, such as parachuting, in *reducing* the stress experienced when the same event is encountered again, is another. In a quite different vein, Elder (1979) reported that some young people gained from their experiences in coping successfully with the many stressors involved in the economic depression. The key question, in all cases, is what determines whether sensitization or steeling occurs?

A second point related to the first is that all children are likely to experience many potentially stressful life events as they grow up, and it is most unlikely that the long-term effects will depend largely on the *number* of such stressors encountered. Rather, it is more probable that the long-term outcome will be determined by *how* the stresses are dealt with at the time, and perhaps especially on whether the outcome of the stress encounter was successful adaptation or humiliating failure.

Another facet of the same point is that certain stressful events are *inevitable*, and one of the developmental tasks is to learn how to deal with them successfully when they occur. Thus, all children will have to separate from their families in order to achieve independence, all will suffer the death of their parents (if they live out their normal span), and all will experience serious illness at some point.

With those considerations in mind, two specific examples of stress events—multiple hospital admissions and the loss of a parent—may be discussed.

Multiple Hospital Admissions

The two key observations, in this connection, with respect to hospital admission are (1) that one admission during the preschool years has *no* association at all with psychiatric disorder some years later; and (2) that the experience of two hospital admissions *is* associated with a markedly increased risk of subsequent disorder (Douglas, 1975; Quinton & Rutter, 1976). The interest in these two findings is that the ill-effects associated with two admissions cannot be due simply to the additive effect of two stressors. This is not possible because there is *no* effect from one admission and hence nothing to summate. Of course, it could be that the risk linked with recurrent hospital admission has nothing at all to do with the admission itself. Perhaps the children experiencing multiple admissions differ in other respects, such as in coming from more disadvantaged homes. Indeed, this proved to be the case to some extent. However, the effect still holds up, even after chronic family adversity has been taken into account. While it is never possible entirely to rule out the operation of variables not measured or not assessed with sufficient discrimination, it does seem that this was not the explanation. Rather, the implication is that, although the first admission does not itself lead to disorder, in some way it predisposes the child to react adversely the second time he is hospitalized.

At present we lack data on how this apparent sensitization effect might operate. There is a total lack of human data, and animal studies are of only limited relevance. However, Spencer-Booth and Hinde (1971) showed that the effects of separating infant monkeys from their mothers for six days was sometimes still evident as long as two years later. But the difference from controls was only evident in a strange situation. The implication is that what persisted was an altered response to stress events rather than any form of generalized disorder. The monkey findings on the possible effects of early separation in altering responses to later separations are somewhat inconclusive, but there is some suggestion that there may be a sensitization effect (Mineka & Suomi, 1978). Of course, hospital admission is much more than just a separation and, in any case, human language skills may mean that the children anticipate and conceptualize the event in ways which make sensitization more likely. The mechanisms involved remain obscure and indeed it is not known whether the effect is due to the admission per se or the altered patterns of parent-child interaction which possibly followed; nor whether the sensitization effect at the time of the second admission resided in the parent's response or the child's reaction.

Loss of a Parent

Brown and Harris (1978a) found that the loss of mother before eleven constituted a vulnerability factor in that it increased the effect of stress events in provoking depression in women. However, whereas loss by death predisposed to psychotic depression only, loss by separation predisposed to neurotic depression only. The suggestion was made that past loss mainly served to influence the symptom pattern rather than to predispose to disorder as such. However, in his theoretical formulations, Bowlby (1969) has attributed a rather greater etiological role to the effects of early loss. He suggests that early loss sensitizes an individual, making him more vulnerable to later setbacks, and especially to loss or threats of loss. On the other hand, he emphasizes that this only happens to some individuals—the likelihood being influenced by the process of mourning at the time and by the pattern of family relationships both before and after the loss.

The hypothesis of a sensitizing effect from early loss is a plausible one, but, apart from Brown and Harris's findings (1978a), there is little empirical evidence in support—at least with respect to death. As several recent reviews have shown (Crook & Eliot, 1980; Tennant, Bebbington, & Hurry, 1980; Lloyd, 1980b), there is only a very weak and inconsistent overall association between parental death in childhood and risk of adult depressive disorder. On the other hand, not only have most of the studies restricted attention to just death (and not other forms of loss), but also few have provided data on the family processes surrounding the loss, and very few have examined interactive effects in conjunction with later losses. However, a recent study by Birtchnell (1980), limited by reliance on case records, suggested that the effects of early loss may be modified (for better or worse) by the quality of the relationship with the mother replacement and by the quality of the later marriage.

Further data are required to resolve the issues. Perhaps it seems unlikely that death of a parent per se plays a very important role as a vulnerability factor, but it remains plausible that certain forms of early loss (including some of those by death) which are associated with unsatisfactory family relationships may serve to sensitize and increase vulnerability to later losses. Once again, the matter warrants further study.

CONCLUSIONS

Undoubtedly the concept of stress has been useful in alerting people to several important sets of phenomena. However, in its most global form, the term "stress" has come to include a far too wide and heterogeneous range of events, which may well have different psychopathological consequences. What is needed now is a more discriminating analysis of the (probably) rather different effects of the various disparate types of life event sometimes considered "stressful." Happenings which reflect some form of loss or disappointment and those involving disturbed interpersonal relationships need to be differentiated from each other and from other types of life events. Calling both of these events "stressors" is unhelpful in drawing misleading parallels with the effects of acute physically noxious stimuli. On the other hand, it is probably useful to retain the term "stressor" for acute events, which do not involve loss or discord but which do lead to immediate physiological arousal and activation. How far such fear-provoking events are important in the genesis of psychiatric disorders in childhood remains quite uncertain, but the matter warrants study. Also, attention needs to be paid to different classes of happenings which are annoying or unpleasant, even though they do not involve fear. Finally, there is the possibly separate class of events which involve lasting life changes or adaptations (such as starting school), but which are not obviously positive or negative in affective tone.

In considering all types of stimuli, individual differences in responsiveness are crucial. Whereas some people develop disorder following adverse experiences, others do not. Indeed, not only may they show resilience in not having succumbed, but the "stresses" may have had a positive and beneficial effect. Our understanding of the processes involved in stress will remain rudimentary until we have gained an appreciation of why and how these individual differences operate. It seems that part of the explanation will lie in the personal qualities and characteristics which an individual brings to the stress interaction, with such variables as age, sex, genetic background, temperament, and problem-solving skills being important. Vulnerability and protective factors may serve as catalysts in increasing or decreasing the likelihood of a maladaptive outcome. A person's cognitive appraisal of the life event is known to be important, but it seems that the crucial elements of this appraisal involve not only perception of the meaning of the event, but also a cognitive set reflecting the anticipation of what can be done about it. Intuitively, it seems that the coping process itself, in terms of active problem solving and of emotional palliation, is likely to influence outcome, but empirical data on the actual importance of coping mechanisms are still lacking.

Last, we need to study the various different ways in which stress events may influence both the developmental process and also later functioning more generally. Traditionally, most attention has been paid to the direct effects of adverse experiences in leading to overt disorder. However, it seems that it may be at least as important to focus on the indirect effects. Thus, early events may operate through their action in altering sensitivities to stress, or in modifying styles of coping which then protect from, or predispose towards, disorder in later life only in the presence of later stress events. Although very little is known about this topic, it is quite possible that the related concepts of stress, coping, and development can be brought together in an interesting and potentially fruitful manner.

REFERENCES

Abramson, L. Y., Seligman, M. E. P., & Teasdale, J. D. Learned helplessness in humans: Critique and reformulation. *Journal of Abnormal Psychology*, 1978, *87*, 49–74.

Andrews, G., & Tennant, C. Life event stress and psychiatric illness. *Psychological Medicine*, 1978, *8*, 545–549.

Anthony, E. J. The syndrome of the psychologically invulnerable child. In E. J. Anthony, & C. Koupernik (Eds.), *The child in his family: Children at psychiatric risk*. New York: Wiley, 1974.

Antonovsky, A. *Health, stress and coping*. San Francisco: Jossey-Bass, 1979.

Bates, J. E. The concept of difficult temperament. *Merrill-Palmer Quarterly*, 1980, *26*, 299–319.

Bebbington, P. Causal models and logical inference in epidemiological psychiatry. *British Journal of Psychiatry*, 1980, *136*, 317–325.

Birtchnell, J. Women whose mothers died in childhood: An outcome study. *Psychological Medicine*, 1980, *10*, 699–713.

Block, J. H., Block, J., & Morrison, A. Parental agreement-disagreement on childbearing orientations and gender-related personality correlates in children. *Child Development*, 1981, 52, 965–974.

Bourne, P. G., Rose, R. M., & Mason, J. W. Urinary 17-OHCS levels: Data on seven helicopter ambulance medics in combat. *Archives of General Psychiatry*, 1967, *17*, 104–110.

Bourne, P. G., Rose, R. M., & Mason, J. W. 17-OHCS levels in combat: Special forces "A" Team under threat of attack. *Archives of General Psychiatry*, 1968, *19*, 135–140.

Bourque, L. B., & Back, K. W. Life graphs and life events. *Journal of Gerontology*, 1977, 32, 669–674.

Bowlby, J. *Attachment and loss: I. Attachment*. London: Hogarth Press, 1969.

Bowlby, J. *Attachment and loss: II. Separation, anxiety and anger*. London: Hogarth Press, 1973.

Bowlby, J. *Attachment and loss: III. Loss, sadness and depression*. New York: Basic Books, 1980.

Brown, G. W., & Harris, T. *Social origins of depression: A study of psychiatric disorder in women*. London: Tavistock Publications, 1978a.

Brown, G. W., & Harris, T. Social origins of depression: A reply. *Psychological Medicine*, 1978b, 8, 577–588.

Brown, G. W., & Harris, T. Further comments on the vulnerability model. *British Journal of Psychiatry*, 1980, *137*, 584–585.

Brown, G., Chadwick, O., Shaffer, D., Rutter, M., & Traub, M. A prospective study of children with head injuries. III. Psychiatric sequelae. *Psychological Medicine*, 1981, *11*, 63–78.

Coelho, G. V., Hamburg, D. A., & Adams, J. E. (Eds.). *Coping and adaptation*. New York: Basic Books, 1974.

Cohen, F. Personality, stress, and the development of physical illness. In G. C. Stone, F. Cohen, N. E. Adler, & Associates (Eds.), *Health psychology: A handbook*. San Francisco: Jossey-Bass, 1979.

Cousins, N. Anatomy of an illness (as perceived by the patient). *New England Journal of Medicine*, 1976, 295, 1458–1463.

Cox, T. *Stress*. London: Macmillan; Baltimore: University Park Press, 1978.

Crook, T., & Eliot, J. Parental death during childhood and adult depression: A critical review of the literature. *Psychological Bulletin*, 1980, 87, 252–259.

Crowe, R. R. An adoption study of antisocial personality. *Archives of General Psychiatry*, 1974, *31*, 785–791.

Curtis, G., Buxton, M., Lippman, D., Nesse, R., & Wright, J. "Flooding in vivo" during the circadian phase of minimal cortisol secretion: Anxiety and therapeutic success without adrenal cortical activation. *Biological Psychiatry*, 1976, *11*, 101–107.

Davies, D. L. Psychiatric illness in those engaged to be married. *British Journal of Preventive and Social Medicine*, 1956, *10*, 123–127.

Dohrenwend, B. P., & Dohrenwend, B. S. Psychiatric disorders and susceptibility to stress. In L. N. Robins, P. J. Clayton, & J. K. Wing (Eds.), *The social consequences of psychiatric illness*. New York: Brunner/Mazel, 1980.

Dohrenwend, B. S., & Dohrenwend, B. P. Overview and prospects for research on stressful life events. In B. S. Dohrenwend, & B. P. Dohrenwend (Eds.), *Stressful life events: Their nature and effects*. New York: Wiley, 1974.

Douglas, J. W. B. Early disturbing events and later enuresis. In I. Kolvin, R. MacKeith, & S. R. Meadow. (Eds.), *Bladder control and enuresis*. Clinics in developmental medicine, Nos. 48/49. London: SIMP/Heinemann, 1973.

Douglas, J. W. B. Early hospital admissions and later disturbances of behaviour and learning. *Developmental Medicine and Child Neurology*, 1975, *17*, 456–480.

Douglas, J. W. B., & Mann, S. Personal communication, 1979. (Cited in M. Rutter, *Changing youth in a changing society*. London: Nuffield Provincial Hospitals Trust, 1979.)

Dunn, J. Individual differences in temperament. In M. Rutter (Ed.), *Scientific foundations of developmental psychiatry*. London: Heinemann Medical, 1980.

Dunn, J., & Kendrick, C. Studying temperament and parent-child interaction: Comparison of interview and direct observation. *Developmental Medicine and Child Neurology*, 1980a, *4*, 484–496.

Dunn, J., & Kendrick, C. The arrival of a sibling: Changes in patterns of interaction between mother and first born child. *Journal of Child Psychology and Psychiatry*, 1980b, *21*, 119–132.

Dunn, J., Kendrick, C., & MacNamee, R. The reaction of first-born children to the birth of a sibling: Mothers' reports. *Journal of Child Psychology and Psychiatry*, 1981, *22*, 1–18.

Dweck, C. S., & Bush, E. S. Sex differences in learned helplessness: I. Differential debilitation with peer and adult evaluators. *Developmental Psychology*, 1976, *12*, 147–156.

Dweck, C. S., Davidson, W., Nelson, S., & Enna, B. Sex differences in learned helplessness: II. The contingencies of evaluative feedback in the classroom, and III. An experimental analysis. *Developmental Psychology*, 1978, *14*, 268–276.

Eaton, W. W. Life events, social supports, and psychiatric symptoms: A re-analysis of the New Haven Data. *Journal of Health and Social Behavior*, 1978, *19*, 230–234.

Elder, G. H. Historical change in life patterns and personality. In P. B. Baltes, & O. G. Brim (Eds.), *Life span development and behavior* (Vol. 2). New York & London: Academic, Press, 1979.

Eme, R. F. Sex differences in childhood psychopathology: A review. *Psychological Bulletin*, 1979, *86*, 574–595.

Everitt, B. S., & Smith, A. M. R. Interactions in contingency tables: A brief discussion of alternative definitions. *Psychological Medicine*, 1979, *9*, 581–584.

Felner, R. D., Stolberg, A., & Cowen, E. L. Crisis events and school mental health referral patterns of young children. *Journal of Consulting and Clinical Psychology*, 1975, *43*, 305–310.

Ferguson, B. F. Preparing young children for hospitalization: A comparison of two methods. *Pediatrics*, 1979, *64*, 656–664.

Furman, E. *A child's parent dies: Studies in childhood bereavement*. New Haven & London: Yale University Press, 1974.

Garmezy, N. The experimental study of children vulnerable to psychopathology. In A. Davids (Ed.), *Child personality and psychopathology: Current topics* (Vol. 2). New York: Wiley, 1976.

Garmezy, N. Children under stress: Perspectives on antecedents and correlates of vulnerability and resistance to psychopathology. In I. A. Rabin, J. Aronoff, A. M. Barclay, & R. A. Zucker (Eds.), *Further explorations in personality*. New York: Wiley, 1981.

Gersten, J. C., Langner, T. S., Eisenberg, J. G., & Orzek, L. Child behaviors and life events: Undesirable change or change per se? In B. S. Dohrenwend, & B. P. Dohrenwend (Eds.), *Stressful life events: Their nature and effects*. New York: Wiley, 1974.

Glass, D. C. *Behavior patterns, stress and coronary disease*. New York: Wiley, 1977.

Gore, S. The effect of social support in moderating the health consequences of unemployment. *Journal of Health and Social Behavior*, 1978, *19*, 157–165.

Haan, N. Proposed model of ego functioning: Coping and defense mechanisms in relation to I.Q. change. *Psychological Monographs*, 1963, *77*, (Whole No. 571).

Haan N. *Coping and defending: Processes of self-environment organization*. New York: Academic Press, 1977.

Haggerty, R. J. Life stress, illness and social supports. *Developmental Medicine and Child Neurology*, 1980, *22*, 391–400.

Hansen, D. S., & Johnson, V. A. Rethinking family stress theory: Definitional aspects. In W. R. Burr, R. Hill, F. I. Nye, & I. L. Reiss (Eds.), *Contemporary theories about the family: research-based theories* (Vol. 1). New York: Free Press; London: Collier Macmillan, 1979.

Heisel, J. S., Ream, S. Raitz, R., Rappaport, M., & Coddington, R. D. The significance of life events as contributing factors in the diseases of children. III. A study of pediatric patients. *Journal of Pediatrics*, 1973, *83*, 119–123.

Hennessy, J. W., & Levine, S. Stress, arousal, and the pituitary-adrenal system: A psycho-endocrine hypothesis. In J. M. Srague, & A. N. Epstein (Eds.), *Progress in psychobiology and physiological psychology*. New York: Academic Press, 1979.

Hess, R. D., & Camara, K. A. Post-divorce family relationships as mediating factors in the consequence of divorce for children. *Journal of Social Issues*, 1979, *35*, 79–96.

Hetherington, E. M. Children and divorce. In R. Henderson (Ed.), *Parent-child interaction: Theory, research and prospect*. New York: Academic Press, 1980.

Hetherington, E. M., Cox, M., & Cox, R. The aftermath of divorce. In J. H. Stevens, Jr., & M. Mathews (Eds.), *Mother-child relations*. Washington, D.C.: N.A.E.Y.C., 1978.

Hetherington, E. M., Cox, M., & Cox, R. Play and social interaction in children following divorce. *Journal of Social Issues*, 1979a, *35*, 26–49.

Hetherington, E. M., Cox, M., & Cox, R. Family interaction and the social, emotional and cognitive development of children following divorce. In V. Vaughn, & T. Brazelton (Eds.), *The family: Setting priorities*. New York: Science and Medicine, 1979b.

Hinde, R. A., & McGinnis, L. Some factors influencing the effect of temporary mother-infant separation: Some experiments with rhesus monkeys. *Psychological Medicine*, 1977, *7*, 197–212.

Hinkle, L. E. The effect of exposure to culture change, social change, and changes in interpersonal relationships on health. In B. S. Dohrenwend, & B. P. Dohrenwend (Eds.), *Stressful life events: Their nature and effects*. New York: Wiley, 1974.

Hofer, M. A., Wolff, C. T., Friedman, S. B., & Mason, J. W. A psycho-endocrine study of bereavement. Parts I and II. *Psychosomatic Medicine*, 1972, *34*, 481–504.

Holmes, T. H., & Rahe, R. H. The social readjustment rating scale. *Journal of Psychosomatic Research*, 1967, *11*, 213–218.

Hudgens, R. W. Personal catastrophe and depression: A consideration of the subject with respect to medically ill adolescents, and a requiem for retrospective life-event studies. In B. S. Dohrenwend, & B. P. Dohrenwend (Eds.), *Stressful life events: Their nature and effects*. New York: Wiley, 1974.

Hultsch, D. F., & Plemons, J. K. Life events and life span development. In P. B. Baltes, & O. G. Brim (Eds.), *Life-span development and behavior* (Vol. 2). New York & London: Academic Press, 1979.

Hunt, J. McV. Psychological development: Early experience. *Annual Review of Psychology*, 1979, *30*, 103–143.

Hutchings, B., & Mednick, S. A. Registered criminality in the adoptive and biological parents of registered male adoptees. In S. A. Mednick, F. Schulsinger, B. Bell, P. H. Venables, & K. O. Christiansen (Eds.), *Genetics, environment and psychopathology*. Amsterdam: North-Holland/American Elsevier, 1974.

Illingworth, R. S., & Holt, K. S. Children in hospital: Some observations on their reactions with special reference to daily visiting. *Lancet*, 1955, *ii*, 1257–1262.

Jacobs, S. C., Prusoff, B. A., & Paykel, E. S. Recent life events in schizophrenia and depression. *Psychological Medicine*, 1974, *4*, 444–453.

Jenkins, C. D. Psychosocial modifiers of response to stress. *Journal of Human Stress*, 1979, *5*, 3–15.

Kanner, A., Kafry, D., & Pines, A. Conspicuous in its absence: The lack of positive conditions as a source of stress. *Journal of Human Stress*, 1978, *4*, 33–39.

Katz, J. L., Weiner, H., Gallagher, T. G., & Hellman, L. Stress, distress, and ego defenses. *Archives of General Psychiatry*, 1970, *23*, 131–142.

Kendall, R. E., Wainwright, S., Hailey, A., & Shannon, B. The influence of childbirth on psychiatric morbidity. *Psychological Medicine*, 1976, *6*, 297–302.

Keogh, B. K., & Pullis, M. E. Temperamental influences on the development of exceptional children. *Advances in Special Education*, 1980, *1*, 239–276.

Kliman, G. W. *Psychological emergencies of childhood*. New York: Grune & Stratton, 1968.

Knight, R. B., Atkins, A., Eagle, C. J., Evans, N., Finkelstein, J. W., Fukushima, D., Katz, J., & Weiner, H. Psychological stress, ego defenses, and cortisol production in children hospitalized for elective surgery. *Psychosomatic Medicine*, 1979, *41*, 40–49.

Lazarus, R. S. *Psychological stress and the coping process*. New York: McGraw-Hill, 1966.

Lazarus, R. S. The self-regulation of emotion. In L. Levi (Ed.), *Emotions—their parameters and measurement*. New York: Raven Press, 1975.

Lazarus, R. S. A strategy for research on psychological and social factors in hypertension. *Journal of Human Stress*, 1978, *4*, 35–40.

Lazarus, R. S., Cohen, J. B., Folkman, S., Kanner, A., & Schaefer, C. Psychological stress and adaptation: Some unresolved issues. In H. Selye (Ed.), *Guide to stress research*. New York: Van Nostrand Reinhold Co., 1980.

Lazarus, R. S., & Launier, R. Stress-related transactions between person and environment. In L. A. Pervin, & M. Lewis (Eds.), *Perspectives in interactional psychology*. New York: Plenum Press, 1978.

Leff, J., & Vaughn, C. The interaction of life events and relatives' expressed emotion in schizophrenia and depressive neurosis. *British Journal of Psychiatry*, 1980, *136*, 146–153.

Levine, S. Comparative and psychological perspectives on development. In W. A. Collins (Ed.), *The concept of development: Minnesota symposia on child psychology* (Vol. 15). Hillsdale, N.J.: Lawrence Erlbaum, 1982.

Levine, S., Chevalier, J. A., & Korchin, S. J. The effects of early shock and handling on later avoidance learning. *Journal of Personality*, 1956, *24*, 475–493.

Lieberman, M. A. Adaptive processes in late life. In N. Datan, & L. H. Ginsberg (Eds.), *Life-span developmental psychology: Normative life crises*. New York: Academic Press, 1975.

Lin, N., Simeone, R. F., Ensel, W. M., & Kuo, W. Social support, stressful life events, and illness: A model and empirical test. *Journal of Health and Social Behavior*, 1979, *20*, 108–119.

Lloyd, C. Life events and depressive disorder reviewed. I. Events as predisposing factors. *Archives of General Psychiatry*, 1980a, *37*, 529–535.

Lloyd, C. Life events and depressive disorder reviewed. II. Events as precipitating factors. *Archives of General Psychiatry*, 1980b, *37*, 541–548.

Marmot, M. Type A behaviour and ischaemic heart disease. *Psychological Medicine*, 1980, *10*, 603–606.

Mason, J. W. A historical view of the stress field. Part I. *Journal of Human Stress*, 1975, *1*, 6–12.

Matheny, A. P., & Dolan, A. B. Persons, situations, and time: A genetic view of behavioral change in children. *Journal of Personality and Social Psychology*, 1975, *32*, 1106–1110.

Mechanic, D. *Students under stress: A study in the social psychology of adaptation*. London: University of Wisconsin Press, 1978.

Meyer, R. J., & Haggerty, R. J. Streptococcal infections in families. *Pediatrics*, 1962, *29*, 539–549.

Miller, E. A discourse on method in child psychiatry. *Journal of Child Psychology and Psychiatry*, 1960, *1*, 3–16.

Mineka, S., & Suomi, S. J. Social separation in monkeys. *Psychological Bulletin*, 1978, *85*, 1376–1400.

Moore, T. Stress in normal childhood. In L. Levi (Ed.), *Society, stress and disease: Childhood and adolescence* (Vol. 2). London: Oxford University Press, 1975.

Moos, R. H. (Ed.). *Human adaptation: Coping with life crises*. Lexington, Mass: D. C. Heath, 1976.

Murphy, L. B., & Moriarty, A. E. *Vulnerability, coping, and growth*. New Haven, Connecticut: Yale University Press, 1976.

Nuckolls, K. B., Cassel, J., & Kaplan, B. H. Psychosocial assets, life crises and the prognosis of pregnancy. *American Journal of Epidemiology*, 1972, *95*, 431–441.

Paykel, E. S. Life stress and psychiatric disorder: Applications of the clinical approach. In B. S. Dohrenwend, & B. P. Dohrenwend (Eds.), *Stressful life events: Their nature and effects*. New York: Wiley, 1974.

Paykel, E. S. Contribution of life events to causation of psychiatric illness. *Psychological Medicine*, 1978, *8*, 245–254.

Paykel, E. S., Emms, E. M., Fletcher, J., & Rassaby, E. S. Life events and social support in puerperal depression. *British Journal of Psychiatry*, 1980, *136*, 339–346.

Pearlin, L. I., & Schooler, C. The structure of coping. *Journal of Health and Social Behavior*, 1978, *19*, 2–21.

Prugh, D. G., Staub, E. M., Sands, H. H., Kirschbaum, R. M., & Lenihan, E. A. A study of the emotional reactions of children and families to hospitalization and illness. *American Journal of Orthopsychiatry*, 1953, *23*, 70–106.

Quinton, D., & Rutter, M. Early hospital admissions and later disturbances of behaviour: An attempted replication of Douglas' findings. *Developmental Medicine and Child Neurology*, 1976, *18*, 447–459.

Robertson, J., & Robertson, J. Young children in brief separation: A fresh look. *Psychoanalytic Study of the Child*, 1971, *26*, 264–315.

Rose, R. M. Endocrine responses to stressful psychological events. *Psychiatric Clinics of North America*, 1980, *2*, 53–71.

Rose, R. M., Jenkins, C. D., & Hurst, M. W. *Air traffic controller health change study: A prospective investigation of physical, psychological and work-related changes*. Report to the Federal Aviation Administration under Contract No. DOT-FA73WA-3211, Boston University School of Medicine, 1978.

Rosenman, R. H., Brand, R. J., Sholtz, R. I., & Friedman, M. Multivariate prediction of coronary heart disease during 8.5 year follow-up in the Western Collaborative Group Study. *American Journal of Cardiology*, 1976, *37*, 903–910.

Roskies, E., & Lazarus, R. S. Coping theory and the teaching of coping skills. In P. Davidson, & S. Davidson (Eds.), *Behavioral medicine: Changing health life styles*. New York: Brunner/Mazel, 1980.

Rutter, M. *Children of sick parents: An environmental and psychiatric study*. Institute of Psychiatry Maudsley Monographs No. 16. London: Oxford University Press, 1966.

Rutter, M. Sex differences in children's responses to family stress. In E. J. Anthony, & C. Koupernik (Eds.), *The child in his family*. New York: Wiley, 1970.

Rutter, M. Parent-child separation: Psychological effects on the children. *Journal of Child Psychology and Psychiatry*, 1971, *12*, 233–260.

Rutter, M. Individual differences. In M. Rutter, & L. Hersov (Eds.), *Child psychiatry: Modern approaches*. Oxford: Blackwell Scientific, 1977.

Rutter, M. Early sources of security and competence. In J. S. Bruner, & A. Garton (Eds.), *Human growth and development*. London: Oxford University Press, 1978.

Rutter, M. Protective factors in children's responses to stress and disadvantage. In M. W. Kent, & J. E. Rolf (Eds.), *Primary prevention of psychopathology: Social competence in children* (Vol. 3). Hanover: University of New England, 1979.

Rutter, M. The long-term effects of early experience. *Developmental Medicine and Child Neurology*, 1980a, *22*, 800–815.

Rutter, M. Attachment and the development of social relationships. In M. Rutter (Ed.), *Scientific foundations of developmental psychiatry*. London: Heinemann Medical, 1980b.

Rutter, M. Emotional development. In M. Rutter (Ed.), *Scientific foundations of developmental psychiatry*. London: Heinemann Medical, 1980c.

Rutter, M. *Maternal deprivation reassessed* (2nd ed.). Harmondsworth: Penguin, 1981a.

Rutter, M. Social/emotional consequences of day care for pre-school children. *American Journal of Orthopsychiatry*, 1981b, *51*, 4–28.

Rutter, M. Epidemiological-longitudinal approaches to the study of development. In W. A. Collins (Ed.), *The concept of development: Minnesota symposia on child psychology* (Vol. 15). Hillsdale, N.J.: Lawrence Erlbaum, 1982.

Rutter, M., Maughan, B., Mortimore, P., Ouston, J., with Smith, A. *Fifteen thousand hours: Secondary schools and their effects on children*. London: Open Books; Cambridge, Mass.: Harvard University Press, 1979.

Rutter, M., Tizard, J., & Whitmore, K. (Eds.). *Education, health and behaviour*. London: Longmans, 1970. (Reprinted, New York: Krieger, 1981).

Schaffer, H. R., & Callender, W. M. Psychological effects of hospitalization in infancy. *Pediatrics*, 1959, *24*, 528–539.

Seligman, M. E. P. *Helplessness: On depression, development and death*. San Francisco: W. H. Freeman, 1975.

Seligman, M. E. P. Comment and integration. *Journal of Abnormal Psychology*, 1978, *87*, 165–179.

Selye, H. *The physiology and pathology of exposure to stress*. Montreal: Acta Inc., 1950.

Selye, H. *The stress of life*. New York: McGraw-Hill, 1956. (Revised, 1976)

Shields, J. Genetics and mental development. In M. Rutter (Ed.), *Scientific foundations of developmental psychiatry*. London: Heinemann Medical, 1980.

Shure, M. B., & Spivak, G. Interpersonal problem solving, thinking and adjustment in the mother-child dyad. In M. W. Kent, & J. E. Rolf (Eds.), *Primary prevention of psychopathology: Social competence in children* (Vol. 3). Hanover: University Press of New England, 1979.

Spencer-Booth, Y., & Hinde, R. A. Effects of brief separations from mothers during infancy on behaviour of rhesus monkeys 6–24 months later. *Journal of Child Psychology and Psychiatry*, 1971, *12*, 157–172.

Stacey, M., Dearden, R., Pill, R., & Robinson, D. *Hospitals, children and their families: The report of a pilot study*. London: Routledge and Kegan Paul, 1970.

Tarnopolsky, A., Barker, S. M., Wiggins, R. D., & McLean, E. K. The effect of aircraft noise on the mental health of a community sample: A pilot study. *Psychological Medicine*, 1978, *8*, 219–234.

Tarnopolsky, A., Watkins, G., & Hand, D. J. Aircraft noise and mental health. I. Prevalence of individual symptoms. *Psychological Medicine*, 1980, *10*, 683–698.

Tarrier, N., Vaughn, C., Lader, M. H., & Leff, J. P. Bodily reactions to people and events in schizophrenics. *Archives of General Psychiatry*, 1979, *36*, 311–315.

Tennant, C., & Andrews, G. The pathogenic quality of life event stress in neurotic impairment. *Archives of General Psychiatry*, 1978, *35*, 859–863.

Tennant, C., & Bebbington, P. The social causation of depression: A critique of the work of Brown and his colleagues. *Psychological Medicine*, 1978, *8*, 565–576.

Tennant, C., Bebbington, P., & Hurry, J. Parental death in childhood and risk of adult depressive disorders: A review. *Psychological Medicine*, 1980, *10*, 289–299.

Tennant, C., Smith, A., Bebbington, P., & Hurry, J. The contextual threat of life events: The concept and its reliability. *Psychological Medicine*, 1979, *9*, 525–528.

Theorell, T. Selected illnesses and somatic factors in relation to two psychosocial stress indices—a prospective study on middle-aged construction building workers. *Journal of Psychosomatic Research*, 1976, *20*, 7–20.

Thompson, W. R., & Grusec, J. E. Studies of early experience. In P. H. Mussen (Ed.), *Carmichael's manual of child psychology* (3rd ed.). New York: Wiley, 1970.

Torgersen, A. M., & Kringlen, E. Genetic aspects of temperamental differences in infants. *Journal of the American Academy of Child Psychiatry*, 1978, *17*, 433–444.

Ursin, H., Baade, E., & Levine, S. *Psychobiology of stress: A study of coping men*. New York: Academic Press, 1978.

Vaillant, G. E. *Adaptation to life*. Boston: Little, Brown, 1977.

Vernon, D. T. A., Foley, J. M., Sipowicz, R. R., & Schulman, J. L. *The psychological responses of children to hospitalization and illness*. Springfield, Ill.: Charles C Thomas, 1965.

Vinokur, A., & Selzer, M. L. Desirable versus undesirable life events: Their relationship to stress and mental distress. *Journal of Personality and Social Psychology*, 1975, *32*, 329–337.

Visintainer, M. A., & Wolfer, J. A. Psychological preparation for surgical pediatric patients: The effects on children's and parents' stress responses and adjustment. *Pediatrics*, 1975, *56*, 187–202.

Wallerstein, J. S., & Kelly, J. B. *Surviving the break up: How children and parents cope with divorce*. New York: Basic Books; London: Grant McIntyre, 1980.

Werner, E. E., & Smith, R. S. *Vulnerable but invincible: A longitudinal study of resilient children and youth*. New York: McGraw-Hill, 1982.

Wolfer, J. A., & Visintainer, M. A. Prehospital psychological preparation for tonsillectomy patients: Effects on children's and parent's adjustment. *Pediatrics*, 1979, *64*, 646–655.

Wolff, C. T., Friedman, S. G., Hofer, M. A., & Mason, J. W. Relationship between psychological defenses and mean urinary 17-hydroxycorticosteroid excretion rates: I. A predictive study of parents of fatally ill children. *Psychosomatic Medicine*, 1964, *26*, 576–591.

Ziv, A., & Israeli, R. Effects of bombardment on the manifest anxiety level of children living in kibbutzim. *Journal of Consulting and Clinical Psychology*, 1973, *40*, 287–291.

CHAPTER 2

STRESSORS OF CHILDHOOD

NORMAN GARMEZY
PROFESSOR OF PSYCHOLOGY
UNIVERSITY OF MINNESOTA

THIS CHAPTER CAN BE viewed as a companion piece to the preceding one in which Rutter has focused on issues and questions posed by the admittedly ambiguous concepts of *stress* and *coping*. But whereas Rutter's assignment was to be evaluative, mine was to be descriptive and to illustrate, by examples drawn from the stress research literature, factors that influence children's adaptations to trying circumstances and events.

It is a somewhat curious task, for it is evident from the preceding chapter, and from those that follow, that many of my colleagues tend to be ambivalent about these twin concepts, despite their intriguing demonstrations of the applicability of these concepts to research areas in which they have made substantial scientific contributions.

Although this seems to be somewhat paradoxical, it is not unusual for those who study stress and its effects. On the one hand there is strong dissatisfaction with the concept of stress: its imprecision of definition, the lack of effective measuring instruments, the inadequacy of a conceptual umbrella that seems to cover too heterogeneous an array of potentiating stimuli, and too overinclusive an aggregation of behavioral and somatic response processes. These shortcomings generate ambivalence in researchers, among whom the less hardy will rarely venture forth into print unless accompanied by a set of quotation marks with which to surround their use of the uncertain concept.

Yet, on the other hand, there is this reality. Contemporary discomfort with the stress concept can be matched against the outpouring of research on the subject. It is a fact of scientific life that despite definitional imprecision, mensurational shortcomings, and conceptual cloudiness, the study of stress is seen as worthy of scientific concern, as evidenced by the thousands of articles and large output of volumes written on the subject.

Thus, the paradox of transposing an evanescent concept into a critical appraisal of several of its relevant research areas. The situation seems akin to one faced by Mark Twain who, when called upon to explain a somewhat murky phenomenon, cheerfully replied: "I was grateful to be able to answer promptly and I did. I said I didn't know."

Efforts to define stress bring to prominence the inherent ambiguity of the concept. It explains Mason's (1975) dictum to use the term "sparingly;" that if one must use it, then define the meaning that has been assigned to it; and try to make as descriptive and as operational as possible the components of stimulus and response that enter into one's interactional definition of stress.

The following definition, offered by Janis and Leventhal (1968) is one attempt to meet Mason's stricture:

> . . . it seems preferable to designate as a 'stressful' event any change in the environment which typically—i.e., in the average person—induces a high degree of emotional tension and interferes with normal patterns of response. . . .
>
> Thus, while the concept of stress is not rigorously defined, it does focus on a broad class of emotional behaviors elicited by antecedent stimulation, ranging from clear cut exposure to painful or injurious physical dangers to purely verbal statements or gestures that convey social disapproval. Moreover, a close examination of stress situations will undoubtedly suggest many common features that are responsible for the similarities of the stress reactions and for parallels in their consequences for adjustment (p. 1043).

The final sentence of the quotation suggests that an explicit taxonomy of stressful events is potentially constructible. Unfortunately this has not been attained primarily because of two factors: (1) the multidimensional nature of most so-called stress situations and (2) "host individuality." (Mason, 1975), i.e., the individual variation in responsiveness to stimulus or environmental conditions considered distressing. These factors compound the taxonomic problem by introducing that unbecoming but omnipresent variable in personality research, "person-situation interaction" (Magnusson & Endler, 1977).

Simplifying categorizations have been found wanting. Schwab and Pritchard (1949) have suggested a triadic category of *mild*, *moderate*, and *severe* stresses for which duration of effect is the major criterion variable. But there are other dimensions to stress experiences which are equally important. For example: *Acute* events may be infinitely more disturbing than are *chronic* conditions to which one has habituated. Events involving loss may be more powerful in their repercussions if the loss involves a single individual than the anonymous thousands lost through natural disasters and man-made wars. For some, the anticipated *pleasure* of a major job promotion may prove to be more fear-arousing than the stressfulness of being unemployed.

It is the inability to control the varied properties of different distressing events that has led researchers to turn to the laboratory for a more precise delineation of stressful stimulation and stress responsiveness. Under such control conditions studies have been conducted that suggest a more general relationship between the severity of a stressful event and the extent of the adaptive demands placed upon normal individuals. Studies of arousal and its consequences for behavioral efficiency (Bartoshuk, 1971) have taken form in the well-known inverted U-shape function which emphasizes that optimal performance is best achieved under a moderate level of arousal. Lindsley (1957) had posited that EEG changes and effective performance were related to a continuum extending from deep sleep to disorganizing states of emotion (Hebb, 1955, 1972). Too high or too low a level of arousal leads to decremental performance.

There has been dispute as to whether or not states of arousal need be experienced as stressful. Levi (1972) argued that both low and high states are so experienced; others have taken the position that a greater degree of independence exists between the two factors (see Cox, 1978, pp. 42–45, for a discussion of the issue). Nevertheless, it is interesting to consider some consequences of hypothesizing that stress, arousal, and performance are indeed interrelated. Such a view would suggest that an inverted U-shape function of performance in relation to intensity of arousal, combined with a comparable U-shaped function of arousal as a function of severity of stress would generate a linear relationship between stress and performance in which increments in stress would produce a progressive decline in behavioral efficiency (Cox, 1978). Studies of soldiers in combat (Grinker & Spiegel, 1945; Marshall, 1947; Sobel, 1949; Stouffer, Lumsdaine, Williams, Smith, Janis, Star, & Cottrell, 1949) and individuals caught up in community disasters (Tyhurst, 1951) would seem to provide support for such a hypothetical construction.

Laboratory studies, however, have the disadvantage of representing only mild analogues of real-world situations. These have included simple deception experiments, the imposition of minor physical discomforts, mild criticism for inadequate performance whether real or falsified, levels of individual performance relative to hypothetical group performance in tasks emphasizing competition and the like. These types of analogue studies enjoyed a vigorous but relatively short life span reaching their peak in the 1940s and 1950s. Their decline can be traced to the many situational criticisms they generated: replications were an infrequent occurrence; the laboratory stressors tended to be pale imitations of real life events and thus had restricted ecological validity; the degree of deception allowed the experimenter was of necessity limited; the coping responses exhibited in these minor and less meaningful situations left untested their generalizations to true-life stressful situations. Then there were the subject criticisms: deceptions that were permitted often were disbelieved by research participants; in addition, there remained a gnawing suspicion that knowledge of the experimenter's purpose revealed in debriefing a subject could result in communication between the tested and to-be-tested participants. There was also the problem of sample bias. Participants were often selected on criteria that reflected convenience rather than meaningfulness as evidenced by the use of subjects drawn from college psychology classrooms who were often atypical in terms of their social class status, intelligence, and willingness to volunteer (Coyne & Lazarus, 1980; Silver & Wortman, 1980). For these many reasons the laboratory analogue began to be replaced by real-life events that were severe, realistic, powerful, and beyond the traditional forms of experimental control since they occurred in natural rather than contrived settings.

This chapter samples the severe end of the stressors of childhood, with reviews of the status of research involving loss and separation, and the effects of war on children. Both are often thought to be representative of stressors that occupy the end point of a dimension of severity. Both are seen as representative of those events that are marked by pervasive threats to individual security. Loss and separation involves the severing of deep-seated attachments through the death of loved ones with accompanying grief and bereavement, or it can be generated by profound neglect and abuse by uncaring parents or surrogates, or by dissolution of the family through divorce. Wars provide all the trappings that accompany malnutrition, dislocation, traumatic injury, death, and separation. Events such as these have an intensity that has assigned them the status of near-universal stressors, experiences that tend to disrupt the behavior of most individuals irrespective of their role status, their geographical locale, or perhaps even the historical era in which they occur. Characteristically, the time period for activation of a response to such a magnitude of threat tends to be more rapid, whereas in markedly less taxing situations a longer period of delay in responding occurs—a period during which the individual presumably engages in a cognitive appraisal of the event, interprets it as threatening or nonthreatening in terms of his or her capability to deal with it, and only when a disparity is found to exist between the demand of the situation and the individual's ability to meet that demand is the stress-induced response with its marked emotional component activated. It is important, however, to realize that even for events that are presumed to evoke a universal distress, reference is only to a modal pattern of response; severity and adequacy of reaction varies considerably from individual to individual in virtually all stressful conditions (Mason's "host individuality"), including the most extreme and demanding. There are many case reports of individuals who function adaptively in the face of the most dire events, while there are others who undergo a marked disruption of behavior even under conditions that most would consider to be minimally threatening.

To return to the prior mention of combat and natural disasters, Marshall (1947), a military historian, reported that most soldiers appear to be immobilized by the stress of combat. But there remained 15–25% of infantrymen who could be counted on to fire their rifles in combat in the direction of the enemy when commanded to do so. A parallel phenomenon has been reported by observers of persons in disaster. Some 15% remain organized and effective in terms of their response to stress; 70% exhibit signs of disorganization but can be mobilized to function with some degree of effectiveness; while 10–25% are totally ineffective, immovable, confused, overly emotional, and aimless or apathetic in their response to the disaster (Tyhurst, 1951, cited in Bindra, 1959).

With regard to the behavior of children under severe stress, although we lack a systematic literature, here too clinical evidence points to individual variations in response to the severe stress of threat of family dissolution (e.g., see Wallerstein, this volume), community disaster whether minor (Blom, 1982), or major (Johnson, 1980), war (Spielberger, Sarason & Milgram, 1982), concentration camp experiences (Langmeier & Matêjcêk, 1975; Freud & Dann, 1951), and the threat of a nuclear accident (Dohrenwend, Dohrenwend, Warheit, Bartlett, Goldsteen, Goldsteen & Martin, 1981).

Differential responses such as these in the face of great misfortune exemplify the second focus of this volume—the concept of coping. Here too there is discomfort with the imprecision of definition, a lack of systematic categorization of coping methods accompanied by a trend toward overinclusiveness in which all responses to a stressful event are defined as coping responses. Although coping behavior is a relative latecomer to the domain of stress research, there has been a rapid escalation in recent years of related studies including: (1) coping patterns in response to a variety of stressors (Antonovsky, 1979; Coelho, Hamburg, & Adams, 1974; Coyne & Lazarus, 1980; Henry & Stephens, 1977; Koocher & O'Malley, 1981; Levine & Ursin, 1980; McCubbin & Boss, 1980; Miller, 1980; Moos, 1976, 1977; Murphy & Moriarty, 1976; NCI, 1980; Silver & Wortman, 1980; Vaillant, 1977); (2) factors that reflect risk and vulnerability to various types of behavior disorders (Anthony & Koupernick, 1974; Gleser, Green & Winget, 1981; Regier & Allen, 1981; Watt, Anthony, Wynne, & Rolf, in press; Wynne, Cromwell, & Matthysse, 1978); and (3) protective factors that may account for resilience and adaptation in the presence of severely threatening events (Baruch & Barnett, 1980; Hartup, 1979; Rathjen & Foreyt, 1980; Rutter, 1979a; Suomi, 1979; Werner & Smith, 1982).

The importance of individual and environmental factors that can influence vulnerability in relation to stress has now gained general acceptance, despite the fact that the specific influences that account for differential responsiveness to stress too often remain speculative. Here is one viewpoint of that relationship as expressed by Appley and Trumbull (1967):

> It is consistently found that these reactions vary in intensity from person to person under exposure to the same environmental event. . . . It has also been noted that, with few exceptions, the *kind* of situation which arouses a stress response in a particular individual must be related to significant events in that person's life. Many people have used the terms "ego-strength," "stress-tolerance," and "frustration-tolerance." It is perhaps doubtful that there is such a thing as a general stress-tolerance in people. There is more likely to be a greater or lesser insulation from the effects of certain kinds of stress-producers rather than others. . . . It seems more likely that there are differing thresholds, depending upon the kinds of threats that are encountered and that individuals must be differentially vulnerable to different kinds of stressors. . . . To know what conditions of the environment are likely to be effective for the particular person, the motivational structure and prior history of the individual would have to be taken into account. Where the particular motives are known—where it is known what a person holds important and not important, what kinds of goals have for him been likely to increase anxiety or lead to aversive or defensive behavior—a reasonable prediction of stress proneness might be made. (pp. 10–11)

The Appley-Trumbull position raises several questions: the first is its seeming neglect of biological predisposition as a significant contribution to stress responsiveness. The growth of interest in children's temperament and its relation to ongoing and future behavior patterns has become a significant aspect of recent research in both normal and psychopathological development (Dunn & Kendrick, 1980; Dunn, Kendrick, & MacNamee, 1981; Graham, Rutter, & George, 1973; Porter & Collins, 1982; Thomas & Chess, 1977), and in children's responsiveness to stressful events (Rutter & Quinton, 1981). The second question is more provocative: Are there persons—adults or children—who are typically stress-resistant or is such behavior invariably situation-specific? At the present time, we lack a solid empirical data base for making an assertion either way. Yet that question is eminently researchable. Third, there is the question as to whether or not we can reasonably predict stress-proneness on the basis of the Appley-Trumbull criteria of a knowledge of life-history factors focused on an individual's motives, goals, and behavioral reinforcements. It is more likely that the prediction of stress proneness or stress-resistance will involve a greater complex of factors, but these can not be clearly specified at this point. What one can safely say is that the moment is ripe for systematic studies of stress responsiveness in adults and children, and until these are in place, the issues raised above can not be adequately treated.

Such research efforts will have to take cognizance of individual predispositional biogenetic and constitutional factors, patterns of family structure and interaction, rearing practices of parents, characteristic personality attributes of the individual and careful analyses of stressful situations and events, modes of coping and outcome, and potentiating and protective factors in the environment.

What we must constantly be alert to is the contemporary reality that even with the disadvantage of a possible genetic loading as diathesis and the stress of a debilitating environment there are many children who never become mentally disordered and instead take their hard won place in society as contributing adults. Children with a potential for mental disorder which fails to be actualized can provide those clues to "protective" factors that enhance resilience in both normal and high risk children (Garmezy, 1981; Rutter, 1979a, 1980; Garmezy & Nuechterlein, 1972; Bleuler, 1978). It is to this point that I will return later in the chapter.

THE STRESSORS OF CHILDHOOD

Children are not strangers to stress. Over a significant span of human history they have been more often the victims of the slings and arrows of an uncaring society than recipients of its beneficient protection. The opening sentences of one attempt to reconstruct the history of childhood refers to it as a "nightmare" from which society has "only recently begun to awaken."

> The further back in history one goes, the lower the level of child care, and the more likely children are to be killed, abandoned, beaten, terrorized, and sexually abused. (de Mause, 1974, p. 1)

Despert (1965), in her history of the "emotionally disturbed" child, noted that the use of this term to denote "problem" children is only a product of the past quarter of our century and reflects an evolution in our attitudes toward maladjusted children. Previous ages provided a different set of labels—"possessed," "wicked," "guilty," "insubordinate," "incorrigible"—in which a burden of guilt was placed on the child for having failed society. Such early beliefs in centuries past scarcely provided a scientific base from which to evaluate whether stressful environments and despairing life events may have played a significant role in the etiology of children's disorders.

The records of 16th, 17th, and 18th century medicine provide few resources for learning about children's emotional and cognitive responses to conflicts, aspirations, reactions to work, and to dreadful workhouse environments that demanded an endurance which children typically lacked. "Difficult as it is," writes Despert, "to recreate in one's mind the physical hardships, it is even more of a challenge to envision the inner feelings of the stunted young beings at work." (p. 15)

Maccoby (1980), in her recent volume on children's social development, begins her account with "the child as victim" in which she provides a graphic portrayal of the stressors of childhood in England and in the American colonies during the 16th to the mid-18th century. Her account is a catalogue of whippings at home and in school, vigorous child abuse, the use of alcohol and opiates as sedatives to quiet young children, garments that were reinforced with "whale bone and iron" to hinder children from creeping, crawling, and standing in their characteristic postures, and the dispatch of children as young as six or seven from their families to work as servants. Such harsh and cruel treatment Maccoby reported had its roots in three factors: Puritan religious values, a lack of medical knowledge, and a perception of children and childhood as a mirrored replica of adults and adulthood.

Although the substance of the treatment accorded children has not been open to dispute, there has been partisan debate over the factors that presumably influenced such ungenerous behavior. On the one hand there is the view that in medieval times child neglect and maltreatment were not motivated by evil intent but rather sprung from a failure of society to achieve a differentiated conception of childhood that was qualitatively and quantitatively different from adulthood (Aries, 1962). By contrast, there are others who dispute this benign view of adult abusiveness and neglect, perceiving in both past and current maltreatment of children either a lack of emotional maturity in significant caretakers (de Mause, 1974; Despert, 1965) or parental perceptions of offspring as encumbrances which justified resentment and the use of corporal punishment (Langer, 1974).

This debate over mechanisms underlying early punitive attitudes and behaviors toward children is quite irrelevant to the central thesis: children throughout history have been subjected to a variety of distressing experiences ranging broadly over malnutrition, physical and sexual abuse, neglect, psychological deprivations, lack of support, separation from and loss of caregivers, forced labor in forbidding factories and mines, and (always) the pervasive handicap through the centuries of powerless role and status assignments.

It is reasonable to suggest that in the wake of such experiences, physiological and behavioral counterparts which today we view as stress responses were also the lot of children in centuries past. Evidence can be drawn from Cannon's (1929, 1932) seminal popular works. When he, more than a half-century ago, first provided the scientific description of the body's response to stressful experience, he described a basic pattern of physiological response that he considered to be pervasively representative of the mammalian species. This response pattern was hypothesized to be innate, primal, and adaptive in preparing the organism for a pattern of fight (i.e., anger) or flight (i.e., fear). It is parsimonious to assume that dangerous, threatening, and fear-arousing situations, in whatever century these occurred, probably produced severe emotional, physiological, and behavioral responses in all humans exposed to them, whether adult or child.

But the systematic study of such reactions had to await necessary developments first in the basic biological sciences and then, in turn, in the basic behavioral sciences. Furthermore, support for such research required a society that had tempered its primitivity and had developed an awareness that there existed a relationship between stress, disease, and adaptation.

Today, having more or less achieved these goals, we witness a striking growth of interest in the study of stress, its antecedents and consequents. Thousands of articles are now published annually attesting to that expanding interest. The preponderance of such investigations, observations, and case accounts have been focused on the physiology of stress, far fewer on its psychological correlates. But in this output of scientific and clinical studies, the effort to observe, record, and study the reactions of children to stressful events has remained an area of neglect in comparison to the many studies of adult responsivity.

The degree of neglect is puzzling in the light of evidence that, in a world of heightened stress, children are frequently among the most affected victims of a range of threatening events. This has been known to clinicians who have observed and treated and reported on children caught up in dire circumstances. Such reports invariably precede more systematic research. Perhaps it is appropriate then to provide first a sample of behavioral observations of distinguished clinicians whose words portray the images of children under specific stressors. Subsequently a restricted segment of the research literature on children exposed to stressful experiences will be appraised—research that clarifies and qualifies children's responsiveness to stress.

Descriptions of the many stressors to which children are exposed would require far more than a single chapter. Constraints of space limit me to a description of two types of stress experience. The first is the psychological threat posed by loss of or separation from a parent or significant caregiver. The second is war and civil strife, with the attendant physical and psychological trauma it evokes in children, its youngest victims.

THE THREAT OF SEPARATION AND LOSS

The trauma for children of potential separation with its accompanying loss of parents or significant surrogates has a near universal stress quality. I have chosen to illustrate the significance of this area from three perspectives: the first, *clinical*, provides a descriptive-behavioral view of the effects of one form of brief separation on very young children; the second, *historical*, examines the transition over decades from social to scientific concern with the problem; the third, *scientific*, examines the contemporary status of research on separation.

The Clinical Perspective

In the volume *Brief Separations*, Heinicke and Westheimer (1965) describe the effects on young children (13–32 months of age) of placement in a residential nursery. In the ten cases studied the reasons for placement were rather ordinary. For eight of the children, their mothers had gone to the hospital to have a baby or to be observed; another mother was hospitalized because of a back injury; placement in one instance occurred because the family was homeless. The stays for most of the children were less than seven weeks. The consequences of the separation have been described by Bowlby (1973) in his volume on *Separation*:

> The children arrived at the nursery in the care of one or both parents. Four of them, brought by father, stayed close to him and seemed already subdued and anxious. Some of the others, who had come with mother or both parents, seemed more confident and were ready to explore the new environment. They ventured forth on short or long excursions and then returned.
>
> When the moment came for the parent(s) to depart, crying or screaming was the rule. One child tried to follow her parents, demanding urgently where they were going, and finally had to be pushed back into the room by her mother. Another threw herself on the floor and refused to be comforted. Altogether eight of the children were crying loudly soon after their parents' departure. Bedtime was also an occasion for tears. The two who had not cried earlier screamed when put in a cot and could not be consoled. Some of the others whose initial crying had ceased broke into renewed sobs at bedtime. One little girl, who arrived in the evening and was put straight to bed, insisted on keeping her coat on, clung desperately to her doll, and cried 'at a frightening pitch.' Again and again, having nodded off from sheer fatigue, she awoke screaming for Mummy. . . .
>
> Oriented as they were to their missing parents, these small children were in no mood either to cooperate with the nurses or to accept com-

> fort from them. Initially the children refused to be dressed or undressed, refused to eat, refused to pot. During the first day all but one child, the youngest, refused to be approached, picked up, or comforted. After a day or two resistance abated, but even at the end of two weeks over one-third of the nurses' requests and demands were still being resisted. . . .
>
> Hostile behavior, though infrequent, tended to increase during the two weeks of observation. It often took the form of biting another child or ill-treating the favourite object brought from home.
>
> A breakdown in sphincter control was usual. Of the eight children who had attained some degree of control before arriving in the nursery, all but one lost it. The exception . . . aged two years eight months was the oldest of the children.

The children's *reactions to reunion* showed the short-term subsequent effects of the separation:

> . . . On meeting mother for the first time after the days or weeks away every one of the ten children showed some degree of detachment. Two seemed not to recognize mother. The other eight turned away or even walked away from her. Most of them either cried or came close to tears; a number alternated between a tearful and an expressionless face.
>
> In contrast to these blank, tearful retreats from mother, all but one of the children responded affectionately when they first met father again. Furthermore, five were friendly to (the observer) as well. . . .
>
> In the Heinicke-Westheimer study one of the two observers who had been present in the nursery visited each child sixteen weeks after his return home. All the children seemed clearly to remember the observer and reacted with strong feeling; all but one made "a desperate attempt" to avoid the observer. The mothers were much surprised that their child should be so afraid, and affirmed that other strangers who visited the house did not arouse such reactions. (Bowlby, 1973, pp. 8–13)

Here indeed is a powerful recital of the effects of separation from parent provided by a carefully wrought clinical investigation of a small sample of very young children. In the previous chapter and elsewhere, Rutter (1981) has discussed separation in the context of the hospitalization of children and has confirmed some of these findings but has advanced others that provide needed qualifications. Young children admitted to hospitals or residential nurseries do show an acute distress reaction, and this may persist after the child returns home. But a view of hospitalization that emphasizes multiple admissions provides a more conditional statement. A single hospital admission lasting a week or less has no long-lasting sequelae. Distress is brief and transitory. But numerous hospitalizations of a young child resulting in long separations which merge into a more chronic pattern have been found to be associated with psychiatric disorder in children in later years. In the case of separation from parents because of maternal illness, if a child can be cared for in a family rather than placed in an institution, a marked tempering of the distress reaction can result (Robertson & Robertson, 1971).

Findings such as these serve to qualify earlier generalizations and represent the typical advance of science. But they provide an even more important role in advancing an understanding of more fundamental processes that underlie the separation—distress reaction. Evidence, as Rutter (1979b) notes, seems to point to the disruption of the bonding or attachment process between mother and child which is a necessary precursor to subsequent healthy adaptation.

All theories of development emphasize the significance of the bonding that takes place between mother and baby, of their reciprocal exchange, of the induction of comfort and the alleviation of the infant's distress that is evident in the course of the loving and affectionate interaction that mother initiates with her baby.

It is the ubiquity of this relationship and the centrality it is accorded in developmental theory that warrants a brief historical look at the century-long concern about psychological (particularly maternal) deprivation and its effects on children.

A Historical Perspective

In 1926 Freud (1959) in *Inhibition, Symptoms and Anxiety* provided almost a first prototypic statement of what we today study as the toddler's response to the experimental Strange Situation (e.g., Ainsworth, 1973, 1979; Ainsworth & Bell, 1970; Ainsworth & Wittig, 1969; Bretherton & Ainsworth, 1974).

> Only a few of the manifestations of anxiety in children are comprehensible to us, and we must confine our attention to them. They occur, for instance, when a child is alone, or in the dark, or when it finds itself with an unknown person instead of one to whom it is used—such as its mother. These three instances can be reduced to a single condition—namely that of missing someone who is loved and longed for. . . .
>
> The child's mnemonic image of the person longed for is no doubt intensely cathected, probably in a hallucinatory way at first. But this has no effect, and now it seems as though the longing turns into anxiety. . . . Here anxiety appears as a reaction to the felt loss of the object. . . .
>
> But a moment's reflection takes us beyond this question of loss of object. The reason why the infant in arms wants to perceive the presence of its mother is only because it already knows by experience that she satisfies all its needs without delay. The situation, then, which it regards as a 'danger' and against which it wants to be safeguarded is that of non-satisfaction of a *growing tension due to need*, against which it is helpless. (pp. 136–137)

Freud's comments are a part of the first phase of a four-period historical sequence in the growth of scientific interest in the problem of "psychological deprivation" in children. That phase sequence reflected the growth of concern about the effects of deprivation events on the adaptation of children. It led to the gradual introduction of better methods for identifying and measuring conditions that evoke deprivational states (of which separation from parent is one of the most powerful) and the consequences for children exposed to such conditions.

What follows is an outline of the four stages of progress in the search to understand the nature and consequences of deprivation events in childhood as depicted by Langmeier and Matêjcêk (1975) in their volume, *Psychological Deprivation in Childhood.*

The first stage has been termed by these authors the *empirical period.* It was a lengthy one extending from the last half of the 19th century through the first three decades of the 20th century. This was a period marked by unsystematized pediatric observations of children living in institutions, particularly orphanages and hospitals. The high incidence of death among children housed in these settings, accompanied by observations of developmental and intellectual retardation, suggested that medical and psychological factors were important determiners of the developmental lags that characterized these children. Hence the stress was placed on the necessity of improving the hygienic care of the children and the physical surround of the institution.

The second period, roughly covering the 1930s and 1940s which the authors identify as the *alarm period,* was triggered by World War II (the aftereffects of World War I initiated the concern for physical debilitation of children as described above). The large numbers of deserted, displaced, and suffering children who wandered over Europe in the closing days of the war generated a concern over their mental, emotional, and physical development after years of suffering, induced by imprisonment, malnutrition, concentration camp experiences, and desertion and loss of parents and family. High mortality rates in institutions in which babies had been fostered, described in the early work of Spitz (1946a, 1946b) and Goldfarb (1943, 1955) comparing institutional children with home-reared children, seemed to suggest that there were unfavorable long-term effects on intellectual and personality development induced by the institutionalization of children.

Another precipitant for concern in this second period was the great social changes that took place after the war. The growth in the number of working mothers, inadequate housing for families, and the dissolution of unstable wartime marriages all brought a heightened awareness that the need for physical reconstruction of war-torn cities was accompanied by a parallel need for the mental and social reconstruction of the families that inhabited them. This dual necessity became one focus of the post-war rehabilitation effort.

In this period a new scientific reconstruction took place involving a reformulation of the nature of children's development and the rise of accompanying theory. Bowlby's (1951) monograph on *Maternal Care and Mental Health* presaged the new era and its message was heralded by Spitz's (1945, 1946a) earlier observations of the severe effects of long-term chronic deprivation in the emergence of the "affectionless character." "Anaclitic depression," "hospitalism," and "deprivation syndrome" were the favored constructs of that era. Its more permanent effects as seen in formulations of the "affectionless character" gave a longitudinal cast to maldevelopment of personality as a consequence of deprivational states.

The third period covered the 1950s and was devoted to correcting and more critically appraising the literature and conclusions of the preceding era. The view that deprivation was inevitable in institutions and that deprivation and its consequences were unerringly correlated gave way to an enlarged conception of children in families rather than in institutions and broadened the context of the environmental roots of deprivation.

There was a recognition that institutions varied in their quality and that the perception of inevitable negative outcomes for institutionalized children was neither valid nor appropriate. Thus, the earlier pessimism of inevitable and tragic developmental outcomes gave way before the reality that many children in institutions more than survived, and were not foreordained victims of developmental, intellectual, and characterological disabilities. Whereas in the previous period the Spitz-Goldfarb emphasis had been on deprivation and deficit, new investigations (e.g., Lewis, 1954; du Pan & Roth, 1955) indicated that only a minority of children were so affected. Rather than institutionalization providing an invariant syndrome of deprivation and deficit, followup studies made clear that this living arrangement too provided a diversity of outcomes. In part this result may have been the consequence of marked changes that took place (because of the findings of earlier studies) in the staffing of institutions, shifts in the formats of residential settings to assure variety, and the development of preventive and therapeutic programs within institutional settings designed to contain negative outcomes. A new and more critical appraisal of investigations of deprivation of maternal care marked the significant correctives of this third era.

The fourth stage, in which we now find ourselves, is one marked by experimental-theoretical advances, in which there has been a marked intensification of a systematic research effort to study separation experiences in a more parametric fashion. For example, in animal research, separation analogues have been developed in the course of which deprivation, separation, and attachment experiences have been manipulated with results that have enhanced our understanding of the effects of maternal and familial separation (e.g., Harlow & Harlow, 1969; Hinde & McGinnis, 1977; Kaufman & Rosenblum, 1967; Levine, this volume; Rosenblum, 1971; Suomi, 1977; Suomi, Harlow, & Novak, 1974).

This period has been one marked by major reviews including Bowlby's classic three-volume work on attachment (Bowlby, 1969, 1973, 1980), as well as other volumes of the same genre (e.g., Emde & Harmon, 1981; Parkes & Stevenson-Hinde, 1982), Rutter's reassessment of maternal deprivation (1972, 1979b, 1981), Foss's (1961, 1963, 1965, 1969) edited four-volume work on the determinants of infant behavior, and studies of the development of emotion in infancy (Dunn, 1977; Emde, Gaensbauer, & Harmon, 1976; Izard, 1978; Izard & Buechler, 1978; Lewis & Rosenblum, 1974, 1978). These works are signposts of an era in which an integration has begun to be recognized as underpinnings for the effort to understand normal and deviant personality development in children. The fruits of the effort can be seen in the current development of attachment models, experimental paradigms (e.g., strange situation) and experimental animal analogues (e.g., Harlow's wire and cloth surrogate mothers); Seligman's (1975) model of learned helplessness applied to poor school achievement (Diener & Dweck, 1978; Dweck, 1975); Kagan's (this volume) model and method of distress evocation in two-year-olds which reflect the beginnings of more systematic studies of stress responsiveness in very young children.

If one were to posit a fifth period in the development of research on psychological deprivation as a stressor in the lives of children it might well take the form of systematic research on the role of three types of factors that affect retention or loss of adaptiveness under stress. The first are factors related to *vulnerability and predisposition*, a diathesis that may be reflected in temperament, somatotype, motivation level, fatigability, biogenetic fragility, and the like. The second group of factors are the *potentiators or triggering events* that are the stress component of diathesis-stress formulations of the etiology of psychopathological states. The third set of factors—and those about which we know least—are the *protective*, *stress-resistant*, or *resilient* factors that assist or foster the maintenance of competence under distressing circumstances.

Research of this sort is more likely to yield significant data through longitudinal-development studies of various high-risk groups in the search for those processes that underlie resilience versus inflexibility, competence versus incompetence, active coping versus passive retreat in the face of stressful experiences.

In the emerging concern with stressors significant for children we can anticipate that fear of loss and separation from loved ones will demonstrate marked staying power through the years of infancy, childhood, and adolescence. From the standpoint of consistency and intensity over time, loss, desertion, and separation constitute universal themes for subsequent despair, grief, and bereavement. It is no wonder then that the strange situation has attained international and cross-cultural status.

What then is the current status of the separation and loss research literature?

Separation

The literature on loss and separation is the most extensive of the multiple stressors that affect children. I lean heavily on Rutter's (1972, 1979b, 1981) reassessment of maternal deprivation to catalogue the more consistent findings of the effects on children of separation from significant caregivers:

1. Admission to hospital or residential nursery evokes an acute distress reaction in children. This is most marked in children between the ages of 6–48 months. Emotional disturbance in children is particularly acute if the child has had a poor relationship with his parents or comes from a home marked by discord. Multiple hospital experiences enhance the probability of later psychiatric disorder. This outcome is greatest in children from disturbed or disadvantaged families.
2. Poor quality institutions can produce intellectual and developmental retardation in children whose period of placement in such a setting is an extended one.
3. Homes marked by discord and/or dissolution tend to relate to subsequent delinquent child behavior.
4. Multiple foster home and institutional placements in early childhood can contribute significantly to the development of later psychopathic and antisocial behavior.
5. The source of privations to which children may be subjected in poor institutions and poor placements requires study in order to learn about the specific effects of specific early life experiences on development.
6. The nature of significant attachments and hence significant separations warrant extension beyond mothers or mother surrogates. Other important figures in the life of infant and child also influence development and these embrace fathers, sibs, teachers, peers, neighbors, and others.
7. "Perhaps the most important recent development in maternal deprivation has been the emphasis on individual differences in vulnerability to deprivation and stress." Factors involved include temperament, sex differences, age at time of stress, strength of prior relationships etc.;

8. Long-range effects in terms of manifest psychological disturbance following separation experiences are not the typical outcome. Those children who do exhibit such consequences are the products of disturbed families prior to separation. When such effects do occur they are more likely to be exhibited by boys and to take the form of antisocial disorder.

There are several inferences suggested by these findings:

Firstly, the foreboding overemphasis on dire outcomes following separation has not been fulfilled on the basis of data gathered from more carefully designed studies. For example, a followup study of the long-term effects on children separated from their parents in the London blitz—20 years later—indicated that these persons, now adults, showed few instances of severe psychopathology. Secondly, a present research concern with the more healthy rather than the more disabled children who have been subjected to separation experiences is clearly warranted. Thirdly, so too is the greater emphasis that has begun to be placed on contextual situational factors. Much is dependent upon the interactions the child has with significant adults in the new settings whether hospital, institution, or foster home.

In general, there would appear to be greater plasticity than had been anticipated in the adaptive capacities of children who have known separation experiences. But data on the age-related effects of separation are meager. Infants under 6 months of age are less affected than are those 6 months and older—a finding that is consistent with the observed wariness of children at that later age (Yarrow & Goodwin, 1973). But more systematic age-related studies extended beyond early and middle childhood are needed.

Bereavement

There are few events more immediately traumatizing for a child than the death of a parent. It is somewhat surprising then that the study of bereaved children has been markedly neglected by researchers. Of the studies that have been performed, many are clinical-descriptive ones (Arthur & Kemme, 1964; Furman, 1974; Schowalter, 1975), others are retrospective case reports, still others have sought to relate childhood loss or separation to adult psychiatric disorders (e.g., Birtchnell, 1970a, 1970b, 1972; Brown, Harris, & Copeland, 1977; Granville-Grossman, 1968). But, as noted by Black (1978) in a recent annotation on the bereaved child, "there are few prospective studies on how children are affected both immediately and later by the death of a parent" (p. 287). Black notes, however, that there are a growing number of large-scale population studies that link parental loss in childhood to later psychiatric disorder, particularly depression (see Brown & Harris, 1978). Rutter (1979a) has performed a similar service for the role of deprivation, discord, and disruption, as opposed to death of a parent, as an antecedent to several forms of psychiatric disorder in affected children.

The effort to establish continuity between bereavement and psychiatric disorder in adulthood has led to a variety of criticisms of such studies: the use of disputed methods of psychiatric evaluation; the failure in some studies to differentiate early separations from early death of a parent; the bias of using adult psychiatric patients in looking backward to the presence of early childhood loss; the failure to control for significant social variables; and the difficulty of ascertaining in a determinate way whether or not severe loss events in childhood play a *causal role* in adult maladaptation (e.g., Costello, 1982; Tennant, Bebbington, & Hurry, 1980, 1982).

Such criticisms have generated an awareness of the importance of creating more adequate studies to answer important questions related to bereavement in childhood. Two will be dealt with in this section. First, what are the psychological consequences, if any, for children following the death of a parent? Second, are there critical age periods in childhood for which, in terms of long-term sequelae, parental death during those periods is more clearly associated with later psychiatric morbidity?

With regard to the first question, two contrasting studies point up the effects of subject sampling and investigative mode on the interpretation of results.

The first study is a clinical investigation conducted in a children's psychiatric hospital. Arthur and Kemme (1964) used an intensive case study approach to the intellectual and emotional problems evidenced by 83 emotionally disturbed children and their families who had experienced the death of a parent. The intensive case study was part of the clinic's assessment procedure and the treatment program which followed. This varied in the cohort from four months of clinic contact to two years. Of the 83 children, 60 were boys and 23 were girls; their ages ranged between 4½ and 17 years. Of the boys 40 had lost their fathers and 20 their mothers; for the girls 9 fathers and 14 mothers had died—61 from natural causes, 12 were accidental, and 10 were suicidal deaths. The results of the clinical study are rather forbidding. The investigators provide a catalogue of troubled behavior, marked personality changes, and manifest increments in the children's sense of vulnerability. The language in which the findings are reported is grim indeed: "the ability to trust may be virtually shattered following the death," "an insecurity of such catastrophic proportions that the reality of the death had to be denied;" "narcissistic self-investment and an elaboration and acting out of infantile omnipotence;" (some children's) "behavior was seemingly ungoverned and unrestricted insofar as impulsive expression was concerned;" "their overt behavior was observed to cover the gamut of impulsive expression of primitive sexual and aggressive urges, ranging from ostensibly unprovoked and unmitigated violence toward peers and adults, 'inexplicable' destructive acts toward property, and overtly seductive invitations for sexual contact with others regardless of age or sex through more attenuated expressions of these same urges" (pp. 44–46).

In addition, many of the children in seeking a cognitive explanation for the parent's death had to contend with the thought that he or she had been the instrument for the event, while in other cases the surviving parent was held to blame. Many of the children's emotional reactions were intensified by the sense of abandonment, despair, hopelessness, and apathy they felt. From the standpoint of coping with stress the children's view of a predictable world had dissolved and had been replaced by a new element of unpredictability and a pervasive fear that such events could recur. Wishes to join the dead parent in death dominated the thoughts of some children; threats of suicide were expressed but never attempted. Phobic reactions occurred in 45% of the cases; almost one-quarter of the group had night terrors and nightmares. Emotional shock was evident in most of the children immediately following the parent's death. But the longer term reactions were equally distressing, including eulogization or idealization of the dead parent, a loss of trust in relationships, a retention of guilt over past hostility to the dead parent accompanied by reactive depressive episodes. Were this study to stand alone, the impact of bereavement on children would suggest the need for psychiatric or psychological treatment for all.

However, a second study of recent origin modifies the picture of acute disturbance. Its sample of children and the research methods employed are quite different (Van Eerdewegh, Bieri, Parrilla, & Clayton, 1982). In the words of the researchers theirs is "the first prospective, controlled study of bereaved children from the general population inquiring systematically about a wide range of psychiatric symptoms, aspects of mental health, and sociodemographic data" (pp. 23–24).

An important aspect of the selection of families to participate in the study was that it consisted of a group of young, white widows and widowers who had been *randomly* selected for the study based upon a review of death certificates from St. Louis city and county (Clayton & Darvish, 1979). Bereaved spouses and controls with children who volunteered to join the study were given a structured interview at one-month and thirteen-month follow-up that was focused on the children's reaction to the death of the parent. Bereaved children included 63 males and 42 females, controls numbered 36 males and 44 females. The mean age was 11 for the bereaved group (range 2–17) and 10 for controls (range 2–17). From each family a maximum of three children between the ages of 2–17 could be selected. Interviews were conducted around such contents as the child's general adaptation to death, school performance, behavior problems at home and at school, behavioral symptoms (depression, anxiety, phobias, hysterical signs), and general health.

Index children and their controls were similar in terms of sex and age distributions, family SES, number of children in the family, and parental psychiatric diagnosis when these were applicable.

In terms of reported mood and symptoms exhibited by the children after a year there were significant differences between the bereaved children and their controls with the former exhibiting a greater frequency of sadness, crying, and irritability. Depressive symptoms that discriminated between the two groups included greater withdrawal, sleep difficulties, and decreased appetite. Significantly more frequent bedwetting marked the bereaved children, as did temper tantrums. In terms of school problems, a significantly greater proportion of the index children (18% to 0%) showed poorer school performance 13 months after the parent's death.

Between the one-month and the thirteen-month follow-up there was a significant decrease in the frequency of depressive mood exhibited by the bereaved children, an increase in the frequency of those fighting with siblings, and an increase in the number of index children who showed continued disinterest in school.

Thus, the data indicated that the immediate reaction of a child to a parent's death was typically mild and of relatively short duration. The only severely depressed bereaved children were primarily adolescent boys who had lost their fathers. Theirs was a grief reaction more like those exhibited by adults.

There are striking differences between the two cited studies. The community study clearly tempers the conclusions described in the clinic study. This may be a function of several factors. Firstly, the selection basis was markedly different. Arthur and Kemme's group was a clinic sample referred either for problems that antedated the parental death or that were precipitated by that event. Either reason for referral would suggest that the clinic children were more disturbed and would be expected to show an intensified symptom picture when compared with the children of widows and widowers who had been selected from the general population and who had not initiated a clinic referral for their children.

Secondly, the interview methods and assessment procedures differed in the two studies. The clinic group had intensive clinical processing, review and treatment that extended in many cases from several months to two years duration. That length of contact suggests that many of the children were probably severely disturbed. How disturbed they were when compared with other clinic children who had not been stressed by the death of a parent can not be assessed since there was no control group in the study.

On the other hand the St. Louis study also has shortcomings, most notable of which is the absence of any investigator contact with the children. It is the surviving grieving parent who is the interpreter of the child's behavior. As the investigators point out, bereavement could have affected the surviving parent's memory. The use of several siblings within a number of the families accentuates the problem. Yet a number of these children were not free of distress. There were some who revealed the possible effects of parental loss in terms of the reduced competency they exhibited in school more than a year following the death of their parent. Another factor may be the self-selection of families who participated in the study. The original acceptance rate for participation in the study was 58% (Clayton & Darvish, 1979). Although there were no differences in death certificate information between volunteers and refusers, factors of grieving, guilt, adaptation, etc. could not be obtained, and thus the nature of sample bias could not be ascertained. However, the direction of the research is commendable.

Future research employing groups of children bereaved by death versus those bereaved by parental divorce has been suggested by the St. Louis investigators and that is desirable. More intensive psychological, psychiatric, and ecological studies with follow-up over a longer period of time would also be helpful in filling in our knowledge gap. In addition severely depressed children being seen in clinics could be compared with other clinic children whose depressed mood and symptoms have been triggered by the death of a parent. These and other more intensive longer term prospective studies would seem to be desirable addenda to bereavement research.

Another question is this: Are there any particular ages of children when parental loss or separation occurs that are related to heightened psychiatric morbidity in adulthood? The data that are available are equivocal. Brown and Harris have suggested that for adult depression the period of 10–14 years of age may be the most vulnerable for daughters when mothers have been the deceased parent. A recently published retrospective study (Tennant, Bebbington & Hurry, 1982) cites the age bracket 5–10 as the most vulnerable age grouping particularly if it occurred for a period exceeding six months separation from parents, siblings, and the family home. But this confounds factors of institutionalization, placement in care, or in the homes of relatives or foster parents with the factor of parental loss.

An earlier study (Munro & Griffiths, 1969) reaffirms the relationship between inpatient depressive illness and an excess of maternal bereavement before the patients' fifteenth birthday but at a marginal level of significance. In general, these investigators report that none of the diagnostic categories of 279 psychiatric patients showed any significant excess of parental bereavement occurring at any particular age in childhood.

It is difficult thus to come to firm conclusions about critical stages, for there are many other factors that can influence the impact of bereavement on children irrespective of age, family closeness preceding the loss, the prior relationship between the affected child and the deceased parent, whether the parent is of the same or opposite sex of the child, the religious beliefs and social class background of the family, and the suddenness as opposed to the gradual onset of the event.

On the side of "steeling" experiences there appears to be an attenuation of the impact of orphanhood on later mental disorder in adulthood if certain protective factors are present of which one of the most important is the quality of care and support bereaved children receive following the parent's death. In general, the risk of psychiatric disorder in relation to parental loss appears to be relatively low, but tends to be heightened by cumulated stressors, whether these occur in childhood or in adulthood.

Perhaps a more general viewpoint is appropriate and it is one that reduces a single-mindedness about the affective consequences of bereavement and introduces the importance of cognitive factors. Younger children (<5 years of age) grieve with less intensity than do older children. This is a consistent finding and it may in part be related to a child's cognitive understanding of the concept of death. Older children have a greater awareness of notions of causality and above all can comprehend the necessary abstraction of death as universal, inevitable, and irreversible. Younger children under six years of age do not understand the concept of universality, whereas by age nine this is comprehended by most children. Irreversibility provides greater ambiguity in that some studies report confusion even in children up to the age 10 (Childers & Wimmer, 1971; White, Elsom, & Prawat, 1978). However, others report that many children, particularly by age eight, can understand that the dead do not return to life. Knowledge of such irreversibility seems to be increased for children who have experienced the death of a family member or of a pet. These data, however, are not inconsistent with a maximization of the effect of loss in children between the ages 5–10 as suggested by Tennant et al. (1982).

The relationship between cognitive understanding of death and the coping responses used by children in bereavement would appear to be a fruitful area for systematic study.

Changing Family Patterns

In considering the effects of threat of separation or loss we are confronted with a broad range of events some of which are fleeting and generate a level of distress which rapidly evaporates over time, while others can present children with the acute trauma of the dissolution of family through death or the more likely event in contemporary society—divorce of the parents (see Wallerstein, this volume). Still others may involve prolonged and repeated hospitalization of a parent because of chronic physical or mental disorder, while other chronic situations may reflect patterns of rejection and neglect in which the desired figure is not so much lost as never gained.

The role of the family and the specific interactions of parent and child are powerful determiners of the social, emotional, and cognitive development of the child. If these relationships are comparatively free of a sustained negative quality, if family life is stable, economic distress minimized, relationships supportive and intimate, affection and love offered and reciprocated, then development can proceed along a normal and comparatively unstressful path. But where such relationships are marked by recurrent threat of separations, a lack of support, or more violently by neglect and abuse, the adaptation of the child is endangered.

This is the more traditional arena of psychopathology. However, in recent years debate has arisen over a cultural transition that is taking place in which some have argued that radical changes are threatening traditional family structure, posing strong threats to the well-being of children. Here are some byproducts of that presumed revolutionary transition as gathered from a variety of reliable sources (Gerbner, Ross & Zigler, 1980; Louis Harris & Associates, 1981; Lasch, 1977; Oakley, 1981; Wallerstein & Kelly, 1980; Zigler & Gordon, 1982).

Divorce rates in the United States and abroad show startling increments. In this country nearly four in ten marriages end in dissolution in divorce courts. Each year from 1972–1979, one million new children below the age of 18 have experienced the trauma of family breakup through divorce. In the first eight months of 1979 the number of divorces and marriages in California neared equality. Other data provide a similar picture:

- In 1980 the number of single-parent families was 8.5 million—approximately 15% of America's families;
- For a variety of reasons (social or economic necessity, self-actualization, to raise the family living standard, escape from household drudgery) the proportion of married women in the work force now stands at 50%, with the projection that the figure will rise to 75% by the end of this decade. In Great Britain in 1911, one in 10 married women had a job; in 1951, one in 5, in 1976, one in 2. In 1980, 2 of 3 employed women are married (Cited in Oakley, 1981).
- Of working mothers in America, the fastest growing segment consists of those with children under two years of age. The number of children under six with working mothers is expected to rise from a current level of 7.1 million to 10.5 million by 1990.
- Such striking changes in the work force require that attention be given to provisions for adequate day care for the children. Unfortunately day

care services, despite the urgent social need for them, are grossly inadequate and marked by an absence of regulations and standards for most of the centers and private homes that care for children of working mothers (Zigler & Gordon, 1982).

There are other stressors in families that can profoundly affect children but these, although less extensive, are sufficiently high in incidence and prevalence to be worrisome. It is difficult to secure reliable data on the extent of child abuse in the United States. Estimates are variable and range from 200,000 to 4,000,000 cases annually. An oft-cited 1975 report from the National Center on Child Abuse and Neglect offers a figure of reported cases that total one million per year (cited in Zigler & Gordon, 1980). Prior reports of the effects of unemployment on family life would suggest that the current recession which has been accompanied by a rise in unemployment toward the 10 million mark, may add further stress in the form of increased alcohol intake by parents, spouse battering, and child abuse.

These are some of the contemporary ills of our time. In many instances, by comparison, they make the earlier and more traditional concerns with separation via hospitalization, illness of parent, etc. seem far less traumatic than they once were. Research of a longitudinal nature in which the impact—short and long term—of various stressors on children could be assessed would provide much needed information on which forms of stress experiences are likely to prove most disruptive to children of different ages, personalities, and types of family settings. Systematic research would provide us with needed clues about predisposing, potentiating, and protective factors in childhood.

CHILDREN AND WAR

Loss and separation are interpersonal traumas to which all individuals are subjected at some point during their lifetime. Although the timing of such an experience is unanticipated, its inevitability is not. There are, however, other events of extraordinary intensity which are sudden, dramatic, difficult to control, unanticipated (but not recognized as inevitable) which induce personal uprooting, loss and separation, family disruption, mental and physical suffering, and enormous social change. Most prominent among these is war, and among its sufferers, least capable of coping with its consequences—hunger, fear, deprivation, and devastation—are children who are caught up in the catastrophe.

In World War II millions of children were uprooted, separated from their parents, and were denied the emotional and physical security they had once known. Estimates of these victims run high: 30 million families displaced by the war, with millions of children left homeless—8 million in Germany, 6½ million in Russia alone. Children came to know the horrors of the holocaust, bombings, malnutrition and starvation, the cruelty of becoming displaced persons, witnesses to murder and to death (Langmeier & Matêjcêk, 1975, p. 50).

How did children meet the stress of displacement and evacuation? With regard to the latter, studies conducted during and after the war produced findings that were unanticipated. Evacuation from the great cities of England (and from parents) under air attack to rural areas produced an estimated prevalence rate of neurotic symptoms ranging from 25–50%. Those who remained in the cities close to their families during the Blitz showed relatively few such neurotic behaviors, suggesting that the security engendered by parents compensated for the traumatic effects of air raids. In Bristol (Bodman, 1941) 4% of the children showed psychological or psychosomatic symptoms. These persisted for only a brief time in children under one year or over 5½ years of age. In describing Bodman's study, Lyons (1971) writes:

> Many children regarded the experience as an adventure and the general impression was of the extraordinary toughness of the child and his flexibility in adapting to potentially dangerous situations. (p. 266)

Freud and Burlingham (1943) in the midst of the war wrote a classic volume, *War and Children*, in which they summarize their major finding of children under war-time stress.

> In this war, more than in former ones, children are frequently to be found directly on the scenes of battle. Though, here in England, they are spared the actual horror of seeing people fight around them, they are not spared sights of destruction, death and injury from air raids. Even when removed from the places of the worst danger there is no certainty, as some of our cases show, that they will not meet new bombing incidents at places to which they were sent for safety. General sympathy has been aroused by the idea that little children, all innocently, should thus come into close contact with the horrors of the war. It is this situation which led many people to expect that children would receive traumatic shocks from air raids and would develop abnormal reactions very similar to the traumatic or war neuroses of soldiers in the last war.
>
> . . . So far as we can notice there were no signs of traumatic shock to be observed in these children. If these bombing incidents occur when small children are in the care either of their own mothers or a familiar mother substitute, they do not seem to be particularly affected by them. Their experience remains an accident, in line with other accidents of childhood. . . . It is a widely different matter when children, during an experience of this kind, are separated from and even lose their parents. (pp. 20–21)

In many cases even the disturbed children adapted well to the change, with outcomes, good or poor, influenced by the quality of foster home care and the atmosphere of the home placement in terms of whether it was consonant or dissonant with the child's personality. Thus, fearful children, it was reported, fitted better into conventional, quiet homes, whereas adventuresome and aggressive children adapted better in less conventional families.

Within the evacuee group, children separated from their families sustained uprooting more poorly than did those who had been evacuated together with their families (Burbury, 1941; Meierhofer, 1949; Sutter, 1952 as cited in Langmeier & Matêjcêk, 1975). Children who were able to handle evacuation best were those who enjoyed "healthy positive relationships with their parents." Children in earlier conflict with their families fared poorly in their new settings. In terms of age factors adolescents and, in some studies, preschool children were more distressed by their change in residence. Most children, however, were able to integrate into their new homes; only a small number (6–7%) adapted poorly (Isaacs, 1941).

Then there were the refugee children who, as might be expected, fared least favorably and whose disturbed behavior was more severe. Those who had been imprisoned in concentration camps, of course, fared worst of all. The behavior of the children, even those from well-adjusted families, quickly deteriorated. They stole, cheated, formed gangs, engaged in varied forms of anti-social behavior. But mental disorders were an infrequent occurrence, and even neurotic symptoms, which a child had shown previously, disappeared. But the longer term effects remained—hostility, anxiety, a desire for vengeance. In some cases, these sometimes came to dominate the children's development (Langmeier & Matêjcêk, 1975, p. 154).

Reports summarized by Langmeier and Matêjcêk, indicate that the children recovered their general physical health rather quickly, but their social behavior posed a longer term problem. Developmental retardation, destructiveness, an inability to learn how to play marked the behaviors of very young children. One report indicated that those children separated from their mothers before the age of three were retarded at age five in the physical, psychomotor, social, and intellectual spheres.

Fifteen thousand Jewish children passed through the Terezin concentration camp in Czechoslovakia. That camp has provided us with one of the most striking clinical case studies of the effects of loss on children. This was a group of six young children whose parents had died in the gas chambers; the infants, when 6–12 months old, were placed in the Terezin camp. At the end of the war, they were flown to England where the staff of Anna Freud's Hampstead Nursery assumed responsibility for their care. Here is a portion of the unique clinical account that Freud and Dann (1951) provided of the behaviors of the children upon entry (The full account can be found in Volume 6 of *The Psychoanalytic Study of the Child*).

> The children's positive feelings were centered exclusively in their own group. It was evident that they cared greatly for each other and not at all for anybody or anything else. They had no other wish than to be together and became upset when they were separated from each other, even for short moments. No child would consent to remain upstairs while the others were downstairs, or vice versa, and no child would be taken for a walk or on an errand without the others. If anything of the kind happened, the single child would constantly ask for the other children while the group would fret for the missing child. . . . (p. 131)
>
> The children's unusual emotional dependence on each other was borne out further by the almost complete absence of jealousy, rivalry and competition, such as normally develop between brothers and sisters or in a group of contemporaries who come from normal families. There was no occasion to urge the children to 'take turns'; they did it spontaneously since they were eager that everybody should have his share. Since the adults played no part in their emotional lives at the time, they did not compete with each other for favors or for recognition. They did not tell on each other and they stood up for each other automatically whenever they felt that a member of the group was unjustly treated or otherwise threatened by an outsider. They were extremely considerate of each other's feelings. They did not grudge each other their possessions, . . . on the contrary lending them to each other with pleasure. When one of them received a present from a shopkeeper, they demanded the same for each of the other children, even in their absence. On walks they were concerned for each other's safety in traffic, looked after children who lagged behind, helped each other over ditches, turned aside branches for each other to clear the passage in the woods, and carried each other's coats. In the nursery, they picked up each other's toys. After they had learned to play, they assisted each other silently in building and admired each other's productions. At mealtimes handing food to the neighbor was of greater importance than eating oneself.
>
> Behavior of this kind was the rule, not the exception. (pp. 133–134)

Initially the children directed strong and uncontrolled aggression toward adults, biting, hitting and striking out at them. Subsequently, a sequence of prosocial behaviors began to emerge: they came to substitute verbal for physical aggression, and then verbal disapproval when they were dissatisfied, and finally, their reactions to staff took a more positive turn of helping them when it was needed and being able to seek their help in turn. They began to treat staff as they treated each other—sharing, growing sensitive to the needs of others, and behaving with consideration for their comfort.

Summing up their extensive clinical report Freud and Dann wrote:

> . . . The six children . . . are, without doubt, 'rejected' infants in this sense of the term. They were deprived of mother love, oral satisfactions, stability in their relationships and their surroundings. They were passed from one hand to another during their first year, lived in an age group instead of a family during their second and third year and were uprooted again three times during their fourth year. . . . The children were hypersensitive, restless, aggressive, difficult to handle. They showed a heightened autoerotism and some of them the beginning of neurotic symptoms. But they were neither deficient, delinquent nor psychotic. They had found an alternative placement for their libido and, on the strength of this, had mastered some of their anxieties, and developed social attitudes. That they were able to acquire a new language in the midst of their upheavels, bears witness to a basically unharmed contact with their environment. (p. 168)

The surprising element in accounts of the many child prisoners of Terezin is that following their liberation many adapted reasonably well in a comparatively short time, with 60% showing no frank symptoms of mental disorder. But a "sensitizing" effect was also evident:

> Almost all of them, however, were scarred in certain ways by their great suffering; this was reflected mainly in their increased vulnerability and mental instability and in the fact that minor changes in their life situations tended to produce breakdowns. (Langmeier & Matêjcêk, 1975, p. 158)

But the critically important factor of individual variation remained, allowing investigators to relate precurser protective factors to patterns of adaptation under extreme circumstances:

> Children from stable families who had happy early lives and who were mentally very healthy withstood these conditions relatively well. Character traits developed in early childhood (notwithstanding a superficial appearance of maladjustment) resisted even the most severe stress to a certain extent. Children who had developed independence also showed higher tolerance of these difficulties. While it is probable that certain long-term anxiety states in all afflicted children could lead to the development of neurosis in later life, actual neurosis during the stay in concentration camps was relatively rare. In more emotionally unstable individuals, however, severe neuroses often developed after liberation. (p. 159)

But even for this latter group, reports indicated that placement in well-run institutions, marked by good care and a responsiveness to the emotional needs of the children, revealed a "high potential for readaptation" that was reflected in a more favorable prognosis even for those children who had been subjected to long-term emotional deprivation.

World War II has faded from our collective awareness and the children of that war have moved into middle age. But new wars and civil strife have reappeared on the world scene, catching up children just as fatefully as it did their predecessors in 1939–1945. In a similar fashion the descriptive literature of the consequences of combat for children in the 1970s and 1980s also bears a striking similarity to its predecessor.

In the Middle East, Israel has been engaged since its founding in a succession of wars or war-like conditions, prompting Lazarus (1982) to refer to that nation as "a great national laboratory, unparalleled in its potential for meaningful research on the psychology and physiology of stress and coping" (p. 34). In Ireland, an equally extraordinary situation has prevailed with chronic civil strife substituted for the more formal trappings of war. From both areas have come forth a series of studies of the impact of war on children (For Israel, see De Shalit, 1970; Jarus, Marcus, Oren & Rapaport, 1970; Kristal, 1975; Spielberger, Sarason, & Milgram, 1982, particularly the chapters by Chen et al., Golan, Halpern, Morawitz, Rofe & Lewin, and Smilansky; Ziv & Israel, 1973; Ziv, Kruglanski & Shulman, 1974). (For Ireland, see Fields, 1976; Fraser, 1974; Harbison & Harbison, 1980; Heskin, 1980; Jahoda & Harrison, 1975.)

These studies too bear the imprint of clinical investigation, and efforts to provide psychological and psychiatric assessments of the children. Here are some of the supportive findings of a number of the studies and volumes cited above.

1. In Belfast, the extraordinary riots that took place over a six-week span in August–September, 1969, resulted in a great deal of destruction and numerous injuries and arrests. In analyzing its psychiatric sequelae, Lyons (1971) reported that of 217 persons seen in the riot areas for psychiatric symptoms, only three were children. They were given a primary diagnosis of Behaviour Disorder (1 enuretic, 1 school refusal, 1 severe nightmares and bouts of screaming). In all three cases a parent had been initially affected and seen for psychiatric care. There is a strong suggestion in these three cases of a modeling of parental distress, and evidence of a behavioral pattern of "communicated anxiety." But Lyons notes that, as a rule, children "appeared to enjoy the excitement (of the riots), and parents described how they played on the barricades with toy guns" (p. 271).
2. The question of communicated anxiety induced by recurrent shelling of border kibbutzim settlements in Israel was studied by Ziv and Israel (1973) who compared children in these settlements with children in other kibbutzim that had never been under enemy fire. Contrary to expectation the investigators found no differences in anxiety level as

measured by a paper and pencil test—the Children's Manifest Anxiety Scale. Explanation for this lack of significant results may be adduced from two related studies. Using similar samples of children who lived under shelling and terrorist attacks in border agricultural settlements with other children who lived on inland settlements that were out of range of such attacks, Kristal (1978) replicated the earlier findings of non-significance in terms of measured anxiety. But another measure that he secured, namely, bruxism (teeth grinding), which has been shown to be correlated with stress and tension level, was higher in the children exposed to shelling as were pre versus post measures of these children's anxiety level after seeing a film depicting an attack on a settlement similar to their own.

Ziv, Kruglanski, & Shulman (1974) in a related study secured additional measures of the children in two similarly contrasted groups of settlements, testing for attitudes toward their residence, sociometric choices of peer favorites, aggressiveness, etc. The children of the shelled settlements exhibited a greater degree of locale patriotism, more covert aggression and a greater positive emphasis on courage as a desirable personality trait of high sociometric choice peers.

These studies suggest several things: Firstly, the importance of multi-method assessments (Nay, 1979) of anxiety including the use of unobtrusive measures (Webb, Campbell, Schwartz, & Sechrest, 1966), analogue enactments, psychophysiological measures, etc. Secondly, the significance of securing multiple measures that can provide an understanding of the role of related factors in the person-situation interaction. For example, a high premium placed by children on courage as a highly valued attribute may well modify their acknowledgement of anxiety in a situation that calls for courage. In that case a rating of diminished anxiety can reflect the operation of a powerful social desirability factor (Block, 1965; Edwards, 1957).

3. The development of mutual support and help networks by bereaved children (Halpern, 1982) and war widows (Morawitz, 1982) is a positive factor in reducing the grief of children and their surviving parents.

4. It would appear that greater attention is now being paid to protective factors that can help to contain the effects of the stress of war (Schwarcz, 1982; Zuckerman-Bareli, 1982). One such factor is the model behavior presented by significant adults in the child's life, including parents, guardians, nurses, teachers, and counselors (De Shalit, 1970; Kurtz & Davidson, 1974).

5. Aggression against and expressed hatred of the "enemy" appears to be tempered in many children caught up in the ravages of war. In some cases this has been explained by reference to communal ideology ex-

pressed by adults, as well as by the efforts of significant adult figures to inculcate a sense of security in the children (Schwarcz, 1982).

If there is any lesson to be derived from these more recent studies, it lies in the reaffirmation of the resilience potential that exists in children under stress. It is this topic to which I now turn in the concluding section of this chapter—the evidence for the presence of stress-resistant qualities in children under the most trying circumstances.

Resilience in Children Under Stress: The "Steeling" Effect

For decades, mental health researchers have devoted their energies to the study of patterns of maladaptation and incompetence. The emphasis has been placed upon symptom patterns characteristic of the various psychopathological states, their etiology, treatment, and outcome. To this end, researchers have sought out those *predisposing* factors, whether biogenetic or experiential, that could be related to the origins of disordered states, and to the *potentiating* factors or the triggering events that produced the final breakdown into that state.

With the growth of risk research in psychopathology (Watt, Anthony, Wynne, & Rolf, in press) attention has shifted from the already disordered individual to the potentially disordered individual, and from the adult patient to the nonpatient child. Abetted by the many contributions of epidemiological research, the previous emphasis on predisposing factors has been joined by a growing concern about "protective" factors (Rutter, 1979a)—those attributes of persons, environments, situations, and events that appear to temper predictions of psychopathology based upon an individual's at-risk status. "Protective" factors provide resistance to risk and foster outcomes marked by patterns of adaptation and competence.

It is quite likely that the next decade will witness a significant growth in research that may pass under many banners: "*stress-resistance*," "*ego-resilience*," "*protective factors*," "*invulnerability*." Whatever its identity tag the identification of such research will probably be marked by several of these elements: (1) an emphasis on prospective developmental studies of children who (2) have been exposed to stressors of marked gravity (3) which can be accentuated by specific biological predispositions, familial and/or environmental deprivations (4) typically associated with a heightened probability of present or future maladaptive outcomes but (5) which are not actualized in some children whose behavior instead is marked by patterns of behavioral adaptation and manifest competence.

The identification of groups such as these will be the starting point of research on protective factors and the processes they activate. At present systematic research in this area lags, but there are pioneering studies available that point the way to a constellation of factors that may play an "inoculative" role in maintaining a child's health and well-being.

I offer a summary of five very different approaches to the study of resilience in children, investigations marked by the use of different methods, applied to different types of disorders, in several cases under disparate conditions of stress, yet with results that are rather congruent.

1. I begin with an epidemiological study by Rutter and his colleagues (1975a, 1975b) who in a series of studies conducted on the Isle of Wight and in an inner London borough isolated six family variables that were found to be associated with an increased incidence of psychiatric disorders in children: marital discord, low socioeconomic status, large family size with overcrowding, paternal criminality, maternal psychiatric disorder, and admission of the child into the care of local authority. The number of familial risk factors were found to be related to a child's risk for psychiatric disorder. But the study also uncovered protective factors which ameliorated a child's risk status. These included temperament factors of a positive sort (e.g., flexibility of response, a positive mood), gender (girls less vulnerable than boys), warmth on the part of a parent toward the child, a distinctively encouraging school environment that enhanced a child's values and competencies. Examination of these "protective" factors provides a triad of categories: (1) positive personality dispositions, (2) a supportive family milieu, and (3) an external societal agency that functions as a support system for strengthening and reinforcing a child's coping efforts.

2. Another effort to identify possible protective factors used an entirely different research method—a literature survey in which the author located studies of competent black children in the urban ghettos who had been exposed to the stressors of poverty and prejudice. This effort (Neuchterlein, 1970; Garmezy & Neuchterlein, 1972; described in Garmezy, 1981) produced a number of correlates that were associated in different studies with these achieving children.

- Teachers and clinicians rated these children as possessing social skills. They were seen as friendly and well-liked by peers and adults, more socially responsive, interpersonally sensitive, less sullen and restless. Teachers reported them to be lower in "defensiveness" and "aggressiveness" and higher on "cooperation," "participation," and "emotional stability."
- They tended to have a positive sense of self, manifesting self-regard rather than self-derogation, and a sense of personal power rather than powerlessness.

• Some studies reported that such students had an internal locus of control and a belief that they were capable of exercising a degree of control over their environment. (The literature of internality suggests that its correlates include a warm, praising, protective, and supportive family environment.)

• Intellectually these children revealed their cognitive skills, but a dominant cognitive style appeared to be one of reflectiveness and "impulse" control.

• An intact family was *not* an identifiable consistent correlate. One was struck by the lack of any consistent evidence in the studies reviewed that father-absence had an adverse effect on academic achievement. Mother's style of coping with and compensating for an absent father appeared to be a powerful redemptive variable.

• The physical and psychological environment of the home was important. One investigative team described the households of these achieving lower-class children as less cluttered, less crowded, neater, cleaner, and marked by the presence of more books.

• Parents were more concerned about their child's education, they assisted willingly with homework, and participated in school-related activities.

• Parents carefully defined their own role in the family as well as the child's. Mothers of underachieving youngsters used their children to meet their own needs and stood more in the role of a pseudosibling than that of parent. The role relationships for the competent children were more structured and orderly.

• Parents accorded their children greater self-direction in everyday tasks and took cognizance of their children's interests and goals.

• The children, several studies suggested, seemed to have at least one adequate identification figure among the significant adults who touched their lives. In turn the achieving youngsters held a more positive attitude toward adults and authority in general.

These attributes of competent black children also suggests a triad of factors: (1) dispositional attributes in the child, (2) family cohesion and warmth, and (3) support figures in the environment and in the schools who can serve as identification models for the child.

3. A third study is a longitudinal-developmental one that extends from birth to early adulthood of a cohort of children born on the island of Kauai in the Hawaiian Islands. The report covers three decades and is reported in three volumes (Werner, Bierman & French, 1971; Werner & Smith, 1977, 1982).

In this research program many of the children when born and subsequently were at risk by virtue of perinatal stress, poverty, family instability, and, in some instances, the parents' serious mental health problems. In the course of their development one of every five children in the cohort developed serious behavior or learning problems. But by early adulthood many in the group had turned things around and had become manifestly competent. In their third volume Werner and Smith have provided a telling title, *Vulnerable But Invincible: A Study of Resilient Children*. This book catalogues the differentiators that marked the resilient children in comparison with peers of the same sex who had problems coping in adolescence. Once again the triad reappears—personality dispositions in infancy and childhood (e.g., "active," "socially responsive," "autonomous"), family milieu (family closeness, rule setting, supportive parents), and the presence of external support from peers, older friends, ministers, and teachers.

4. A fourth study is also a longitudinal-developmental one of children in which the central theme is "ego resilience" (Block & Block, 1980). These investigators perceive resiliency to be based in genetic and constitutional factors as seen in the way the infant responds to environmental change, can be comforted, equilibrates physiological responses, and modifies sleep-wakefulness states. Of equivalent importance is the nature of the family. Ego-resilient children have competent, loving parents who have shared values; ego-brittle children are exposed to discord and conflict in their homes.

5. Finally, I turn back to studies of children in war. These studies from the basic observations of Freud and Burlingham to the more recent studies in Israel have indicated that the prime factor in how children respond to the stress of war is based to a large extent on the behavior of their parents, guardians, and other significant adults. Such adults provided for the children a representation of their efficacy and ability to exert control in the midst of upheaval. From that standpoint the confidence of the adult community is in itself a support system of enormous importance to the well-being of children. Zuckerman-Bareli (1982) attempted to identify specific stress-resistance factors in those children exposed to border incidents in Israel. Citing attributes anchored in the individual the author noted "anxiousness" as a "comprehensive mental attitude that precedes the actual response to stress." Other factors included *age* (the younger, the greater the reservoir of energy), level of education (for the flexibility of problem-solving), sex (a greater emphasis in the kibbutzim that men are expected to be the defenders of the settlement), and a sense of identification and satisfaction with the community and its goals. Here too the triad of protective factors appeared.

Such evidence of resilience in children under stress is far more ubiquitous a phenomenon than mental health personnel ever realized, largely because of their long-term attention to behavior pathology. The aura of the old lingers on and, as an example, I turn to civil strife in Ireland and its effects on children in concluding this chapter.

Morris Fraser in *Children in Conflict* wrote a poignant description of the stress that marks the lives of the children of Belfast. His recital conveys a background to the civil strife that goes far beyond bullets and bombings.

> Environment, for a Belfast working-class child, means a decaying terrace, a high flat or a concrete housing estate with less than one-third the Government recommended playing space. He will mix, play, and be educated exclusively with his own religious group, and may never see a child of the 'other' group, except across a barricade. His home area is divided from other areas by armed sentries and steel barriers; he cannot leave this area, and to go out even in his own street after dusk is to court injury or death. The street is in pitch darkness at night, carpeted with stones and broken glass, littered with burnt-out, rusted skeletons that, perhaps a year ago, were cars, buses and lorries. His home is overcrowded, his father has a high chance of being unemployed, and poverty may be acute. He is brought up with a fear and hatred of members of the other religion that will last him all his life. (pp. 40–41)

Despite the uniformity of these stressful experiences, Fraser provided a context for a finding in his study that is ubiquitous in stress research, namely the variation in adaptation evident in children exposed to similar traumatic circumstances.

> In Belfast . . . the way in which each child reacted to riot stress seemed to depend on three main factors. There was, first, the degree of emotional security enjoyed by the child both before and during the period of acute stress. This related not only to his *own* psychological resources, but also to those of his immediate family. Secondly, there was the role of the stressful experience itself. Thirdly, each child's response was idiosyncratic, or unique, depending on his own usual way of responding to new experiences. (pp. 99–100)

The constellation of factors noted by Fraser is consistent with the studies of resilience in children that have been described. But what of the long-term consequences for the children who have been exposed to such a lengthy period of civil strife? An American psychologist, Dr. Rona Fields (1977) looked at Ireland in a volume, *Society Under Siege*, and wrote despairingly of the future of its children. Her volume refers to "psychological genocide," and indicates that in the absence of "massive rehabilitation efforts . . . the children of Northern Ireland—those who survive physically, those who do not emigrate—will be militaristic automatons, incapable of participating in their own destiny." (p. 55)

An Irish psychologist Dr. Ken Heskin (1980) in *Northern Ireland: A*

Psychological Analysis concluded his recent volume on this wholly different note:

> The people of Northern Ireland have suffered much in the past decade but they have come thus far with characteristic human fortitude and resilience in the face of adversity. Despite the prophets of doom, the evidence is that societal norms in Northern Ireland have not deteriorated and will not deteriorate to a level at which peace might be only marginally better than conflict. There remains in Northern Ireland a community of people whose strengths and similarities far outweigh their weaknesses and differences. (p. 157)

Which view shall we heed? The literature of stress, the evidence for the adaptive potential of children, their resilience, patterned in part out of personal disposition, the nature of their families, and that community of people whose strengths and similarities provide support for them places me in Heskin's corner. There is little gained by those who cry havoc while failing to heed the recurrent findings of our research literature on the ability of children to meet and to conquer adversity.

REFERENCES

Ainsworth, M. D. S. The development of infant-mother attachment. In B. M. Caldwell, & H. N. Ricciutti (Eds.), *Review of child development research* (Vol. 3). Chicago: University of Chicago Press, 1973.

Ainsworth, M. D. S. Infant-mother attachment. *American Psychologist* 1979, 34, 932–937.

Ainsworth, M. D. S., & Bell, S. M. Attachment, exploration, and separation: Illustrated by the behavior of one-year-olds in a strange situation. *Child Development*, 1970, *41*, 49–67.

Ainsworth, M. D. S., & Wittig, B. A. Attachment and exploratory behavior of one-year-olds in a strange situation. In B. M. Foss (Ed.), *Determinants of infant behavior* (Vol. 4). London: Methuen, 1969.

Anthony, E. J., & Koupernik, C. (Eds.), *The child in his family: Children at psychiatric risk* (Vol. 3). New York: John Wiley and Sons, 1974.

Antonovsky, A. *Health, stress and coping*. San Francisco: Jossey-Bass, 1979.

Appley, M. H., & Trumbull, R. *Psychological stress*. New York: Appleton-Century-Crofts, 1967.

Ariès, P. *Centuries of childhood*. New York: Vintage Books, 1962.

Arthur, B., & Kemme, M. L. Bereavement in childhood. *Journal of Child Psychology and Psychiatry*, 1964, *5*, 37–49.

Bartoshuk, A. K. Motivation. In J.W. Kling & L. A. Riggs (Eds.), (Woodworth & Schlosberg's) *Experimental psychology* (3rd ed.). New York: Holt, Rinehart & Winston, 1971.

Baruch, G. K., & Barnett, R. C. On the well-being of adult women. In L. A. Bond, & J. C. Rosen (Eds.), *Competence and coping during adulthood*. Hanover, New Hampshire: University Press of New England, 1980.

Bindra, D. *Motivation: A systematic reinterpretation*. New York: The Ronald Press Co., 1959.

Birtchnell, J. Early parent death and mental illness. *British Journal of Psychiatry*, 1970a, *116*, 281–288.

Birtchnell, J. The relationship between attempted suicide, depression and parental death. *British Journal of Psychiatry*, 1970b, *116*, 307–313.

Birtchnell, J. Early parental death and psychiatric diagnosis. *Social Psychiatry*, 1972, *7*, 202–210.

Black, D. Annotation: The bereaved child. *Journal of Child Psychology and Psychiatry*, 1978, *19*, 287–292.

Bleuler, M. *The schizophrenic disorders: Long-term patient and family studies*. New Haven: Yale University Press, 1978.

Block, J. *The challenge of response sets*. New York: Appleton-Century-Crofts, 1965.

Block, J. H., & Block, J. The role of ego-control and ego-resiliency in the organization of behavior. In W. A. Collins (Ed.), *Development of cognition, affect, and social relations. The Minnesota symposia on child psychology* (Vol. 13). Hillsdale, N.J.: Lawrence Erlbaum Associates, 1980.

Blom, G. E. Psychological reactions of a school population to a skywalk accident. In C. D. Spielberger, I. G. Sarason (Eds.), & N. A. Milgram (Guest Ed.), *Stress and anxiety* (Vol. 8). Washington, D.C.: Hemisphere Publishing Corporation, 1982.

Bodman, F. War conditions and the mental health of the child. *British Medical Journal*, 1941, *ii*, 486–488.

Bowlby, J. *Maternal care and mental health*. Geneva: World Health Organization, 1951.

Bowlby, J. *Attachment and loss: Attachment* (Vol. 1). New York: Basic Books, 1969.

Bowlby, J. *Attachment and loss: Separation, anxiety and anger* (Vol. 2). New York: Basic Books, 1973.

Bowlby, J. *Attachment and loss: Loss, sadness and depression* (Vol. 3). New York: Basic Books, 1980.

Bretherton, I., & Ainsworth, M. D. S. Responses of one-year-olds to a stranger in a strange situation. In M. Lewis, & L. A. Rosenblum (Eds.), *The origins of fear*. New York: John Wiley & Sons, 1974.

Brown, G. W., & Harris, T. *Social origins of depression: A study of psychiatric disorder in women*. New York: The Free Press, 1978.

Brown, G. W., Harris, T., & Copeland, J. R. Depression and loss. *British Journal of Psychiatry*, 1977, *130*, 1–18.

Burbury, W. M. Effects of evacuation and of air raids on city children. *British Medical Journal*, 1941, *ii*, 660–662.

Cannon, W. B. *Bodily changes in pain, hunger, fear and rage* (2nd ed.). New York: Appleton-Century Co., 1929.

Cannon, W. B. *The wisdom of the body*. New York: W. W. Norton & Company, 1932.

Childers, P., & Wimmer, M. The concept of death in early childhood. *Child Development*, 1971, *42*, 1299–1301.

Clayton, P., & Darvish, H. S. Course of depressive symptoms following the stress of bereavement. In J. E. Barrett (Ed.), *Stress and mental disorder*. New York: Raven Press, 1979.

Coelho, G. V., Hamburg, D. A., Adams, J. E. (Eds.), *Coping and adaptation*. New York: Basic Books, 1974.

Costello, C. Social factors associated with depression: A retrospective community study. *Psychological Medicine*, 1982, *12*, 329–339.

Cox, T. *Stress*. Baltimore: University Park Press, 1979.

Coyne, J. C., & Lazarus, R. S. Cognitive style, stress perception, and coping. In L. Kutash, L. B. Schlesinger and Associates (Eds.), *Handbook on stress and anxiety*. San Francisco: Jossey-Bass Publishers, 1980.

de Mause, L. (Ed.) *The history of childhood*. New York: The Psychohistory Press, 1974.

De Shalit, N. Children in war. In A. Jarus, J. Marcus, J. Oren, & Ch. Rapaport (Eds.), *Children and families in Israel: Some mental health perspectives*. London: Gordon & Breach, 1970.

Despert, J. L. *The emotionally disturbed child—then and now*. New York: Robert Brunner Inc., 1965.

Diener, C. I., & Dweck, C. S. An analysis of learned helplessness: Continuous changes in performance strategy, and achievement cognitions following failure. *Journal of Personality and Social Psychology*, 1978, *36*, 451–462.

Dohrenwend, B. P., Dohrenwend, B. S., Warheit, G. J., Bartlett, G. S., Goldsteen, R. L., Goldsteen, K., & Martin, J. L. Stress in the community: A report to the President's Commission on the accident at Three Mile Island. *Annals of the New York Academy of Sciences*, 1981, *365*, 159–174.

Dunn, J. *Distress and comfort*. Cambridge, Mass.: Harvard University Press, 1977.

Dunn, J., & Kendrick, C. The arrival of a sibling: Changes in the pattern of interaction between mother and first-born child. *Journal of Child Psychology and Psychiatry* 1980, *21*, 119–132.

Dunn, J., Kendrick, C., & MacNamee, R. The reaction of first-born children to the birth of a sibling: Mothers' reports. *Journal of Child Psychology and Psychiatry* 1981, *22*, 1–18.

Dweck, C. S. The role of expectations and attributions in the alleviation of learned helplessness. *Journal of Personality and Social Psychology*, 1975, *31*, 674–685.

Edwards, A. L. *The social desirability variable in personality assessment and research*. New York: The Dryden Press, 1957.

Emde, R. N., Gaensbauer, T. J., & Harmon, R. J. Emotional expression in infancy: A biobehavorial study. *Psychological Issues*, 1976, *10* (1, Monograph 37). New York: International Universities Press.

Emde, R. N., & Harmon, R. J. (Eds.), *The development of attachment and affiliative systems*. New York: Plenum, 1981.

Fields, R. M. *Society under siege: A psychology of Northern Ireland*. Philadelphia: Temple University Press, 1977.

Forman, E. *A child's parent dies: Studies in childhood bereavement*. New Haven: Yale University Press, 1974.

Foss, B. M. (Ed.), *The determinants of infant behaviour* (4 volumes). London: Methuen, 1961–1969.

Fraser, M. *Children in conflict*. Harmondsworth, Middlesex: Penguin Books, 1974.

Freud, A., & Burlingham, D. T. *War and children*. London: Medical War Books, 1943.

Freud, A., & Dann, S. An experiment in group upbringing. In *The psychoanalytic study of the child* (Vol. 6). New York: International Universities Press, 1951.

Freud, S. Inhibitions, symptoms and anxiety. In *The standard edition of the complete psychological works of Sigmund Freud* (Vol. 20). London: The Hogarth Press and The Institute of Psychoanalysis, 1959. (Original publication date: 1926)

Garmezy, N. Children under stress: Perspectives on antecedents and correlates of vulnerability and resistance to psychopathology. In A. I. Rabin, J. Aronoff, A. M. Barclay, & R. A. Zucker (Eds.), *Further explorations in personality*. New York: Wiley Interscience, 1981.

Garmezy, N., & Neuchterlein, K. Invulnerable children: The fact and fiction of competence and disadvantage. *American Journal of Orthopsychiatry*, 1972, *42*, 328–329. (Abstract)

Gerbner, G., Ross, C. J., & Zigler, E. (Eds.), *Child abuse: An agenda for action*. New York: Oxford University Press, 1980.

Gleser, G. C., Green, B. L., & Winget, C. *Prolonged psychosocial effects of disaster: A study of Buffalo Creek*. New York: Academic Press, 1981.

Goldfarb, W. The effects of early institutional care on adolescent personality. *Journal of Experimental Education*, 1943, *12*, 106–129.

Goldfarb, W. Emotional and intellectual consequences of psychological deprivation in infancy: A reevaluation. In P. H. Hoch, & J. Zubin (Eds.), *Psychopathology of childhood*. New York: Grune & Stratton, 1955.

Graham, P., Rutter, M., & George, S. Temperamental characteristics as predictors of behavior disorders in children. *American Journal of Orthopsychiatry* 1973, *43*, 328–339.

Granville-Grossman, K. L. The early environment of affective disorder. In A. Coppen, & A. Walk (Eds.), *Recent developments in affective disorders*. London: Headley Brothers, 1968.

Grinker, R., & Spiegel, J. *Men under stress*. Philadelphia: Blakiston, 1945.

Halpern, E. Children's support systems in coping with orphanhood: Child helps child in a natural setting. In C. D. Spielberger, I. G. Sarason (Eds.), & N. A. Milgram (Guest Ed.), *Stress and anxiety* (Vol. 8). Washington, D.C.: Hemisphere Publishing Corporation, 1982.

Harbison, J., & Harbison, J. *A society under stress: Children and young people in Northern Ireland*. London: Open Books, 1980.
Harlow, H. F., & Harlow, M. K. Effects of various mother-infant relationships on rhesus monkey behaviours. In M. B. Foss (Ed.), *Determinants of infant behaviour* (Vol. 4). London: Methuen, 1969.
Harris, Louis and Associates, Inc. Families at work: Strengths and strains. *The American Family Report, 1980–1981*. Minneapolis, Minn.: General Mills, 1981.
Hartup, W. W. Peer relations and the growth of social competence. In M. W. Kent, & J. E. Rolf (Eds.), *Primary prevention of psychopathology: Social competence in children* (Vol. 3). Hanover, N.H.: University Press of New England, 1979.
Hebb, D. O. Drives and the conceptual nervous system. *Psychological Review*, 1955, *62*, 243–254.
Hebb, D. O. *Textbook of psychology* (3rd ed.). Philadelphia: W. B. Saunders Co., 1972.
Heinicke, C. M., & Westheimer, I. *Brief separations*. New York: International Universities Press, 1965.
Henry, J. P., & Stephens, P. M. *Stress, health, and the social environment: A sociobiologic approach to medicine*. New York: Springer-Verlag, 1977.
Heskin, K. *Northern Ireland: A psychological analysis*. New York: Columbia University Press, 1980.
Hinde, R. A., & McGinnis, L. Some factors influencing the effect of temporary mother-infant separation: Some experiments with rhesus monkeys. *Psychological Medicine*, 1977, *7*, 197–212.
Holmes, T. H., & Rahe, R. H. The Social Readjustment Rating Scale. *Journal of Psychosomatic Research*, 1967, *11*, 213–218.
Isaacs, S. *Cambridge evacuation survey: A wartime study in social welfare and education*. London: Methuen, 1941.
Izard, C. E. On the development of emotions and emotion-cognition relationships in infancy. In M. Lewis, & L. Rosenblum (Eds.), *The development of affect*. New York: Plenum Press, 1978.
Izard, C. E., & Buechler, S. Emotion expressions and personality integration in infancy. In C. E. Izard (Ed.), *Emotions in personality and psychopathology*. New York: Plenum Press, 1978.
Jahoda, G., & Harrison, S. Belfast children: Some effects of a conflict environment. *Irish Journal of Psychology*, 1975, *3*, 1–19.
Janis, I. L., & Leventhal, H. Human reactions to stress. In E. F. Borgatta, & W. W. Lambert (Eds.), *Handbook of personality theory and research*. Chicago: Rand McNally & Co., 1968.
Jarus, A., Marcus, J., Oren, J., & Rapaport, Ch. (Eds.), *Children and families in Israel: Some mental health perspectives*. London: Gordon & Breach, 1970.
Johnson, W. *Adults' and children's reactions to disasters and other extreme situations*. Unpublished summa cum laude thesis, University of Minnesota, 1980.
Kaufman, I. C., & Rosenblum, L. A. The reaction to separation in infant monkeys: Anaclitic depression and conservation-withdrawal. *Psychosomatic Medicine*, 1967, *29*, 648–675.
Koocher, G. P., & O'Malley, J. E. *The Damocles Syndrome: Psychosocial consequences of surviving childhood cancer*. New York: McGraw-Hill Book Co., 1981.
Kristal, L. Bruxism: An anxiety response to environmental stress. In C. D. Spielberger, & I. G. Sarason (Eds.), *Stress and anxiety* (Vol. 5). New York: Halsted Press, 1975.
Kurtz, H., & Davidson, S. Psychic trauma in an Israeli child: Relationship to environmental security. *American Journal of Psychotherapy*, 1974, *28*, 17–25.
Langer, W. L. Foreward. In L. de Mause (Ed.), *The history of childhood*. New York: The Psychohistory Press, 1974.
Langmeier, J., & Matêjcêk, Z. *Psychological deprivation in childhood*. New York: Halsted Press, 1975.
Lasch, C. *Haven in a heartless world*. New York: Basic Books, 1977.
Lazarus, R. S. The psychology of stress and coping: With particular reference to Israel. In C. D.

Spielberger, I. G. Sarason (Eds.), & N. A. Milgram (Guest Ed.), *Stress and anxiety* (Vol. 8). Washington, D.C.: Hemisphere Publishing Corporation, 1982.

Levi, L. *Stress and distress in response to psychosocial stimuli*. Oxford: Pergamon Press, 1972.

Levine, S., & Ursin, H. (Eds.), *Coping and health*. New York: Plenum Press, 1980.

Lewis, H. *The Mersham experiment*. New York: Oxford University Press, 1954.

Lewis, M., & Rosenblum, L. A. (Eds.), *The origins of fear*. New York: John Wiley & Sons, 1974.

Lewis, M., & Rosenblum, L. A. (Eds.), *The development of affect*. New York: Plenum Press, 1978.

Lindsley, D. B. Psychophysiology and motivation. In M. R. Jones (Ed.), *Nebraska symposium on motivation*. Lincoln: University of Nebraska Press, 1957.

Lyons, H. A. Psychiatric sequelae of the Belfast riots. *British Journal of Psychiatry*, 1971, *118*, 265–273.

Maccoby, E. E. *Social development: Psychological growth and the parent-child relationship*. New York: Harcourt Brace Jovanovich, 1980.

Magnusson, D., & Endler, N. *Personality at the crossroads: Current issues in interactional psychology*. Hillsdale, N.J.: Lawrence Erlbaum Associates, 1977.

Marshall, S. L. A. *Men against fire*. New York: Morrow, 1947.

Mason, J. W. A historical view of the stress field: Part II. *Journal of Human Stress*, 1975, *1*, 22–36.

McCubbin, H. I., & Boss, P. G. (Guest Eds.), Family stress, coping, and adaptation. *Family Relations*, 1980, 29, No. 4 (Special Issue).

Meierhofer, M. First experience in medical-psychological work at the Pestalozzi children's village at Trogen, Paris. UNESCO, Mimeographed, 1949. (Cited in Langmeier & Matêjcêk, 1975.)

Miller, S. M. Why having control reduces stress: If I can stop the roller coaster, I don't want to get off. In J. Garber, & M. E. P. Seligman (Eds.), *Human helplessness: Theory and applications*. New York: Academic Press, 1980.

Moos, R. H. *Human adaptation: Coping with life crises*. Lexington, Mass.: D. C. Heath Co., 1976.

Moos, R. H. (Ed.), *Coping with physical illness*. New York: Plenum Press, 1977.

Morawitz, A. The impact on adolescents of the death in war of an older sibling. In C. D. Spielberger, I. G. Sarason (Eds.), & N. A. Milgram (Guest Ed.), *Stress and anxiety* (Vol. 8). Washington, D.C.: Hemisphere Publishing Corporation, 1982.

Munro, A., & Griffiths, A. B. Some psychiatric non-sequelae of childhood bereavement. *British Journal of Psychiatry*, 1969, *115*, 305–311.

Murphy, L. B., & Moriarty, A. E. *Vulnerability, coping and growth: From infancy to adolescence*. New Haven: Yale University Press, 1976.

National Cancer Institute (NCI) *Coping with cancer*. (NIH Publication No. 80-280) Washington, D.C.: U. S. Department of Health and Human Services, 1980.

Nay, W. R. *Multimethod clinical assessment*. New York: Gardner Press, 1979.

Nuechterlein, K. H. *Competent disadvantaged children: A review of research*. Unpublished summa cum laude thesis. Minneapolis: University of Minnesota, 1970.

Oakley, A. *Subject women*. New York: Pantheon Books, 1981.

Pan, R. M. du, & Roth, S. The psychologic development of a group of children brought up in a hospital type residential nursery. *Journal of Pediatrics*, 1955, *47*, 124–129.

Parkes, C. M., & Stevenson-Hinde, J. (Eds.), *The place of attachment in human behavior*. New York: Basic Books, 1982.

Porter, R., & Collins, G. (Eds.), *Temperamental differences in infants and young children*. London: Pitman Books, 1982.

Rathjen, D. P., & Foreyt, J. P. *Social competence: Interventions for children and adults*. Oxford: Pergamon Press, 1980.

Regier, D. A., & Allen, G. (Eds.), *Risk factor research in the major mental disorders*. (DHHS Publication No. ADM81-1068, National Institute of Mental Health) Washington, D.C.: U.S. Government Printing Office, 1981.

Robertson, J., & Robertson, J. Young children in brief separations: A fresh look. *The Psychoanalytic Study of the Child*, 1971, *26*, 264–315.

Rosenblum, L. A. Infant attachment in monkeys. In H. R. Schaffer (Ed.), *The origins of human social relations*. London: Academic Press, 1971.

Rutter, M. Protective factors in children's responses to stress and disadvantage. In M. W. Kent, & J. E. Rolf (Eds.), *Primary prevention of psychopathology: Social competence in children* (Vol. 3). Hanover, New Hampshire: University Press of New England, 1979a.

Rutter, M. Maternal deprivation, 1972–1978: New findings, new concepts, new approaches. *Child Development*, 1979b, *50*, 283–305.

Rutter, M., *Scientific foundations of developmental psychiatry*. London: William Heinemann Medical Book, Ltd., 1980.

Rutter, M. *Maternal deprivation reassessed* (2nd ed.). Harmondsworth, Middlesex: Penguin Books, 1981. (1st ed., 1972)

Rutter, M., Cox, A., Tupling, C., Berger, M., & Yule, W. Attainment and adjustment in two geographical areas: I. The prevalence of psychiatric disorder. *British Journal of Psychiatry*, 1975a, *126*, 493–509.

Rutter, M., & Quinton, D. Longitudinal studies of institutional children and children of mentally ill parents (United Kingdom). In S. A. Mednick, and A. E. Baert (Eds.), *Prospective longitudinal research: An empirical basis for the primary prevention of psychosocial disorders*. Oxford: Oxford University Press, 1981.

Rutter, M., Yule, B., Quinton, D., Rowlands, O., Yule, W., & Berger, M. Attainment and adjustment in two geographical areas: III. Some factors accounting for area differences. *British Journal of Psychiatry*, 1975b, *126*, 520–533.

Schwab, R., & Pritchard, J. Situational stresses and extrapyramidal disease in different personalities. In *Life stress and bodily disease*. Association for Research in Nervous and Mental Disease, 1949.

Schwarcz, J. H. Guiding children's creative expression in the stress of war. In C. D. Spielberger, I. G. Sarason (Eds.), & N. A. Milgram (Guest Ed.), *Stress and anxiety* (Vol. 8). Washington, D.C.: Hemisphere Publishing Corporation, 1982.

Schowalter, J. E. Parent death and child bereavement. In B. Schoenberg, I. Gerber, A. Wiener, A. H. Kutscher, D. Peretz, & A. C. Carr (Eds.), *Bereavement: Its psychosocial aspects*. New York: Columbia University Press, 1975.

Seligman, M. E. P. *Helplessness: On depression, development, and death*. San Francisco: W. H. Freeman & Co., 1975.

Silver, R. L., & Wortman, C. B. Coping with undesirable life events. In J. Garber, & M. E. P. Seligman (Eds.), *Human helplessness: Theory and applications*. New York: Academic Press, 1980.

Sobel, R. Anxiety-depressive reactions after prolonged combat experience: The old sargeant syndrome. *Bulletin of the U. S. Army Medical Department*, 1949, *9*, 137–146.

Spielberger, C. D., Sarason, I. G. (Eds.), & Milgram, N. A. (Guest Ed.), *Stress and anxiety* (Vol. 8). Washington D.C.: Hemisphere Publishing Corporation, 1982.

Spitz, R. A. Hospitalism: An inquiry into the genesis of psychiatric conditions in early childhood. *The Psychoanalytic Study of the Child*, 1945, *1*, 53–74.

Spitz, R. A. Hospitalism: A follow-up report. *The Psychoanalytic Study of the Child*, 1946a, *2*, 113–117.

Spitz, R. A. (with the assistance of K. M. Wolf). Anaclitic depression. *The Psychoanalytic Study of the Child*, 1946b, *2*, 313–342.

Stouffer, S., Lumsdaine, A., Williams, R., Smith, M., Janis, I., Star, S., & Cottrell, L., Jr. *The American soldier: Combat and its aftermath* (Vol. 2). Princeton, N.J.: Princeton University Press, 1949.

Suomi, S. J. Adult male–infant interactions among monkeys living in nuclear families. *Child Development*, 1977, *48*, 1255–1270.

Suomi, S. J. Peers, play, and primary prevention in primates. In M. W. Kent, & J. E. Rolf (Eds.), *Primary prevention of psychopathology: Social competence in children* (Vol. 3). Hanover, New Hampshire: University Press of New England, 1979.

Suomi, S. J., Harlow, H. F., & Novak, M. A. Reversal of social deficits produced by isolation rearing in monkeys. *Journal of Human Evolution*, 1974, *3*, 527–534.

Tennant, C., Bebbington, P., & Hurry, J. Parental death in childhood and risk of adult depressive disorders: A review. *Psychological Medicine*, 1980, *10*, 289–299.

Tennant, C., Bebbington, P., & Hurry, J. Social experiences in childhood and adult psychiatric morbidity: A multiple regression analysis. *Psychological Medicine*, 1982, *12*, 321–327.

Tyhurst, J. S. Individual reactions to community disaster. *American Journal of Psychiatry*, 1951, *107*, 764–769.

Vaillant, G. E. *Adaptation to life*. Boston: Little, Brown and Co., 1977.

Van Eerdewegh, M. M., Bieri, M. D., Parrilla, R. H., & Clayton, P. J. The bereaved child. *British Journal of Psychiatry*, 1982, *140*, 23–29.

Wallerstein, J. S., & Kelly, J. B. *Surviving the breakup: How children and parents cope with divorce*. New York: Basic Books, 1980.

Watt, N. F., Anthony, E. J., Wynne, L. C., & Rolf, J. (Eds.), *Children at risk: A longitudinal perspective*. New York: Cambridge University Press, in press.

Webb, E. J., Campbell, D. T., Schwartz, R. D., & Sechrest, L. *Unobtrusive measures: A survey of non-reactive research in the social sciences*. Chicago: Rand McNally, 1966.

Werner, E. E., Bierman, J. M., & French, F. E. *The children of Kauai: A longitudinal study from the prenatal period to age ten*. Honolulu: University of Hawaii Press, 1971.

Werner, E. E., & Smith, R. S. *Kauai's children come of age*. Honolulu: University of Hawaii Press, 1977.

Werner, E. E., & Smith, R. S. *Vulnerable but invincible: A study of resilient children*. New York: McGraw-Hill Book Company, 1982.

White, E., Elsom, B., & Prawat, R. Children's conceptions of death. *Child Development*, 1978, *49*, 307–310.

Wynne, L. C., Cromwell, R. L., & Matthysse, S. (Eds.), *The nature of schizophrenia: New approaches to research and treatment*. New York: John Wiley & Sons, 1978.

Yarrow, L. J., & Goodwin, M. S. The immediate impact of separation: Reactions of infants to a change in mother figures. In L. J. Stone, H. T. Smith, & L. B. Murphy (Eds.), *The competent infant: Research and commentary*. New York: Basic Books, 1973.

Zigler, E. F., & Gordon, E. W. (Eds.), *Daycare: Scientific and social policy issues*. Boston: Auburn House Publishing Company, 1982.

Ziv, A., & Israel, R. Effects of bombardment on the manifest anxiety level of children living in kibbutzim. *Journal of Consulting and Clinical Psychology*, 1973, *40*, 287–291.

Ziv, A., Kruglanski, A. W., & Shulman, S. Children's psychological reactions to wartime stress. *Journal of Personality and Social Psychology*, 1974, *30*, 24–30.

Zuckerman-Bareli, Ch. The effect of border tension on the adjustment of kibbutzim and moshavim on the northern border of Israel. In C. D. Spielberger, I. G. Sarason (Eds.), & N. A. Milgram (Guest Ed.), *Stress and anxiety* (Vol. 8). Washington, D.C.: Hemisphere Publishing Corporation, 1982.

CHAPTER 3

NEUROCHEMICAL ASPECTS OF STRESS

ROLAND D. CIARANELLO, M.D.
PROFESSOR OF PSYCHIATRY AND CHIEF
DIVISION OF CHILD PSYCHIATRY AND CHILD DEVELOPMENT
DEPARTMENT OF PSYCHIATRY AND BEHAVIORAL SCIENCES
STANFORD UNIVERSITY SCHOOL OF MEDICINE

THE HISTORY OF stress research is interwoven with that of neurochemistry. Indeed, some of the first contributions on the physiology of stress were made by investigators studying the responses of the autonomic nervous system. Beginning with Cannon's work over a half-century ago, the fundamental importance of the "involuntary nervous system" in maintaining organismic viability in the face of stressful stimuli has been uncontested. Yet despite this understanding, and a concerted and dedicated effort by scores of modern-day investigators, there is much about stress and neurochemistry that remains undiscovered.

Cannon's work initially focused on bodily changes in pain, hunger, fear, and rage (Cannon, 1963), with the aim of understanding how stress could lead to disease. Cannon showed that rats which had been adrenalectomized remained well, provided they were not stressed, but the same animals could not survive stressful stimuli. He attributed this to a chemical which he had recently discovered and named "sympathin." This material was normally present in the adrenal medulla and was released into the circulation in copious quantities during stress. Cannon postulated that sympathin, which we now recognize as norepinephrine, was essential for the animal's survival. In addition to the responses to physiologic stimuli, Cannon showed that sympatho-adrenal medullary mechanisms were also involved in psychic events, such as the challenges of a cat by a barking dog (Henry, 1980).

Cannon's discoveries were momentous, and have become the cornerstone of modern neuroendocrinology and neurochemistry.

The expansion of our knowledge about the central nervous system, and particularly the rapid growth of neurochemistry, has stimulated many researchers to examine the cellular and molecular events in stress. Neurochemical systems are influenced by stress as both *responders* and *effectors*, that is, they are both stimulated by stress, and in turn act upon other systems to provoke secondary and tertiary responses. The result is a cascade of biochemical and neuronal responses that begin with the perception of a stressful event and result in a complex array of behaviors. In between, a multitude of physiologic responses has been provoked, each of which acts in some way to mobilize the organism: secretion of hormones, acceleration of heart rate, vasoconstriction and rerouting of blood flow, contraction of muscles, immunologic responses, alerting and arousal reactions, and alterations in mood and emotional state. In each of these, and in probably others as well, neurotransmitters, and particularly the catecholamines, play an important role.

CATECHOLAMINES

The catecholamines are so named because they are aromatic amines with a dihydroxybenzene (catechol) nucleus. They are synthesized in neuronal cells of the brain, sympathetic nervous system, and adrenal medulla. The catecholamines are derived from the amino acid tyrosine by a series of enzymatic conversions. The members of this family are dopamine, norepinephrine (noradrenalin), and epinephrine (adrenalin). L-DOPA, another important member of this family, is technically not a catecholamine, but a catechol amino acid. Because of their diffuse distribution in neurons, the catecholamines occur throughout the body, where they act as both hormones and neurotransmitters. Outside the brain, the catecholamines regulate blood pressure, heart rate, fat breakdown, and sugar metabolism. In the brain, catecholamine-containing neurons project to limbic, cortical, cerebellar, and hypothalamic structures. In these regions, they act as neurotransmitters, and are involved primarily in the expression of certain behaviors (arousal, affect, rage, reward, motor function), and in the regulation of neuroendocrine secretion. The catecholamines interact with a number of other neurotransmitter and neurohormonal systems; in so doing, they play a critical role in the biological response to stress.

CATECHOLAMINES AS HORMONES

The adrenal medulla synthesizes the bulk of the catecholamines which subserve hormonal roles. Embryologically, the adrenal gland consists of a glucocorticoid-secreting cortex of mesenchymal origin and a catecholamine-secreting medulla derived from the neural crest. The adrenal medulla is innervated by the splanchnic nerves, which play a major role in regulating the levels of medullary catecholamines. The splanchnic axons have cell bodies in the lateral horn of the spinal cord, and form cholinergic synapses directly onto the adrenal medullary chromaffin cells. Thus, the adrenal medulla is actually a modified sympathetic ganglion in which the splanchnic neurons are the presynaptic, and the adrenal medullary cells the postsynaptic, elements. Epinephrine is the principal catecholamine synthesized in the adrenal medulla. Once synthesized, epinephrine is released via the adrenal venous effluent into the general circulation. All of the epinephrine and a small portion of the norepinephrine found in the peripheral circulation comes from the adrenal medulla. Epinephrine has important hormonal actions on the heart, regulates lipolysis and glycogenolysis, and interacts with thyroid hormones to potentiate their action.

CATECHOLAMINES AS NEUROTRANSMITTERS

Dopamine and norepinephrine appear to function primarily as central and peripheral neurotransmitters. The peripheral sympathetic neurons synthesize norepinephrine for direct release onto the smooth musculature of blood vessels, digestive tract organs, various secretory glands, and structures in the face and head. Norepinephrine is the neurotransmitter in the sympathetic nervous system, where it facilitates smooth muscle contraction, which leads to vasoconstriction, cardiac acceleration and glandular secretion. Circulating norepinephrine is derived almost exclusively from peripheral sympathetic nerve terminals innervating the vasculature.

The brain synthesizes and degrades a substantial portion of the total body content of catecholamines. Catecholamines in the brain are synthesized mainly within central nervous system neurons, since the peripherally formed catecholamines cross the blood-brain barrier only to a limited extent. These central catecholamines, principally dopamine and norepinephrine, act as neurotransmitters.

ANATOMY AND DEVELOPMENT OF CATECHOLAMINE PATHWAYS

Cells of the peripheral sympathetic nervous system arise in the lateral horn of the spinal cord. The axons project a short distance to two chains of paravertebral sympathetic ganglia, where they make synaptic contact with cells within the ganglia. The axons of the ganglion cells then course to blood vessels, exocrine glands, and a variety of other organs and structures, where they make synaptic connections with smooth muscle or secretory cells. These terminals utilize norepinephrine as their transmitter.

Central adrenergic tracts arise from cell bodies in discrete brainstem nuclei. Detailed information about the distribution of dopamine and norepinephrine comes primarily from histofluorescence procedures. Recently it has been possible to differentiate clearly norepinephrine pathways from dopamine pathways, using specific fluorescent-labelled antibodies directed against dopamine β-hydroxylase (Watson, 1977; Watson, Richard, Ciaranello, & Barchas, 1980).

Brainstem nuclei project axons throughout the brain. The terminals of these cells each contain a specific transmitter (Figure 3-1). For example, the cells of the locus ceruleus project norepinephrine-containing axons, while dopamine is present in terminals originating from cells in the substantia nigra. Noradrenergic cells arising from the locus ceruleus project caudally to the spinal cord, dorsally to the cerebellum, and rostrally to a wide variety of structures, including cortex, hippocampus, hypothalamus, and septum. Dopamine neurons arise from mesencephalic nuclei and from the substantia nigra: they project rostrally to the caudate-putamen and cortex, and to limbic structures, such as nucleus accumbens, olfactory tubercle, and septum.

The development of adrenergic neurons is a rich and complex field, and a comprehensive review cannot be attempted here. Studies have been conducted in several animal species as well as in human fetuses. Obviously the time in gestation when cells appear and tracts develop differs according to the experimental animals, but the basic details do not differ much between species.

Developing noradrenergic cells may be seen as early as 11.5 days gestation in the rat fetus, halfway through the normal gestation time of 21 days (Black, Coughlin, & Cochard, 1979). By 14 days, the tracts are well demarcated and the course of the axons to their target organs is plainly visible (Olson, 1970). Between 11.5 and 14 days the developing adrenal medullary chromaffin cells begin to show the appearance of catecholamines (Hervonen, 1971). In the human fetus, central catecholamine and indoleamine (serotonin) tracts can be easily visualized between 3 and 4 months gestation (Nobin, & Bjorklund, 1973).

Development and maturation of biochemical function occurs a short time after the neuronal tracts are laid down. In the brain, noradrenergic regions show maturation of the enzymes of catecholamine synthesis beginning at 15 days gestation, while development of uptake, release, and reuptake properties occurs around 18 days (Coyle, 1973).

Development of the adrenergic tracts is under complex biochemical regulation. At least three major influences may be identified: (1) regulation

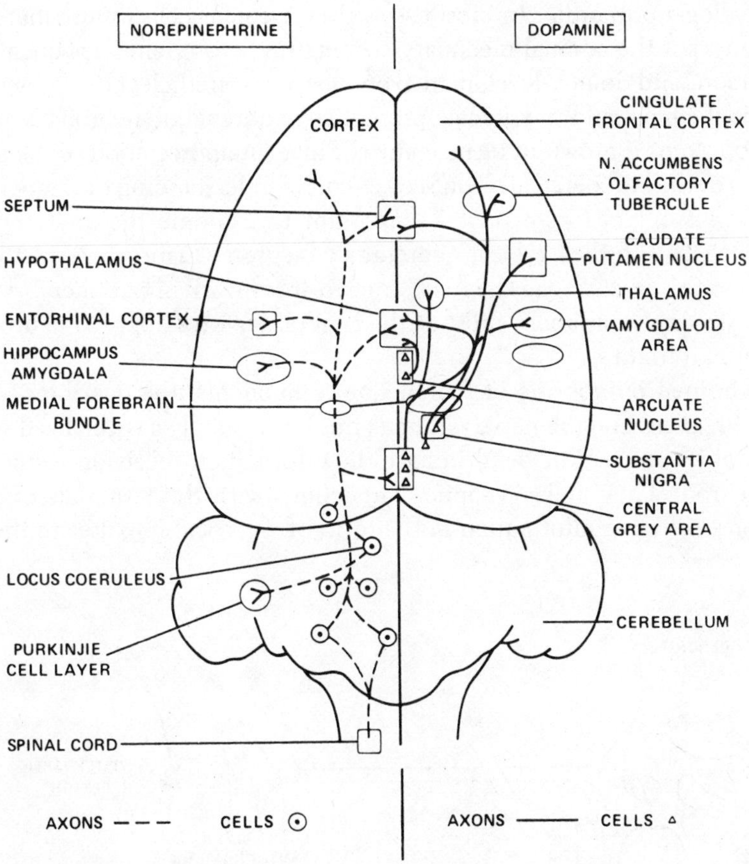

Figure 3-1. Schematic Representation of Dopaminergic and Noradrenergic Pathways in the Rat Brain

Norepinephrine pathways and cell bodies are indicated on the left side of the illustration, while dopamine projections are shown on the right side.

by other neurons making synaptic connections with the developing nerve cell; (2) regulation by the target organ, which in some way influences the final stages of neuronal maturation; and (3) regulation by the neuronal microenvironment, which includes trophic factors, nerve growth factors, hormones, and nutrients (Black et al., 1979).

AN OVERVIEW OF THE ADRENERGIC NEURON

All catecholamine-releasing cells, whether of adrenal medullary, peripheral sympathetic, or central adrenergic origin, are derived from neuronal embryologic primordia. In most cases, the precursor cells differentiate into neurons, but the adrenal medullary chromaffin cells retain a spherical configuration, and do not develop an axon *in situ*. Nonetheless they possess all the biochemical and physiologic properties of adrenergic neurons, and will develop axons if grown in tissue culture. Since an appreciation of the architecture of the adrenergic neuron is essential to understanding the response of neurotransmitters to stress, it is important to examine the anatomy and biochemistry of the "typical" adrenergic neuron (Figure 3-2). Although much of this picture has been constructed from work in peripheral sympathetic systems of animals, most of the general features apply to neurons in the human brain.

The neuron consists of four major components: the dendrites, a cell body, an axon, and the nerve terminal; this last is simply a specialized subdivision of the axon. The dendrites are the information-receiving segment of the neuron. They make synaptic connections with the terminals of other neurons, bringing information in the form of electrical impulses to the cell

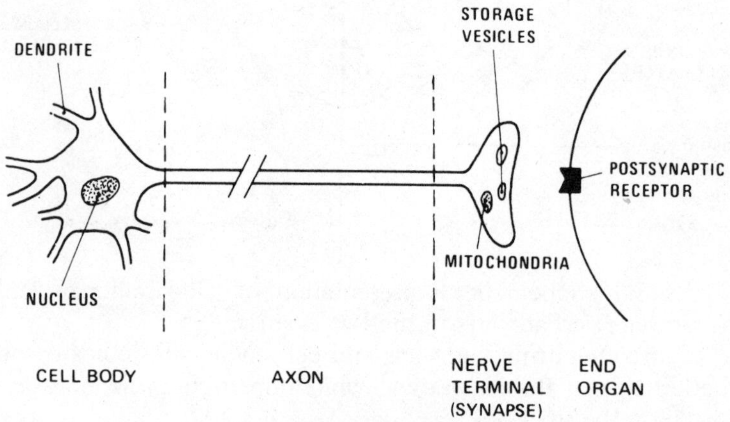

Figure 3-2. Schematic Representation of a Neuron

The cell body is the site of synthesis for synthetic and degradative enzymes and for storage vesicles. In addition, precursors are taken up into the cell from the surrounding milieu by specific uptake mechanisms. The axon transports enzymes, vesicles, and precursors from the cell body to the nerve terminals. In addition, it conducts electrical impulses of nervous transmission. The nerve terminal is the site of transmitter synthesis and storage. With electrical excitation, the transmitters are released into the synaptic cleft, where they activate the postsynaptic receptors. Transmitters are then degraded or taken back up into the nerve terminal by active reuptake mechanisms, thus ending the synaptic transmission (Ciaranello & Patrick, 1977).

body. The cell body has the general function of integrating and processing incoming information, and maintaining overall neuronal integrity. How the cell body integrates this diverse information, which may include data from thousands of other cells, remains one of the exquisite mysteries of neurobiology. Its nucleus contains DNA, in which is encoded genetic information for manufacturing all the materials needed in normal cell function. Among the enzymes made in the cell body are those involved in the synthesis and degradation of the specific transmitter for that neuron. Cell bodies also contain membrane pump mechanisms specifically to take up the appropriate neurotransmitter precursor (such as tyrosine, choline, or tryptophan) from the surrounding milieu.

The axon is the output arm of the neuron. Information, again in the form of surface-conducted electrical impulses, travels down its length until it arrives at the nerve terminal. The axon also serves as a conduit for transporting materials from the cell body to the nerve terminal. Specific transport systems conduct different materials at different rates. Thus enzymes travel at rates that differ markedly from those for mitochondria or for amino acids. The transport systems require energy and can be blocked by colchicine and vinblastine, drugs that disrupt microtubular architecture.

The nerve terminal is the "business end" of the neuron. In this specialized axonal outcropping, there are all the neuronal functions pertinent to neurotransmission: uptake of neurotransmitter precursors, synthesis, release, and reuptake of the neurotransmitter. The terminal contains subcellular membranous structures called vesicles that are specialized for the uptake, storage, and release of neurotransmitters. Terminal endings are also rich in mitochondria. These organelles generate the metabolic energy required for neuronal function, and also contain important degradative enzymes, such as monoamine oxidase.

NEUROTRANSMITTER DYNAMICS

Depolarization of the nerve cell membrane by an action potential results in changes in the flux of sodium, potassium, and calcium. Calcium appears to be critical in the transmitter-release process. Following depolarization, the transmitter is released from its storage vesicle. Although precise release mechanisms have still not been entirely elucidated, the first step appears to involve fusion of the vesicle to the membrane of the nerve terminal. The vesicular contents are then extruded into the synaptic cleft by a process known as exocytosis. In addition to the neurotransmitter, other associated materials are also released. Thus, peripheral adrenergic nerves release norepinephrine, adenosine triphosphate (ATP), and dopamine β-hydroxylase.

Once released, the neurotransmitter diffuses across the synaptic cleft, where it interacts with the postsynaptic receptor. Receptor-dynamics is currently one of the most actively investigated areas in neurobiology, and our understanding of it is far from complete. Receptor protein molecules are intimate constituents of the cell membrane. Their structure is highly specific for a particular transmitter, which they bind in a lock-and-key arrangement. Binding of the transmitter appears to alter the receptor conformation, resulting in changes in the membrane permeability for sodium and potassium, which permit propagation of the action potential. In addition, receptor-transmitter binding initiates a complex chain of intracellular reactions within the postsynaptic effector cell. In some neurons, this is mediated via a coupling between the receptor and the enzyme adenylate cyclase. When the receptor is stimulated, adenylate cyclase is activated and the production of cyclic AMP (cAMP) is increased. Cyclic AMP acts as a "second messenger," stimulating a variety of metabolic reactions with the cell. Not all neurotransmitter receptors are coupled to adenylate cyclase, however, so our understanding of how neurotransmitter receptor stimulation is transduced into stimulation of cell reactions in these neurons is incomplete.

The association of transmitter to receptor is an equilibrium process in which transmitter molecules are constantly dissociating from the receptor, freeing it to be restimulated. In the cholinergic system, neurotransmitter action is terminated at the postsynaptic membrane by acetylcholinesterase. For catechol- and indoleamines, termination of transmitter action depends upon washout of the synaptic cleft by microcirculatory perfusion, postsynaptic degradation, or reuptake of the transmitter into the presynaptic neuron, the last being the most important. The reuptake process is highly dependent on sodium, and is an active transport system which can be saturated by high concentrations of transmitter.

REGULATION OF CATECHOLAMINE SYNTHESIS

The metabolic pathways involved in catecholamine synthesis and degradation are shown in Figure 3-3. Catecholamines are derived from the amino acid tyrosine, which undergoes a series of enzymatic transformations into active neurotransmitter. The enzymes catalyzing these reactions are found in the adrenal gland, in neurons of the sympathetic nervous system, and in adrenergic and dopaminergic neuronal tracts in the brain (for review, see Ciaranello & Patrick, 1977).

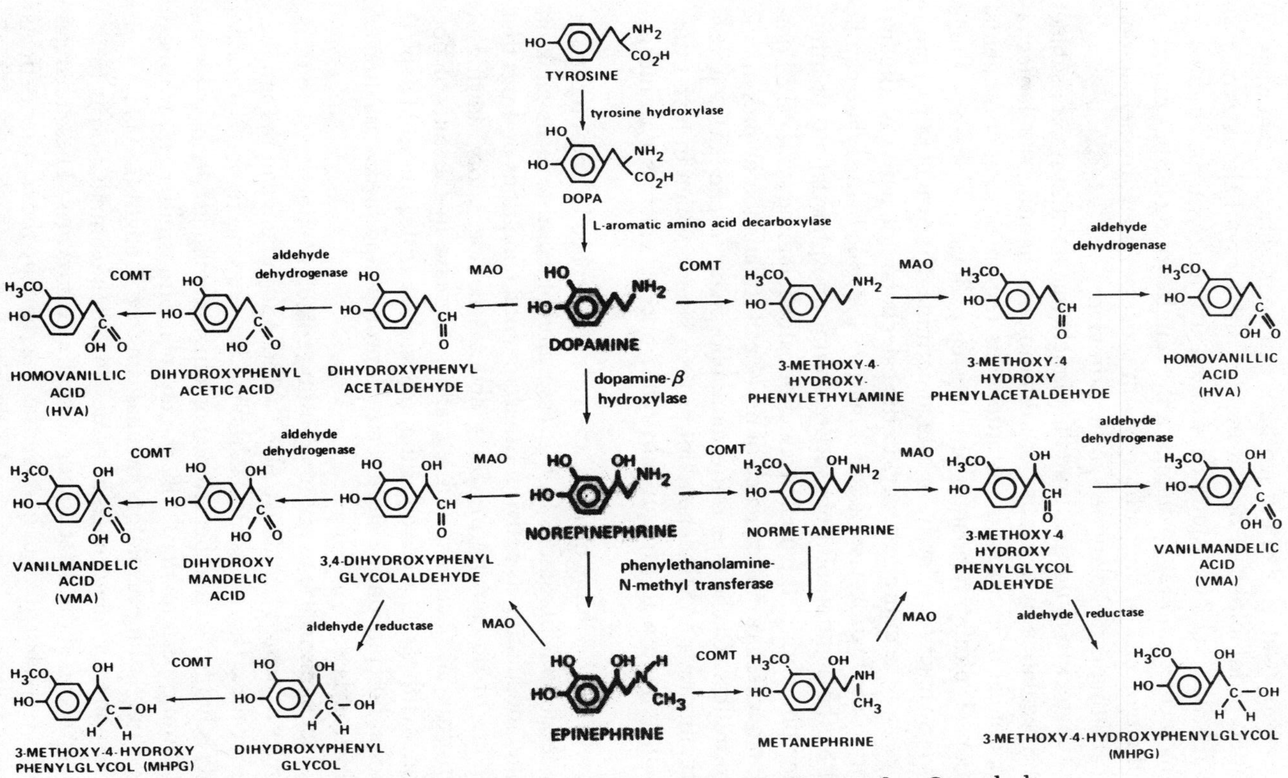

Figure 3-3. Synthetic and Degradative Pathways for Catecholamines (Ciaranello & Patrick, 1977)

The rate at which catecholamine production and inactivation proceeds is a major factor in the regulation of neurotransmitter processes, and therefore of behavior. Catecholamine synthesis can be modified in two ways: (1) by activation or inhibition of one or more of the biosynthetic enzymes, so that the reaction velocity is altered without a change in the number of enzyme molecules; and (2) by changing the number of molecules of one or more of the enzymes in the pathway. Both processes are extremely important in regulating catecholamine synthesis in vivo.

The enzymes in multistep, branched biochemical pathways are subject to complex regulation by activating or inhibiting mechanisms. Such mechanisms are critical in controlling instantaneous responses to environmental perturbation. Typically, regulation of multistep pathways occurs at a single enzyme whose reaction velocity, or rate, determines the overall rate of product synthesis for the entire pathway. In the catecholamine pathway, the first enzyme, tyrosine hydroxylase, is rate-limiting. Tyrosine hydroxylase can be activated by the addition of a phosphate group (phosphorylation) or inhibited by norepinephrine, the final product of catecholamine synthesis. Phosphorylation occurs as a consequence of nerve cell stimulation by presynaptic neurotransmitters. Cyclic adenosine monophosphate (cyclic AMP) is produced, stimulating a cAMP-dependent protein kinase, which in turn transfers phosphate groups to protein substrates, one of which is tyrosine hydroxylase.

The activity of tyrosine hydroxylase is also controlled by end-product or "negative-feedback" inhibition. In this case, norepinephrine feeds back on the enzyme, modulating its activity. Environmental conditions or drugs that cause buildup of norepinephrine bring about a compensatory slowing of tyrosine hydroxylase activity, and a gradual decrease in the rate of norepinephrine synthesis. Conversely, situations such as acute stress that deplete intraneuronal norepinephrine stores cause a prompt and brisk activation of tyrosine hydroxylase.

Such mechanisms are useful in adjusting catecholamine levels to transient changes in demand, and take place without any change in the number of tyrosine hydroxylase molecules. Although the enzyme responds rapidly, its capacity is limited so that persistence of a high-demand state for catecholamines (chronic perturbation) will deplete neurotransmitter stores unless other more long-lasting regulatory mechanisms are brought into play.

The response of noradrenergic tissues to chronic stimulation is to increase the levels of all the catecholamine synthetic enzymes. These changes occur more slowly, but are much longer-lasting than are the transient effects of enzyme activation or inhibition. All the catecholamine enzymes are affected by these processes, so that the tissue levels of each enzyme are increased. Two such mechanisms jointly regulate the levels of the catecholamine synthetic enzymes: neuro-transmitter released from the presynaptic neuron and glucocorticoid hormones from the adrenal cortex. Increased firing of the presynaptic neuron causes responses in the postsynaptic adrenergic cell, which include expressing the genes coding for specific enzymes, and the production of new messenger RNA complementary to the DNA of the genome. New enzyme molecules are rapidly synthesized from the mRNA template and shipped to the nerve terminal. This process is termed "induction," and is an essential means of producing new catecholamine enzyme molecules in response to persistent stimulation. In the rat, induction of new enzyme molecules occurs as rapidly as 24 hours after the onset of persistent stress, and achieves maximal levels 5–7 days later. Induction is the major route whereby long-lasting increases in catecholamine enzyme levels above normal (steady-state) can be achieved, and seems to operate in all adrenergic tissues.

Steady-state levels of the catecholamine enzymes seem to be determined primarily by the levels of adrenal glucocorticoid hormones (Ciaranello, 1979a). In the adrenal medulla, steady-state levels of tyrosine hydroxylase, dopamine β-hydroxylase, and phenylethanolamine N-methyltransferase are controlled by adrenal glucocorticoids. Reduction of glucocorticoids, as occurs with pituitary removal or destruction, profoundly reduces the levels of these three enzymes by accelerating their in vivo degradation by proteolysis. Glucocorticoids inhibit this degradation, probably by controlling the levels of enzyme cofactors, whose binding to the enzymes protects them against intracellular destruction. However, the glucocorticoids seem to control only steady-state enzyme levels, since neither exogenous administration of glucocorticoids nor excessive endogenous glucocorticoid production increase the level of these enzymes.

The role of glucocorticoids, in regulating biosynthetic enzyme levels in the peripheral sympathetic neuron and in the brain, is not well understood. There is some evidence that circulating glucocorticoids may play a role in maintaining tyrosine hydroxylase activity in sympathetic ganglia, but practically nothing is known about the importance of glucocorticoids to catecholamine synthesis in the brain. In these latter two systems, regulation of catecholamine synthesis is predominantly determined by activity of the nerves making synaptic formations with the catecholaminergic neurons. Increased presynaptic input induces the synthesis of tyrosine hydroxylase and dopamine β-hydroxylase in peripheral sympathetic ganglia and in central adrenergic neurons.

Nerve impulses and adrenal glucocorticoids may work cooperatively to maintain the level of catecholamine enzymes at times of increased demand (for review, see Ciaranello, 1980a). Neuronal stimuli increase the synthesis of tyrosine hydroxylase, dopamine β-hydroxylase, and phenylethanolamine

N-methyltransferase, while glucocorticoids inhibit in vivo proteolysis of these same enzymes. Such cooperativity has direct relevance to stress. Under stress situations, both splanchnic neuronal firing and pituitary ACTH secretion increase. Accelerated nerve firing stimulates adrenal cortical and medullary cholinergic receptors. In the cortex, cholinergic stimulation may facilitate ACTH-mediated glucocorticoid production, while in the medullary cell induction of catecholamine enzyme synthesis occurs. The increase in cortical glucocorticoid production results in synthesis of S-adenosylmethionine and ascorbic acid, stabilizing the medullary enzymes against intracellular breakdown. Thus, the synthesis of the enzymes is increased, and their breakdown is slowed under stress conditions. In this fashion, production of catecholamines at maximum rates is ensured.

When the stressful stimulation ceases, the system operates in the reverse fashion. Firing of the splanchnic neuron is reduced, and pituitary ACTH output falls. This decreases glucocorticoid production, at the same time removing the inducing stimulus to catecholamine enzyme synthesis. Thus enzyme synthesis is slowed while enzyme degradation is enhanced. The result is a fall in catecholamine production.

GENETIC REGULATION OF CATECHOLAMINES

The importance of the catecholamines in both normal and abnormal behaviors has prompted examination of their genetic regulation. Studies in inbred mice have demonstrated that the steady-state level of each of the catecholamine biosynthetic enzymes is controlled by a single autosomal codominant genetic locus (Ciaranello & Axelrod, 1973; Ciaranello, Hoffman, Shire, & Axelrod, 1974). A striking feature of these studies is the finding that the levels of all the enzymes are similar in different mouse strains; analysis of hybrid and segregating progeny suggests that concordant inheritance of enzyme phenotypes occurs, and that a single genetic control over steady-state levels of the enzyme pathway is exerted (Ciaranello, 1979b, 1980b).

Studies dealing with genetic control of enzyme responsiveness to stress and environmental perturbation have shown a complex degree of genetic control. So far, genetic regulation is thought to exist on the rate of enzyme responsiveness to stress, the type of stimulus to which the enzyme will respond, and the presence of different receptor types on adrenergic cells which mediate the enzyme response (Ciaranello, Dornbusch, & Barchas, 1972). Genetic control of dopamine receptors (Boehme & Ciaranello, 1981a, 1981b; Ciaranello, 1981) and of the number of neurons in dopaminergic regions of the brain (Baker, Joh, & Reis, 1980) has also been demonstrated.

The results of these studies strongly suggest that the catecholamine system in the brain and in the adrenal is under genetic control. Genetic control can be expressed in various ways: (1) on neuron number in certain brain regions; (2) on *steady-state* enzyme levels, through mechanisms regulating their rates of synthesis or degradation; and (3) on the responsiveness of the enzymes to stimulation. In part, this is mediated through (1) changes in the rate of enzyme response, and (2) the hormonal and neuronal receptors eliciting that response. Observations made on other enzyme systems show a multiplicity of genetic controls: on enzyme structure, on rate of synthesis or degradation, on rate of intercalation into membranes, and on rate of release from secretory cells. Clearly other genetic regulators in the catecholamine system are awaiting discovery.

CATECHOLAMINES AND STRESS

Despite the profusion of cellular responses initiated by the catecholamines, they themselves do not respond in a random or nonspecific fashion to stimulation. For many years, investigators working with the peripheral sympathetic-adrenal medullary system have differentiated the stimuli provoking norepinephrine release from those causing mainly adrenaline release. Not only do specific circumstances cause preferential release of one or the other catecholamine, but personality type seems to be an important determinant as well, at least in experiments with human subjects.

Individuals who are competitive and aggressive have larger vasomotor responses, excrete more norepinephrine, and are more prone to coronary artery disease. They respond to defeat by becoming depressed. In general, such persons fit the description of the well-known "Type A" personality. Such persons strive for achievement, are impatient, and have accelerated time-urgency. They cope well, and as long as they cope successfully, are protected against some of the deleterious consequences of stress: depression and defective immune response mechanisms. However, when they lose control of their situation, this protection is lost, and stress responses develop (Glass, 1977).

Anger, irritation, frustration, and sexual intercourse all have been shown to cause (or at least be associated with) an increase in plasma norepinephrine (Henry, 1980). In general, norepinephrine levels in plasma increase in individuals who are challenged by their environment, who are striving to achieve a particular goal, and for whom the behavioral repertoire relevant to goal-satisfaction are available (Mandler, 1967). Such conclusions drawn from human experimentation also seem generalizable to experimental animals, such as the rat. Henry (1980) has shown that the plasma norepinephrine level of mice experiencing prolonged social interaction is greater than those who have suffered repeated defeats in fighting. In contrast, adrenaline release from the adrenal is associated more with anxiety and helplessness. Frankenhaeuser's studies have demonstrated that adrenaline excretion is greater in students taking critical examinations (Frankenhaeuser, 1978).

Elsewhere in this volume, Levine has summarized the role of the pituitary-adrenocortical system in stress. This review has made reference to an integration of adrenocortical and adrenomedullary systems in response to stress. Although both hormonal systems show profound sensitivity to stress, there is some data to indicate that these responses depend on the stimuli provoking them. Ursin's work (reviewed in Henry, 1980) differentiates cortisol secretion from an increase in plasma catecholamines and free fatty acids in parachutist trainees, and suggests the responses are nearly independent of one another. Cortisol correlated negatively with performance and positively with fear, while norepinephrine was associated with activity and successful coping. These studies and others contrasting catecholamine with cortisol responses have led Henry to develop the model of stress, neuroendocrine response, and coping, shown in Figure 3-4.

According to this conceptualization, how an individual perceives a stimulus is critical in determining the outcome of his neuroendocrine response. This, in turn, is influenced by a complex interaction of genetic, early experiential, and learned coping patterns. If a stimulus is perceived as a challenge to control, then the "fight-flight" mechanism is triggered. This is mediated through the amygdala, a portion of the brain limbic system particularly associated with noradrenergic arousal systems. Activation of the amygdala ultimately provokes a response in the peripheral sympathetic adrenal medullary system, resulting in an increased secretion of norepinephrine and epinephrine. Significantly, corticosterone remains unaffected by this stimulus, while testosterone increases.

If the stimulus is associated with loss of control, i.e., helplessness, then routing of neuronal impulses is postulated to occur via the hippocampus and septum. These are also important components of the limbic system, but these are associated more with the neurotransmitters serotonin and dopamine, as well as with norepinephrine. Activation of this system results in stimulation of the hypothalamic-pituitary-adrenal system, of ACTH production, and finally, of secretion of corticosterone. Testosterone secretion is reduced in this case, while secretion of catecholamines is unaffected.

Henry's model makes reference to activation of certain brain regions, particularly the amygdala and the septal nuclei. These regions receive rich innervation from noradrenergic and dopaminergic neurons arising elsewhere in the brainstem. There have been several studies which have described changes in discrete brain regions of rats after acute stress. Palkovits has developed an elegant procedure for isolating discrete brain nuclei, and has refined the technique so that chemical assay can be performed on thin sections of brain nuclei. This has allowed subdivision of the ventral medial hypothalamus, for example, into 17 discrete regions, some of which show marked differences after stress, compared with other regions (Palkovits, Mezey, & Feminger, 1980; Kiss, Culman, Juraj, Mitro, Kvetnansky, & Palkovits, 1980). Dopaminergic, noradrenergic, serotonergic, and adrenergic neurons all participate in central responses to stress. Individual nerve terminals respond to stress by altering their neurotransmitter levels at different rates, and not all are affected equally, so it is not possible to describe a uniform stress response in the central nervous system. It is likely that the catecholamines and indoleamines act locally as neurotransmitters or neuromodulators, and, at a distance, as neurohormones.

CONCLUSIONS AND SPECULATIONS

The papers in this volume have wrestled with the myriad facets of stress and its related terminologies. As one reads the reports, one is struck with the valiant efforts being made in other fields to consider what stress is, whether stress and stressor are synonymous, the meaning of coping, etc. Neurochemistry, despite achieving brilliant insights into the chemical workings of neurons, has not considered stress in so comprehensive a fashion.

Stress research in neurochemistry has instead focused primarily on the response of neurochemical systems to stressful stimuli, i.e., stress and stressor are synonyms. This approach has yielded a rich lode of information on which systems respond, how they respond, and the interrelations between systems. So far, however, there has been less appreciation of the importance that the properties of the stressor (acute vs. chronic; novel vs. familiar; single vs. repetitive) bring to bear. In large part, this is because most researchers have been intent on studying the details of a particular biologic system, rather than its relation to stress. Stress has been a convenient tool to force a system response, but understanding the mechanism of response has generally been the primary goal.

We have seen that the catecholamine system is intimately involved in the response of an organism to stress, and that, in responding, it causes other metabolic and cellular events to occur. Although the system is responsive to a wide variety of stimuli, it is not nonspecific or unselective. Most environmental perturbations will provoke a response in some part of the adrenergic/noradrenergic/dopaminergic systems. A loud noise, for example, will cause an animal to startle and turn (noradrenergic arousal and alerting). If the stimulus represents a danger, other physiologic changes will occur: accelerated heart rate, vasoconstriction, and outpouring of adrenal hormones. However, stimuli which cause activation of one transmitter system may not activate others, or may trigger opposing responses in them. Different parts of a transmitter system may respond differentially to a given stimulus. Thus the levels of organization that determine a response to a stimulus occur between transmitter systems (e.g., noradrenaline and dopamine), within components of a given system (e.g., peripheral vs. central), and within individual structures (e.g., nuclei of the hypothalamus).

At the molecular level, similar differential response capabilities exist. In general, the various components of the catecholamine system respond to stress at different rates. Activation of adrenergic neurons and release of catecholamines from nerve terminals and the adrenal medulla occur virtually instantaneously after exposure to a stressor. Response of cellular target organs varies from very fast (contraction of muscles) to somewhat slower (fat breakdown). Doubtless this has something to do with the biologic function being served by the metabolic process. The most slowly responding part of the catecholamine system seems to be replenishment of the spent neurotransmitter by enzyme action.

Thus, at all levels, differential response capability exists to modulate, amplify, or attenuate responses to stress. The function of this system is quite basic: it serves to keep the animal alive. This is so fundamental that the kinds of questions preoccupying behavioral scientists (why is this important? what is its value to the organism?) are likely to be met by a cynical lifting of the neurochemist's eyebrow. If survival isn't important, what is? This system is so intimately related to so many metabolic systems that it is difficult to find one with which it does not interact.

In light of this, it is puzzling that more work has not been done to address questions about stress being asked by workers in other fields. As one reviews the field, one is struck by how much attention is paid to the neurochemical response to a stressor, to the exclusion of other equally interesting questions. I have made the point above, but perhaps it bears repeating, that most neurochemists concerned with stress have equated stress and stressor and have investigated the system response for its own sake. Their concern has been with the mechanism of response, not with stress.

Much of this work has been done with animals. It would be helpful, indeed critical, to know about the generalizability of these findings to humans. Another gap in our knowledge concerns development, particularly of the stress response. There have been very few neurochemical studies of stress and development in animals, and almost none in children. Thus, such issues as coping, mastery, and adaptation are not addressed in the neurochemical literature except inferentially: where a familiar stimulus initially provoked a neurochemical response, and now fails to elicit that response, we say "adaptation" has occurred. Whether this is a biochemical equivalent of the same process our psychological colleagues are describing is not certain. It is of interest, however, that Henry's work, perhaps the most comprehensive of any in this field, demonstrates that the dominant animal in a hierarchy has the least catecholamine secretion, whereas the subordinate animal has the greatest.

Henry's work offers further opportunities for some interesting speculations. It is clear from Figure 3-4 that there exists an important interplay between the genetic "hard-wiring" of an organism, its environment, and how the organism perceives its environment. This last, of course, depends heavily on prior experience. Depending on the organism's perception of the threatening nature of a stimulus, it will activate one or another central neuronal pathway, utilizing different neurotransmitters, resulting in different sympathetic and hormonal responses. We know from much animal data that the development, basal functioning, and ability of these systems to respond is subject to genetic regulation. The gene controls on these functions are varied and complex. Their effect is to place natural limits on the ability of an organism to respond to environmental stimuli. If the constraints are too

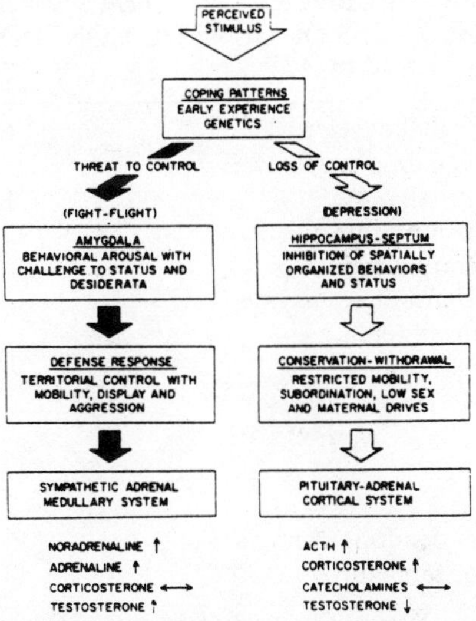

Figure 3-4. Depending on an individual's coping abilities, a stimulus is perceived either as a challenge to control with ensuing arousal of the fight-flight defense response or as an inducement to conservation-withdrawal with depression and arousal of the pituitary adrenal-cortical system. The ensuing hormonal patterns emphasize the catecholamines in the fight-flight state and the corticoids in the helpless-depressed state. (J.P. Henry, 1980)

severe, vulnerability to environmental stressors can result. This vulnerability takes place within an otherwise neutral environment, so that nonthreatening events may have harmful consequences. Maldevelopment of neuronal tracts, failure of synaptogenesis or confusion in neuronal "wiring," where neurons establish contact with the wrong neurons, can occur either as a genetic (mutation in a temporal gene), or a congenital, event (infection during pregnancy with a neurotropic virus). Regardless of the mechanism, vulnerability to stress and behavioral disorders might easily result.

Table 3-1 lists those aspects of neurochemical functioning for which genetic variability has already been described, or where preliminary evidence supports its existence, and the four major types of genes involved in biochemical systems. The total number of variants that can occur in this system could be as great as the product of the number of items in each column, but probably it is somewhat less in practice, since not all mutants are viable. If we expand this table to include other neural systems (indolaminergic, peptidergic, cholinergic, GABAergic, purinergic, etc.) and other physiologic processes (immunologic, endocrinologic), we begin to appreciate the complexity of the problem.

TABLE 3-1
SPECIFIC NEUROTRANSMITTER PROCESSES AND TYPES OF GENETIC CONTROL

*Specific Neurotransmitter Process**	*Type of Gene Control**
Neurotransmitter synthetic enzymes	Structural genes
Neurotransmitter degrading enzymes	Processing genes
Rate of enzyme synthesis	Regulator genes
Uptake of neurotransmitter precursor	Temporal genes
Transport of neurotransmitter	
Transport of neurotransmitter enzymes	
Release of neurotransmitter	
Reuptake of neurotransmitter	
Neurotransmitter receptors	
Neuronal number	
Neuronal architecture:	
Membrane stability	
Three-dimensional dendritic configuration	
Enzyme response to stimulation	

* The first column lists those neurotransmitter functions for which some evidence already supports a genetic control. The second column lists the major types of genes which are known to regulate biochemical processes. The total number of genetic variants that might exist in this system is somewhat less than the product of the number of items in the two columns. Let us use as an example dopamine-β-hydroxylase (DBH), one of the three enzymes of norepinephrine synthesis. The amino acid sequence of DBH is determined by at least one structural gene. The enzyme contains a copper atom at the active site; thus at least one processing gene is also involved. The rate of production of DBH is determined by a regulator gene, while the developmental appearance of the enzyme is under control of a temporal gene. Mutations may occur in any of these genes, but some might not be viable, and would not be discovered. Unraveling the biochemistry of a system such as this would provide a lifetime of fascinating work for a genetically inclined neurochemist.

But the genetic wiring is only one component determining the vulnerability of an organism to stress. Clearly the environment itself is important, but neurochemists have so far not paid detailed attention to the kinds and qualities of stressors or stimuli. The third component in determining the organism's response, according to Henry's model, is the perception of the environment by the organism. Here is where learning and developmental experiences come into play and exert a crucial impact on the type of biologic response. We know relatively little about the impact of learning and experience on the expression of neurochemical systems, or on their response to stimuli. This, too, is an important area of investigation on which more effort should be focused in the future.

Translating the results of studies in animals into concepts or conclusions applicable to humans may be difficult. Moreover, it may be impossible to conduct parallel studies in humans, where the only materials to which we have ready access are urine, blood, and cerebrospinal fluid. The animal work has taught us that the brain is vastly more complex than we believed, that its level of organization is more discrete than we learned in graduate neuroanatomy courses, and that individual parts of a brain region may react quite differently to the same stimulus. How can we ever explore this in humans using conventional neurochemical measurements, that usually require bits of brain tissue? How useful is it to measure compounds in the CSF, which, after all, receives its constituents from the entire central nervous system? If these are complex questions to pose in adults, how much more difficult are they to apply to children? In light of this, should we be surprised that practically no neurochemical studies have been done with children?

Real headway in linking animal work in neurochemistry to progress in understanding human stress-related events may come only when noninvasive methods to investigate neurochemical systems *in situ* become available. The positron emission tomogram (PET) scan is one such device. Certain compounds can be tagged with short-lived isotopes that can be detected by scanners outside the body. When given to human subjects, they are taken up in various parts of the brain, where the chemical reactions in which they participate can be followed externally. Such instrumentation is almost unimaginably expensive and is limited in availability, but already there are various centers in the United States where cooperative efforts are underway.

Where, then, are we? In this writer's view, stress work is an important area of neurochemical investigation. We particularly need to focus on developmental and genetic issues. These have not been actively investigated, despite growing evidence that they are critical in determining individual vulnerability to stress. Although there is much yet to be learned about neurochemical systems and how they are related, the data that currently exist more than amply permits the design and testing of sophisticated models for understanding the relationship of neuronal systems to stress. The challenge will come in integrating the data and in making the next higher conceptual leap—the translation of biochemical events into behavioral processes.

REFERENCES

Baker, H., Joh, T. H., & Reis, D. J. Genetic control of number of midbrain dopaminergic neurons in inbred strains of mice: Relationship to size and neuronal density of the striatum. *Proceedings of the National Academy of Science* (*USA*), 1980, *77*, 4369–4373.

Black, I. B., Coughlin, M. D., & Cochard, P. Factors regulating neuronal differentiation. In J. A. Ferrendelli (Ed.), *Aspects of developmental neurobiology*. Bethesda: Society for Neuroscience, 1979.

Boehme, R. E., & Ciaranello, R. D. Dopamine receptor binding in inbred mice: Strain differences in mesolimbic and nigrostriatal dopamine binding sites. *Washington D.C. Proceedings of the National Academy of Science* (*USA*), 1981a, *78*, 3255–3259.

Boehme, R. E., & Ciaranello, R. D. Strain differences in mouse brain dopamine receptors. In E. S. Gershon, S. Matthysse, X. O. Brakefield, & R. D. Ciaranello (Eds.), *Genetic strategies in psychobiology and psychiatry*. Pacific Grove: Boxwood Press, 1981b.

Cannon, W. B. *The wisdom of the body*. New York: Norton, 1963.

Ciaranello, R. D. Regulation of phenylethanolamine N-methyltransferase degradation by S-adenosylmethionine. In E. Usdin, R. Borchardt, & C. R. Creveling (Eds.), *Transmethylation*. New York: Elsevier Press, 1979a.

Ciaranello, R. D. Genetic control of the catecholamine biosynthetic enzymes. In J. Shire (Ed.), *Genetic variation in hormone systems*. Boca Raton, Fla.: CRC Press, 1979b.

Ciaranello, R. D. Regulation of adrenal catecholamine biosynthetic enzymes: Integration of neuronal and hormonal stimuli in response to stress. In E. Usdin, R. Kvetnansky, & I. J. Kopin (Eds.), *Catecholamines and stress*. New York: Elsevier Press, 1980a.

Ciaranello, R. D. Regulation of the synthesis and degradation of phenylethanolamine N-methyltransferase. In S. Parvez, & H. Parvez (Eds.), *Biogenic amines in development*. New York: Elsevier Press, 1980b.

Ciaranello, R. D. Biochemical genetics in mice: Implications for psychiatric research. In E. S. Gershon, S. Matthysse, X. O. Brakefield, & R. D. Ciaranello (Eds.), *Genetic strategies in psychobiology and psychiatry*. Pacific Grove: Boxwood Press, 1981.

Ciaranello, R. D., & Axelrod, J. Genetically controlled alteration in the rate of degradation of phenylethanolamine N-methyltransferase. *Journal of Biological Chemistry*, 1973, *248*, 5616–5623.

Ciaranello, R. D., Dornbusch, J. N., & Barchas, J. D. Regulation of adrenal phenylethanolamine N-methyltransferase activity in three inbred mouse strains. *Molecular Pharmacology*, 1972, *8*, 511–520.

Ciaranello, R. D., Hoffman, H., Shire, J. G. M., & Axelrod, J. Genetic regulation of the catecholamine biosynthetic enzymes. *Journal of Biological Chemistry*, 1974, *249*, 4528–4534.

Ciaranello, R. D., & Patrick, R. L. Catecholamine mechanisms. In J. D. Barchas, P. A. Berger, R. D. Ciaranello, & G. R. Elliott (Eds.), *Psychopharmacology: From theory to practice*. New York: Oxford University Press, 1977.

Coyle, J. T. Development of the central catecholaminergic neurons of the rat. In E. Usdin, & S. H. Snyder (Eds.), *Frontiers in* catecholamine research. New York: Pergamon, 1973.

Frankenhaeuser, M. Clinical psychoneuroendocrinology in reproduction. In L. Carenza, P.

Pancheri, & L. Zichella (Eds.), *Proceedings of the Serono Symposia* (Vol. 22). New York: Academic Press, 1978.

Glass, D. D. *Behavior patterns, stress, and coronary disease*. Hillsdale, N.J.: Lawrence Erlbaum Associates, 1977.

Henry, J. P. Present concepts of stress theory. In E. Usdin, R. Kvetnansky, & I. J. Kopin (Eds.), *Catecholamines and stress: recent advances*. New York: Elsevier Press, 1980.

Hervonen, A. Development of catecholamine-storing cells in human fetal paraganglia and adrenal medulla. *Acta Physiologica Scandinavica*. 1971, Suppl. 368.

Kiss, A., Culman, J., Mitro, A., Kvetnansky, R., & Palkovits, M. Distribution of catecholamines and serotonin in some subdivisions of hypothalamic ventromedial nucleus in rats: Effect of acute stress. In E. Usdin, R. Kvetnansky, & I. J. Kopin (Eds.), *Catecholamines and stress: Recent advances*. New York: Elsevier Press, 1980.

Mandler, G. The conditions for emotional behavior. In D. C. Glass (Ed.), *Neurophysiology and emotion*. New York: Rockefeller University Press, 1967.

Nobin, A., & Bjorklund, A. Topography of the monoamine neuron systems in the human brain as revealed in fetuses. *Acta Physiologica Scandinavica*. 1973, Suppl. 388.

Olson, L. *Growth of sympathetic adrenergic nerves*. Stockholm: Grafikon, 1970.

Palkovits, M., Mezey, E., & Feminger, A. Neuroanatomical basis for the activation of brain monoaminergic systems under stress. In E. Usdin, R. Kvetnansky, & I. J. Kopin (Eds.), *Catecholamines and stress: Recent advances*. New York: Elsevier Press, 1980.

Watson, S. J. Hallucinogens and other psychotomimetic biological mechanisms. In J. D. Barchas, P. A. Berger, R. D. Ciaranello, G. R. Elliot (Eds.), *Psychopharmacology: From theory to practice*. New York: Oxford University Press, 1977.

Watson, S. J., Richard, C. W., III, Ciaranello, R. D., & Barchas, J. D. Interaction of opiate peptide and noradrenaline systems: Light microscopic studies. *Peptides*, 1980, *1*, 23–30.

CHAPTER 4

A PSYCHOBIOLOGICAL APPROACH TO THE ONTOGENY OF COPING

SEYMOUR LEVINE

PROFESSOR, DEPARTMENT OF PSYCHIATRY AND BEHAVIORAL SCIENCES
STANFORD UNIVERSITY SCHOOL OF MEDICINE

COPING: AN ATTEMPT AT A DEFINITION

Whenever one attempts to define or clarify the concept of coping, the initial problem that needs to be confronted is the issue that *coping* normally refers to an active process which occurs in the course of attempting to adapt to environmental conditions that have stress as a major component. However, the concept of stress is itself ubiquitous in physiology and psychology, and precise definition has remained elusive. The notion of stress is diffuse, referring to many different kinds of stimulus variables which produce a constellation of responses (Ursin, Baade, & Levine, 1978). Selye (1936, 1950) conceptualized stress as a nonspecific process which represents the intersection of symptoms produced by a wide variety of noxious stimuli. Nonspecificity, according to Selye, refers to the diversity of agents which can bring about the same syndrome. The agents were called *stressors*, and *stress* referred to the pattern of responses which occurred as a consequence of the stressor. The primary measure of stress was an increased activity in the pituitary-adrenal system. Since then, the adrenocortical system has received much attention, presumably because the activity of this system has utility as a measure of stress. Some writers have treated the two as being synonomous (Ganong, 1963). The response characteristics of the pituitary-adrenal system seem to meet the criterion of nonspecificity (Mason, 1971); a large number of variables are capable of inducing an increase in adrenocorticotropic hormone (ACTH) followed by glucocorticoid secretion. Although Selye did propose that emotional factors might act as stressors, the emphasis in his classic work on the stress syndrome was oriented toward the study of the effects of physical insult.

More recently, the notion of stress has been put into a more psychobiological perspective, and the effects of psychological factors on neuroendocrine function are being taken into account more frequently. There is now an abundant body of information which would indicate that most of the stimuli which activate the pituitary-adrenal system stem from changes in environmental events that are mainly psychogenic. Over the past twenty to thirty years there has been an increasing awareness that psychological and social factors can have effects which are similar to, and perhaps even more potent than, those of physical stresses, and that the pituitary-adrenal system is particularly sensitive to these psychological variables. In many instances, it appears that even under conditions in which severe physiological insult is imposed, there exists an important emotional component which contributes to the activation of the pituitary-adrenal system (Gann, 1969; Mason, 1971). In studies on mice, for example, it has been observed that many of the physical effects in experiments on fighting are due more to psychological factors than to factors such as wounding or attack. Previously defeated mice placed in the presence of a trained fighter show as much pituitary-adrenal activation as mice that are attacked and defeated (Bronson & Eleftheriou, 1965). Further, rats exposed to electric shock in pairs, and less able to fight in response to shock, show significantly lower levels of ACTH than animals that are prevented from fighting (Conner, Vernikos-Danellis, & Levine, 1971). Other studies have shown that exposing animals to a novel chamber can produce plasma corticoid elevations as great as those produced by exposure to painful shock (Bassett, Cairncross, & King, 1973; Friedman & Ader, 1967). Our current understandings of psychological variables suggest that the initial mediators in many of Selye's experiments may have been the central nervous system substrates involved in emotional arousal. This basically alters the Selye concept of nonspecificity, at least in terms of the pituitary-adrenal response to stress. Instead of viewing the hormonal response as being elicited by a great diversity of stimuli, the current prevailing view is that the hormonal responses are being stimulated largely by a single stimulus, or stimulus configuration, common to a variety of situations. The component which is common to these situations appears to be some aspect of emotional arousal.

It has been proposed that activation of the pituitary-adrenal system by environmental events which do not involve tissue damage is best accounted for by a two-stage model involving expectancies. Thus, either the lack of any previously established expectancies about the environment, or a change in expectancies, can result in an increased output of ACTH from the pituitary, which leads to subsequent increase in circulating glucocorticoids. It has been further proposed that the processes involving neuroendocrine activation from lack of expectancies are best explained by a model elaborated by Sokolov (1960), which originally was intended to account for the general processes of habituation. The Sokolov model, in essence, is based on a matching system and the representation in the central nervous system of prior events, whereby the organism has either habituated or gives an alerting reaction. This matching process is defined as the development of expectancies (Pribram & Melges, 1969). Thus, the organism which has become habituated has a set of prior expectancies with which to deal with the environment, and if the environment does not contain any new contingencies, the organism does not respond with the syndrome of physiological responses related to the orienting response.

However, there is further evidence that one of the conditions that will activate neuroendocrine mechanisms leading to subsequent release in ACTH is a change in expectancy developed during previously well-established behavior. Thus, the absence of reinforcement under conditions where reinforcement has been continuously present will lead to an adrenocortical response which is equivalent in magnitude to that observed when the organism is initially exposed to noxious stimuli. Although this expectancy hypothesis does make a valiant attempt at trying to specify the sets of conditions that will reliably lead to activation of the pituitary-adrenal system, and therefore would be considered stressful, as yet it does not provide a precise definition of stress.

Perhaps it is not possible to come up with such a clear definition, since, to a very large extent, stress is idiosyncratic. The response to such noxious stimuli as electric shock, cold, or hemorrhaging, are themselves markedly modified by the environmental conditions under which these stimuli are presented. Yet, in spite of the many attempts to provide experimental and theoretical underpinnings to the concept of stress, the fact remains that, on an intuitive level, stress is a fact of life. To some extent, current interests in stress have depicted stress as the twentieth-century plague responsible for a variety of psychosomatic disturbances, as well as contributing to the manner in which many pathogens are capable of producing pathophysiological states. It would follow, therefore, if the concept of stress is difficult to define, that the definition of coping would be almost as elusive as the definition of stress.

Coping has been inferred either by alteration in behavior or by changes in the physiological response to threatening or aversive stimulation. The term has been used to denote a process utilized by an individual to deal with significant threats to his psychological stability and to enable him to function more effectively (Hamburg, Hamburg, & DeGoza, 1953). Most of the major theories in coping, at least in humans, have been concerned primarily with alterations in behavior. The individual is presumed to be coping if his behavior consists of responses that permit him to master the situation. Coping also includes intrapsychic processes that contribute to successful adaptation to psychological stress (Friedman, Mason, & Hamburg, 1963). Success or failure of coping may be evaluated in many ways. The first is behavioral; judgments are made as to whether the behavior allows the individual to continue to carry out the personally or socially defined goals and to tolerate stressful situations without disruptive anxiety or depression, regardless of whether the behavior is socially desirable. The second way of examining coping is whether there are changes in internal states, particularly hormone levels. For example, the excretion rates of cortisol appear to be stable if the coping behavior is effective in protecting the individual from anxiety and depression (Friedman et al., 1963). Since there appear to be two somewhat mutually exclusive criteria that define coping with aversive stimuli, there is considerable confusion concerning the best index of coping.

Most of the human literature has defined coping in terms of behavioral responses, whereas the research on coping using animals has defined coping both in behavioral and physiological terms. There is little problem with using both criteria if these measures are consistent. For example, in a series of studies examining both behavioral and physiological changes when animals were learning an active-avoidance response, Coover, Ursin, and Levine (1973) reported that there was a significant drop in plasma corticosterone following repeated avoidance training, and furthermore, that certain behavioral indices of fear also tended to disappear systematically. However, it appears that there are many instances in which the behavioral and physiological indices of coping are dissociated. Using a similar avoidance paradigm to that reported by Coover et al., Weinberg and Levine (1980) report that animals that fail to learn an active-avoidance response, and consequently are shocked on every trial, also show a similar drop in plasma corticosteroids. Using a behavioral definition of coping, these animals appear to be showing maladaptive behavior, but in terms of the physiological indices, the response of being able to escape the shock and also terminate the signal appear to be sufficient to reduce circulating corticosteroids.

Other clear examples of the dissociation between behavioral and physiological coping responses are evident in several studies which have examined the response of infant squirrel monkeys when separated from their mothers. If the animal is separated into a novel environment, there are marked signs of behavioral distress, such as heightened vocalization and activity, accompanied by markedly elevated plasma cortisol values. However, if the mother is removed, leaving the infant with familiar conspecifics in its home environment, the infant appears to show very few signs of behavioral agitation and distress, but the elevations in plasma cortisol as a consequence of removing the mother are still very apparent. In yet another study (Coe & Levine, unpublished), infant squirrel monkeys were separated from their mothers for a 6-hour period. It was found that the infants showed an initial heightened behavioral distress, in terms of the usual criteria of marked increase in vocalization and activity. However, these responses tended to gradually diminish so that by the end of the 6-hour period the animals were showing few signs of the behavioral agitation which follow separation from the mother. When one examined the plasma cortisol response to separation, the response increase was linear, and by the end of the 6-hour period the animals were showing values of plasma cortisol that were higher than we had ever seen in any other experimental situation with these monkeys.

It is our firm belief that the biological responses to aversive situations and the alterations of biological responses as a function of coping are more sensitive indices of cognitive and perceptual changes that occur when an animal is utilizing appropriate coping mechanisms. Further, the capacity to reduce the endocrine response to persistently aversive stimuli is of enormous biological utility, since heightened corticoids have a number of deleterious biological effects. They interfere with the action of insulin and exacerbate diabetes, cause loss of calcium from the bones, suppress growth, contribute to peptic ulcers, are involved in menstrual irregularities, and appear to induce hypertension. Another important effect of the corticoids is to suppress the immune mechanisms. Thus, heightened corticoids result in the involution of lymphoid tissue, suppress gamma globulin formation, reduce the eosinophil count, and interfere with the action of the white blood cells. There are many other reactions which are also attributed to elevated corticoids. Thus, there appears to be a very high biological cost to an animal if continued elevated corticoids are sustained. Therefore, from a biological perspective, it would appear essential that coping mechanisms should have as their major consequence the reduction of continued hypersecretion of neuroendocrine systems that can affect a multitude of physiological responses (Miller, 1980).

We stated previously that stress is a fact of life. Perhaps more important is that coping is a fact of life. What has perplexed many investigators is the fact that it is extremely difficult to create a situation, for animals or humans, either in the laboratory or the field, in which chronic elevations of corticoids can be established. It has been reported that cortisol secretion in depressed patients is markedly different from that of normal subjects. Cortisol is normally secreted episodically, with the secretion virtually ceasing during the late evening and early morning hours. In depressed patients, there is an increase in the number of episodes of plasma cortisol secretion and in the concentration of plasma cortisol, both at the beginning and at the end of the episodic periods. The patients' secretion of cortisol actively continues throughout both day and night. In rhesus monkeys that were separated from the mother, there was an elevation of cortisol for at least 24 hours following the separation, and cortisol remained slightly elevated for at least 5 days. These are only a few instances, however, where chronic elevation has been observed. For the most part, even under what appear to be severe experimental conditions (i.e., chronic shock), it is difficult to maintain elevations of plasma cortisol (Murison, 1980).

MECHANISMS OF COPING

It has been clearly demonstrated that psychological factors lead not only to increased arousal—and therefore to increased pituitary-adrenal responses—but also to decreased arousal, as indexed by decreased pituitary-adrenal activity (Levine, Weinberg & Brett, 1979). The response to noxious stimuli is markedly altered by psychological factors. The psychological variables that have been studied most often related to (1) control, or the ability to make coping responses during stress; (2) the amount of feedback or information which the organism receives following a noxious stimulus, or the response to that stimulus; and (3) predictability of the stressor. The most important single determinant, however, which appears to be involved in the capacity of an animal to reduce its hormonal responses to pervasive aversive stimuli, is control.

Control can best be defined as the capacity to make active responses during the presence of an aversive stimulus. These responses are frequently effective in allowing the animal to avoid or escape from the stimulus, but might also provide the animal only with the opportunity to change from one set of stimulus conditions to another, rather than to escape the shock entirely. Control in and of itself appears to be a factor which can reduce an organism's physiological responses to a stimulus such as shock. It has been observed that rats able to press a lever to avoid shock show less severe physiological disturbance, e.g., weight loss and gastric lesions, than yoked controls which cannot respond, even though both animals received the same amount of shock (Weiss, 1968). Animals able to escape from shock show reduction in plasma corticosterone following repeated experience with controllable shock (Davis, Porter, Livingstone, Herrmann, MacFadden, & Levine, 1977). Control over high-intensity shock produces a reduction in plasma cortisol levels. Similarly, Hanson, Larson, and Snowdon (1976) found that rhesus monkeys that had control over noxious noise showed plasma cortisol levels which were similar to animals that were not exposed to noise, and that both of these groups were significantly less elevated when compared to animals which had no control over the aversive stimuli. When animals were in a group which had suddenly lost control—lever-pressing no longer terminated the noise—cortisol levels rose to those of the "no control" group.

The effects of control on plasma cortisol level in dogs was demonstrated very clearly in a recent experiment conducted by Dess-Beech et al. (1981) in the laboratory of Bruce Overmier. In this experiment, animals were subjected to a standard procedure which has been used to produce the phenomenon of learned helplessness. Animals are placed in a hammock and given uncontrollable, unpredictable shock. For other dogs, however, the shock could be controlled by the animal's capacity to terminate the shock by making a panel-press response with its head. The effects of predictability were also studied in this experiment, and animals were given either controllable (C) or uncontrollable ($\bar{C}$) shock, with (P) or without ($\bar{P}$) predictability. The results indicated that predictability and controllability affect the severity of the aversive events. Having neither maximizes the cortisol response; having both minimizes the impact of the shock. However, the controllability main effect suggested a larger role of controllability in the response to shock as compared to the response of animals receiving predictable shock in the absence of control (Table 4-1).

There have been a number of studies using human subjects which suggest that a similar process is involved, and that the effects of control can lead to a reduction in the pituitary-adrenal response to both acute and chronic stressful conditions. Frankenhaeuser (1980) demonstrated that when individ-

TABLE 4-1

GROUP MEAN POSTSESSION CORTISOL LEVELS EXPRESSED AS A PERCENT OF PRESESSION BASELINE AVERAGED ACROSS TWO TREATMENT SESSIONS

		P	$\bar{P}$
Controllability	C	240.5	280.0
	$\bar{C}$	339.0	418.5
Non-Shock			274.5

uals performed a task at their "preferred work pace," and when the subjects were given an opportunity to modify rate and maintain an optimal pace throughout a one-hour session, pituitary-adrenal activity decreased from baseline. Further evidence for the view that control was important in modifying pituitary-adrenal activity in humans was obtained in an experiment in which the subjects performed mental arithmetic under noise exposure (Lundberg & Frankenhaeuser, 1978). Subjects were offered a choice between the noise intensities, while the comparison subjects served as yoked controls and were subjected to the same noise levels. The group experiencing lack of control showed more subjective discomfort and secreted higher levels of cortisol.

More recently Rodin (1980) has presented an elegant series of studies which have demonstrated the importance of control in aged individuals. She argued very succinctly that the transition from adulthood to old age may represent loss of control, both physiologically and psychologically (Birren, 1958; Gould, 1972). She further argued that the ability to sustain a sense of personal control in old age may be greatly influenced by societal factors, and that this, in turn, may affect the physical well-being of the aged individual. In order to investigate this problem, she introduced a program of "coping skill training," which, in part, was intended to reintroduce control to a group of individuals in which she hypothesized that helplessness and lack of control were present. There were two impressive aspects of the cortisol data presented by Rodin. First, among the aged in institutions, cortisol levels appeared to be chronically elevated, similar to that observed in depressed individuals. Perhaps more important, however, when individuals received training with certain aspects of coping skills, including control, there was a marked and significant suppression of these elevated cortisol levels.

The importance of control is obvious from many different aspects. First, there is clear evidence that many organisms prefer control (Overmier, Patterson, & Wielkiewicz, 1980). Second, the loss of control also has a profound effect on the pituitary-adrenal system. One interesting example of the effects of having and then losing control can be observed using the conditioned taste aversion situation. In the version of this task which has been developed in our laboratory (Smotherman, Hennessy, & Levine, 1976), animals are given 5 exposures to a sweetened milk solution; immediately following the fifth exposure they are injected with LiCl (an i.p. injection of 0.40 M LiCl). This treatment makes them ill, and a single injection will cause the animals to avoid the milk solution when reexposed to it several days later. Furthermore, we have observed that the physiological response to the reexposure session depends upon the animals' food and water intake during the interval between conditioning and reexposure. If the animals are maintained on ad lib food and water during this interval, plasma corticoid levels measured at the end of the 30-minute reexposure session are similar to basal levels. If, however, animals are deprived during this interval, plasma corticoid levels are markedly elevated. It has been suggested that this corticoid elevation reflects the fact that deprived animals are in a conflict situation (Smotherman, Margolis, & Levine, 1980; Weinberg, Smotherman, & Levine, 1978). That is, they are hungry and thirsty, yet are presented only with a substance which has been paired with illness. Under these conditions they are, in a sense, forced to consume a small amount of the milk solution. The arousal produced by this approach-avoidance conflict is reflected in elevated corticosteroid levels. Nondeprived animals, on the other hand, do not experience such conflict, and thus do not exhibit any steroid elevations. We suggest that one can also interpret these data in terms of control and loss of control. Animals in the nondeprived condition have control in this situation. Because they are neither hungry nor thirsty, they can effectively avoid the milk solution on the reexposure day. Once animals are deprived, however, they lose control. When reexposed to the milk solution they can no longer make an effective avoidance response, and this loss of control produces elevated levels of plasma corticosterone.

One can also view extinction of an established operant response as loss of control. For example, Coover et al. (1973) observed that during extinction of a shuttlebox avoidance response, plasma corticoid elevations occurred whether extinction was accomplished by punishing the ongoing crossing response or by blocking the crossing response with a Plexiglas barrier, and presenting only the conditioned stimulus (CS). The fact that corticoid elevations occurred in the latter case, where the response was simply prevented from occurring, clearly indicates that it was not the physical stimulus of shock itself which was causing the increased arousal. It is possible that the psychological factor—loss of control—may have been one of the factors which produced the plasma corticoid elevations observed. In this situation, animals had learned the task, and thus had established a high level of control, i.e., they could make an effective avoidance response. When this control was suddenly removed by blocking the ongoing response, plasma corticoids became elevated. Furthermore, this phenomenon is not limited to loss of control over noxious stimuli. Extinction of an appetitive response can also activate the pituitary-adrenal system. For example, if an animal has learned to bar-press for food in an operant chamber, and food is suddenly withdrawn in this situation, there is a marked elevation of plasma corticoids (Coover, Goldman, & Levine, 1971; Davis, Memmott, MacFadden, & Levine, 1976). Once again, these data can be viewed within the context of loss of control.

Thus, having control is helpful; losing control is aversive; and previous experience with control can significantly alter the ability to cope with subsequent aversive stimuli (Overmier et al., 1980).

FEEDBACK

Although it is clear that control appears to be a major factor responsible for coping, the ability or efficiency with which an organism can cope is also dependent on another factor—feedback. *Feedback* is defined as stimuli occurring after a response and not associated with the noxious stimulus (Weiss, 1971a,b). These stimuli do have the capacity to convey information to the responding organism, indicating that it has done the right thing, or that the aversive stimulus is terminated, at least for some interval of time (time out). According to Weiss, the amount of stress an animal actually experiences when exposed to noxious stimuli depends upon (1) the number of coping attempts the animal makes (control), and (2) the amount of relevant feedback that the coping responses produce. As the number of coping responses increase and/or the amount of relevant feedback decreases, the amount of stress experienced increases. In an extensive (and now classic) series of studies, Weiss demonstrated that if two groups of rats were subjected to the same amount of shock, the aversive effects of shock in terms of ulceration were ameliorated if the animal could respond—that is, avoid or escape—and if the situation had some feedback information, i.e., a signal following the termination of shock. Although in general, feedback information usually occurs in the context of control, namely that information is available about the efficacy of a response, it has been reported that feedback information per se, even in the absence of control, does have the capacity to reduce the pituitary-adrenal response to noxious stimuli. Hennessy, King, McClure, and Levine (1977) reported that the presence of a signal following the delivery of shock resulted in a reduced adrenal response to the noxious stimulus, even in the absence of control. In contrast, the effects of a warning signal were ineffective, and the pituitary-adrenal response of animals given a warning signal, and then shocked, was not significantly different from animals given a random signal.

PREDICTABILITY

Although the evidence regarding the effects of control and of control plus feedback on the ability of the animals to make appropriate coping responses under conditions of aversive stimuli appears unequivocal, the effects of predictability are less clear-cut. When given a choice, humans and animals appear to choose signaled rather than nonsignaled shock, even when no escape from shock is possible (Averill, 1973; Badia & Culbertson,

1972; Badia, Culbertson, & Harsh, 1973; Seligman, Maier, & Solomon, 1971). The same physical stressor had different consequences depending on the psychological variable of predictability. Gliner (1972) found that signaled or predictable shock was less destructive in terms of somatic reactions to stress. In this case, rats were given a choice of predictable or unpredictable shock. Animals which chose predictable shock developed fewer ulcers under this condition than animals not given this choice but which received the same amount of shock unpredictably.

In contrast, however, there are a number of reports which indicate that either predictable shock has no effect or that, in fact, presenting a signal prior to the onset of inescapable shock appears to increase the pituitary-adrenal response to noxious stimuli (Bassett et al., 1973). More recently, the Bassett et al. study was replicated by this author in their laboratory. The length of the signal was systematically increased from the original 4 seconds (which was used by Bassett et al.) to 30 seconds. It was found that as the length of the signal increased, the levels of circulating plasma corticoid also increased systematically, so that the circulating levels of plasma corticosterone were significantly higher following the presentation of a 30-second warning signal as compared to the 4-second warning signal. Both warning signal conditions, however, produced higher corticosterone responses than were present under the "no signal" condition. Thus, whereas predictability is often cited as an important psychological variable which can ameliorate the stress response, a careful review of the studies that have tested the effects of predictability reveals that the results are both complex and confusing. While many investigators claim that predictable shock is less aversive for an organism, based primarily on the fact that organisms tend to prefer predictable to unpredictable shock, others find that predictable shock is more aversive and produces an increase in plasma corticosterone over the nonpredictable conditions.

A close and critical scrutiny (Weinberg & Levine, 1980) of many of the studies dealing with preference for predictability shows that, in addition to the major variable of predictability, other variables have been introduced into the experimental design. It is likely that these other variables were primarily responsible for the results obtained. Most of the studies on predictability have stated that they were investigating the influence of predictability. Yet, in many of the experiments, the animals not only had predictability, but also had control, even though control was not considered a parameter in the experiment. In several studies, animals could choose either one side or the other of an experimental chamber (Gliner, 1972; Lockard, 1963). Thus, the availability of the choice actually gave the animals control over the stimulus conditions. In the studies by Badia and co-workers (1972, 1973), where a bar-press was required so that the animals could change over from signal to nonsignal conditions, this bar-press provided control over the test conditions. In addition, the changeover procedure presented the animal with an asymmetrical choice; that is, an active bar-press response produced a signal, while a passive response produced unsignaled shock (Furedy & Biederman, 1976). Thus, not only was predictability of the shock varied in these experimental situations, but so too the availability of an active versus a passive response. Thus, one of the major contributors to the so-called effect of predictability appears to be some element of control.

In attempting to relate the concept of feedback to predictability, it has been argued that if shock is inescapable, predictability may only be effective in reducing stress if it provides feedback for an organism. This notion is best exemplified by the safety-signal hypothesis (Seligman, 1968) which states that in situations where reliable CS predicts shock, the absence of the CS is also a reliable predictor of safety, and what regulates behavior in these shock situations is, in fact, the ability of the animal to predict safe or shock-free periods. It appears that the animal prefers signaled shock because of the information value imbedded in the signal. Thus, when shock is unpredictable, the entire test session is probably spent in anticipation of shock. With predictable shock, however, a safety signal exists, and animals show a response only during the CS and not in the absence of the signal. Although the safety signal hypothesis does have some appeal in attempting to account for some of the data on predictability, we are still faced with the fact that there are sets of circumstances in which the variables are as yet not totally explicable, and that a warning signal, in fact, causes a striking increase in plasma corticosterone. To the extent that feedback is an important variable in accounting for the effects of predictability, it may also be related to the fact that control is also present in most of these experiments.

We have defined coping, in terms of reductions in neuroendocrine activity, as a function of control and feedback. It should be apparent that the behavior of the individual is an important contributor to the coping process. Control is more often dependent on some aspect of the organism's behavior that makes control possible. It seems obvious that control is biologically and psychologically important to an organism. The absence of control or the loss of control apparently leads to an increased stress response. There is extensive evidence suggesting that restrictions in control are indeed stress-inducing. Seligman and his co-workers (1975) have shown that decreased control increases feelings and behaviors associated with helplessness. Increased feelings of helplessness, or lack of control, have been associated with the etiology of disease and death (Glass, 1977; McMahon & Rhudick, 1964). Perhaps the most concise statement that control processes may be related to health and survival was presented by Lefcourt (1973) when he concluded in his article on perception of control, "The sense of control, the illusion that one can exercise personal choice, has a definite and positive role in sustaining life." (p. 424)

ONTOGENY OF COPING

The importance of control has been recognized as a salient feature of the ontogeny of coping. For the infant, its initial experience with contingencies and control are within the context of the mother-infant relationship (Seligman, 1975; Watson, 1967). As Lewis and Goldberg (1969) have stated,

> . . . contingency is important not only because it shapes the acquisition of specific behaviors, but because it enables the child to develop a motive which is the basis for all future learning. The main characteristic of this motive is the infant's belief that his actions affect his environment. . . . The mother is important because it is the contingency between the infant's behavior and her responses that enables the infant to learn that his behavior does have consequences. (p. 82)

Mason (1978), in discussing the difference between infant rhesus monkeys that were reared with stationary surrogates and infant rhesus monkeys raised with dogs, comments:

> I believe that the critical distinction between attachment figures in these experiments is the presence or absence of response-contingent stimulation. Stationary surrogates and hobby horses surely provide few opportunities for the developing individual to experience the fact that his behavior has effects on the environment and to learn that the events going on around him are amenable to his control. Inert mother substitutes make no demands, occasion no surprises, do not encourage the development of attentional processes and the acquisition of simple instrumental behaviors that are the fabric of social interactions. (p. 249)

That mothers are the prime source of contingent stimulation in the primate needs little elaboration. These early contingent relationships are required in order for the infant to learn certain cogent aspects of its environment which permit it to acquire adaptive coping responses. These early coping responses appear to be essential for normal infant development, and they also permit the infant to become an adaptive functioning adult as compared to surrogate-reared infants who show many behavioral aberrations as adults.

Although there are striking species-specific differences in mother-infant interactions among nonhuman primates, in general the initial relationship between the primate mother and the neonate is continuous, with the infant playing an active role in the maintenance of dyadic interaction. The maintenance of contact between mother and infant monkey, for example, is largely dependent upon the infant's clinging and following behaviors. Thus, the squirrel monkey infant assumes a position upon the dorsal surface of the mother almost immediately after birth. It maintains that position actively for a considerable period of time until it ultimately begins to leave the mother, initially for brief periods of time, and finally, for sustained periods of time. However, observations of squirrel monkey mothers and infants indicate very clearly that although the infant may be spending time away from the mother, the presence of stimuli which may signal threat or elicit distress results in the infant almost immediately seeking the mother, and once again resuming the clinging position. Although squirrel monkey mothers are also active in maintaining proximity to the infant, they do not retrieve their infants in the usual sense; however, under conditions of stress, they will seek the infant and present themselves so that the infants can more easily assume the clinging position. In other primates, such as the rhesus, the expressions of the mother-infant relationship are different in that the infant spends considerably more time in a ventral-ventral position. But, once again, observations of mother-infant pairs in a group living situation indicate very clearly that the infant, when distressed, will actively seek the mother and achieve proximity either by clinging or by maintaining a position close to the mother. The mother also responds to the infant's distress signals by actively seeking the infant and retrieving it vigorously.

In a group living situation in which mothers and infants are not separated at weaning, this process appears to go on for a considerable length of time. Year-old infants seek proximity to the mother when conditions in the environment appear to be unstable or when the infant is subject to some distressful experience. The response of the mother and infant to achieve proximity or contact under conditions of stress appears to be characteristic of most primate species, including humans. With a few notable exceptions (Rosenblum & Kaufman, 1968), the only salient animal in the environment to which the infant will respond in such a manner is the mother. Conversely, the mother appears to respond only to those signals emitted by her own infant. This selective preference has been dealt with extensively by attachment theorists and is one of the criteria for the presence of an attachment relationship. A second major criterion is response to the loss of the attachment figure.

Perhaps the most widely used method of studying attachment has been the separation procedure. Both the behavioral and the physiological responses of mothers and infants have been examined in reaction to the loss of either figure from the normal environment. The earlier studies of separation (Kaufman, 1973; Seay, Hansen, & Harlow, 1962; Seay & Harlow, 1965) primarily examined the behavioral responses of the infant to loss of the mother. The initial response to loss of the mother has been described as protest, involving distress vocalizations and agitated activity. Upon sustained separation, however, it has been noted that the infant moves from this protest phase to a phase of despair and "depression" which is manifested by extremely low levels of activity, a general lethargy, and apparent withdrawal from the environment.

The protest reaction following separation is, however, dependent upon the species and the conditions of separation. Whereas squirrel monkey infants show protest responses following total separation and isolation from the stimuli of other conspecifics, protest responses of the macaque infant are almost absent when all cues of the social group are removed. However, the squirrel monkey infant is quite capable of differentiating social cues, and shows much more distress vocalizations following separation if it is adjacent to the mother, than when totally isolated. The expression of depression is closely dependent upon the conditions of separation (Mineka & Suomi, 1978). Depression is most likely to occur when the infant remains behind in the social group after the mother has been removed. The responses of the mother have not been examined in as much detail, although one of the major theories of attachment, that of Bowlby (1969, 1973), does predict that the response of both mother and infant should be similar under conditions of separation.

More recently, our own laboratory has been investigating the effects of separation on the endocrine responses of both mother and infant squirrel and rhesus monkeys. In general, we have found that both infant and mother squirrel monkeys show a vigorous endocrine response to brief (30 minute) periods of separation (Mendoza, Smotherman, Miner, Kaplan, & Levine, 1978). The squirrel monkey mother shows a striking elevation in plasma cortisol following separation from her infant. This response occurs whether the mother is permitted to remain in her own cage, permitted to remain with her group, or removed from the group. The uniformity of this response is striking (Coe, Mendoza, Smotherman, & Levine, 1978). Every mother in at least a dozen different studies has responded with a marked increment in cortisol values following the separation procedures. The effects of separation occur under conditions when the infant is removed to another room and the infant cues are not available to the mother. Thus, the primate mother appears to be responding to the absence of the infant, and not to the particular stimulus emitted by that infant as a consequence of the agitation caused by separation. Furthermore, the plasma cortisol response of the mother squirrel monkey following separation from her infant is at least as high as that which has been observed using more traditional types of stressful stimuli in non-pregnant squirrel monkeys.

In our initial studies of the influence of brief periods of separation on the infant's endocrine response, separation of the infant from the mother resulted in a striking elevation in plasma cortisol. In these studies, it was difficult to assess whether the effects of separation were a consequence of the separation per se, or were confounded by the additional variable that the infant is both separated and in a novel environment.

In a subsequent experiment, we attempted to partial out the effects of separation from the effects of novelty. A group of squirrel monkey mother-infant pairs were tested under the standard conditions utilized in our laboratory for assessing the effects of separation. The conditions involve obtaining a basal blood sample from the mother and infant upon immediate removal from the group; another sample is obtained following separation-reunion in which the mother and infant are separated briefly and immediately reunited; a third blood sample is taken 30 minutes later. Other blood samples were taken when the infant was removed, leaving the mother in a group with her social partners. Under some circumstances, female squirrel monkeys without infants will show maternal behavior in that they will permit infants to ride dorsally, and also will attempt to retrieve infants. This phenomenon is particularly evident in late pregnant females. In our group living situation, there was one late pregnant female who, when the mother was removed, "aunted" the separated infants. The infants, when aunted by the female, showed few signs of the usual protest behavior observed immediately following separation.

The phenomenon of reduced behavioral agitation, when an infant is with an aunt, has been interpreted by Rosenblum (1972) as indicating that aunting reduces the effect of separation. Our data (Coe et al., 1978) indicate that although aunting does tend to reduce the behavioral agitation that is observed in separated infants, the infant still shows a striking pituitary-adrenal response which is significantly elevated over basal and separation-reunion conditions, and just as elevated as when the infants were removed from their mothers and from their social group. We interpreted these data as indicating that the infant shows specific recognition of its mother, and that only the mother has the capacity to serve the function of arousal reduction for the infant. Since normal mothers do not usually aunt other infants, it is difficult to assess whether the infant also has the same specific arousal reduction function for the mother.

Although we have focused largely on the effects of separation and the stressful consequences of separation, perhaps the more important finding in this series of studies is not the influence of separation, but the effects which were observed under our separation-reunion condition. Recall that the separation-reunion condition involved removing the mother and infant, separating them (which clearly appears to be disturbing in view of the excessive vocalizations that are emitted by both infant and mother), and immediately reuniting the pair and returning them to their home cage. Under these conditions we observed no change in plasma cortisol in either the mother or infant, even though the procedure appeared to be extremely disturbing. These data were somewhat surprising since we had previously demonstrated that removing a nonlactating female from her cage, and immediately returning her to the home cage, does lead to a significant elevation of plasma cortisol as measured 30 minutes later. This is consistent with the use of handling by some investigators (Ader, 1970) as a standardized procedure for activating the pituitary-adrenal system.

Two hypotheses were entertained to account for these data. The first was that the mother and infant have the capacity to buffer each other from stress; therefore, under some conditions, the presence of the mother and infant prevents an increase in arousal as measured by activity of the pituitary-adrenal system. However, an alternate explanation of these data is that both mother and infant cortisol levels could have been significantly elevated initially, but, by 30 minutes, could have returned to basal levels. Thus separation could indeed have constituted a stress, both for the 30-minute separated condition and for the separated-reunited condition. However, contact between the mother and infant in the immediate reunion condition could have reduced that stress to permit a return to basal values by 30 minutes.

A study designed to evaluate this question (Levine, Coe, Smotherman, & Kaplan, 1978) indicated that the first hypothesis more accurately described the process. Blood samples were obtained from mothers and infants under the separation-reunion condition 5, 10, and 30 minutes after being reunited. Under no circumstances did the observed rises of plasma cortisol approach that seen under 30-minute separation. These data indicated that the mother and infant serve a mutual function to reduce the response to stress under the experimental circumstances used in this situation. Another aspect of this experiment also demonstrated an additional functional consequence of being reunited. Following 30 minutes of separation, when both mother and infant showed elevated cortisol levels, the infant was reunited with the mother, and 30 minutes later another blood sample was taken. These data indicated that the infants continued to show elevated cortisol levels as high as after 30-minute separation, but that the mother actually showed a reduction. These data were difficult to interpret until the results of a prolonged (6-hour) separation experiment were obtained. Although the infants' cortisol levels do not appear to return to basal levels quickly after being reunited, they do not continue to show elevations which were observed following prolonged separation. The mother, in contrast, shows a significant drop, whereas following a prolonged separation she tends to maintain elevated levels. It therefore appears that even following a brief separation, being reunited can once again modulate and reduce the response that was observed as a consequence of separation.

These data suggest that the nature of the mother-infant interaction leads to differential effects on each member of the dyad. The effects of reunion are more immediately observable in the mother following a 30-minute period of separation. It appears as though the mother's plasma cortisol returns to basal level during the period of time in which the infant is still showing a vigorous pituitary-adrenal response. This interpretation has some appeal from an ethological point of view since it may be argued that the stability of the mother is essential in maintaining the mother-infant relationship. If the mother were to remain disturbed following reunion, her capacity to provide adequate care for the infant could indeed be impaired.

We have recently demonstrated a phenomenon similar to the buffering of the response to disturbance in rhesus macaques (Gunnar, Gonzalez, & Levine, 1980). Mothers and infants (5–7 months of age) were removed from their social group and housed as dyads in standard laboratory primate cages. The capture procedure was most stressful. As a control group, adult multiparous females who did not have an infant during that breeding season were also captured and rehoused in individual cages. Following capture and rehousing, blood samples were taken in 3 hours, 3 days, and 5 days, while the monkeys were adapting to the new housing conditions. Three hours following capture, all adult females showed highly elevated levels of plasma cortisol. However, by the third day, the females with their infants had returned to basal levels whereas the other adult females were still showing elevated levels. Thus, the presence of the infant facilitated the adaptation to the novel housing condition. Perhaps more striking was that the infants with their mothers showed no change in plasma cortisol levels at any time during the capture and rehousing procedure. These findings are similar to those reported by Smotherman, Hunt, McGinnis, and Levine (1979).

These data suggest that under conditions of stress, proximity and contact with the mother result in the modulation and reduction of the infant's arousal levels. Since coping requires control as a mechanism for reducing stress, proximity-seeking behavior that results in arousal reduction can best be viewed within the context of coping.

SURROGATE-REARED INFANTS

The hypothesis that the infant is involved in a contingent relationship between its responses and their outcomes bears directly on the interpretation of the long-term consequences of surrogate rearing. The original paper by Harlow and Zimmerman (1959) disproved the hypothesis that rhesus infantile attachment was based solely on the pleasures of feeding. This experiment argued that the overriding factor in such attachment was contact comfort, and was based on the finding that young monkeys formed a clear preference for cloth surrogates over wire surrogates, regardless of which surrogate was involved with feeding. Nevertheless, all of the available evidence indicates that surrogate rearing results in widespread long-term deficits (Sackett & Ruppenthal, 1974). Surrogate-reared infants appear to fail to deal with even subtle changes in the environment. A very elegant demonstration of this process was presented in an experiment by Sackett (1972). He demonstrated that when young rhesus monkeys are presented with a series of visual stimuli ranging from very complex to most simple, the mother-reared infants spent more time exploring the more complex stimuli. In contrast, surrogate-reared animals spent most of their time exploring the least complex of the stimuli.

There are very clear differences between the surrogate-reared infant's response to its surrogate, and to the loss of its surrogate, when compared to the response of mother-reared infants. A recent experiment (Hennessy, Kaplan, Mendoza, Lowe, & Levine, 1979) indicates that, in contrast to mother-reared infants, the removal of the surrogate from the home cage resulted in a significant increase in behavioral agitation, but under no circumstances did the infant exhibit a change in plasma cortisol levels. The surrogate-reared infant squirrel monkey does have the capacity to show significant elevations of plasma cortisol when exposed to novelty, but does not appear to show changes in plasma cortisol following removal of the surrogate from its home environment. Here again, we have an interesting dissociation between behavior and the physiological response. This dissociation is paradoxical to the dissociations we have reported upon previously. Here we have indication of behavioral distress with no indications of physiological arousal.

Other investigators have also shown similar differences between mother rearing and surrogate rearing. Using other physiological measures, Reite, Short, and Seiler (1978) found an increase in heart rate and body temperature compatible with a state of hyperarousal in separated group-living pigtail monkeys. But, when infant pigtail monkeys were reared on surrogate mothers, and the surrogate mothers were then removed, the changes in the physiological responses observed were quite different. These animals failed to show any of the physiological changes that were observed when mother-reared infant pigtails were separated from their mothers.

Another aspect of these separation studies also revealed a marked difference between surrogate- and mother-reared infants when certain experimental conditions were imposed following removal of the surrogate. These conditions were designed to determine the specificity of the response of the infants reared on surrogate cloth mothers. Thus, following removal of the surrogate, either the infant was left alone, or, on separate occasions, one of a variety of surrogates was placed in the cage—its own surrogate, a clean cloth surrogate, or a surrogate from another infant. All of these surrogates were capable of reducing behavioral agitation in response to surrogate removal, although the presence of the strange surrogate was not sufficient to reduce a plasma cortisol response in the surrogate-reared infant. In contrast, mother-reared infants, even when in proximity to their mothers and not showing behavioral agitation, do show a marked elevation of plasma cortisol when exposed to a stranger. This cortisol response was present only in the infant, not in the mother (Vogt & Levine, 1980).

CONCLUSION

Mother-infant relationships are truly dyadic. The mother certainly imposes control over the infant's behavior and the infant, by use of certain specific signals, is capable of controlling its mother's behavior. Research on rodents has indicated that the signals emitted by the young influence the behavior of the mother (Bell, 1974; Noirot, 1972; Smotherman, Bell, Starzec, Elias, & Zachman, 1974). The neonatal infant rodent emits very specific ultrasonic signals that lead to an increase in certain aspects of maternal behavior, particularly retrieving. The infant rodent, however, is limited in its motor responses and therefore requires a different set of stimuli that are capable of modifying the mother's behavior. In the primate, the more advanced motor development permits the infant actively to seek proximity and to achieve contact in addition to emitting vocal signals which elicit both retrieval and proximity-seeking behavior on the part of the mother. Thus, the infant is functioning in a contingent environment in which it can control outcomes through the specific responses it emits.

We have noted the importance of contingent relationships for the normal development of the human infant. It remains to consider the appropriateness of our models for normal human function and dysfunction. There is one particular area of development to which these models may have particular relevance—that is, the long-term consequences of prematurity. It seems that the maternal responses to premature infants, even when these infants are returned home, are different from responses to normal full-term infants (Barnett, Leiderman, Grobstein, & Klaus, 1970; Seashore, Leifer, Barnett, & Leiderman, 1973). A number of investigators have reported a greater incidence of maternal disorders among mothers not able to experience frequent contact with their infants during the first weeks of life. One could postulate that one of the consequences of the enforced separation early in life as a consequence of prematurity, together with the developmental sequelae of the premature infant, results in a deficiency of the infant's capacity to emit the appropriate signals that would elicit a contingent maternal response. In turn, the absence of such signals could lead to inappropriate maternal behavior in addition to preventing the infant from learning these early coping responses as a function of the proposed contingent mother-infant response relationship. Thus, the observations of Klaus, Kennell, Plumb, and Zuehlke (1970) and of Faranoff, Kennell, and Klaus (1972) of greater maternal abuse could be a result of this dysynchrony between the infant's capacity to elicit the appropriate response and the mother's own inability to elicit behaviors in response to her infant.

It is apparent that in contemporary western society many well-established patterns of family structure and mother-infant relationships are changing dramatically. There is an increasing tendency for mothers to remain in the work force and to spend long periods of time away from their infants, leaving them in day-care centers (Zigler & Gordon, 1981). As yet, it is difficult to ascertain what, if any, long-term consequences could result as a function of this increasingly common practice. The hypothesis that the development of the coping responses is dependent upon early experience, with control on the part of the infant, does have important implications for the practices involving day-care centers. The hypothesis does not preclude the use of day-care centers, but does prescribe that certain characteristics of such installations be carefully structured so that the infant is not deprived of these early experiences with control that could inhibit the acquisition of later appropriate coping responses.

REFERENCES

Ader, R. The effects of early experience on the adrenocortical response to different magnitudes of stimulation. *Physiology and Behavior*, 1970, *5*, 837–839.

Averill, J. R. Personal control over aversive stimuli and its relationship to stress. *Psychological Bulletin*, 1973, *80*, 286–303.

Badia, P., & Culbertson, S. The relative aversiveness of signalled vs. unsignalled escapable and inescapable shock. *Journal of the Experimental Analysis of Behavior*, 1972, *17*, 463–471.

Badia, P., Culbertson, S., & Harsh, J. Choice of longer or stronger signalled shock over shorter or weaker unsignalled shock. *Journal of the Experimental Analysis of Behavior*, 1973, *19*, 25–32.

Barnett, C. R., Leiderman, P. H., Grobstein, R., & Klaus, M. H. Neonatal separation: The maternal side of interactional deprivation. *Pediatrics*, 1970, *45*, 197–205.

Bassett, J. R., Cairncross, K. D., & King, M. G. Parameters of novelty, shock predictability and response contingency in corticosterone release in the rat. *Physiology and Behavior*, 1973, *10*, 901–907.

Bell, R. W. Ultrasounds in small rodents: Arousal-produced and arousal producing. *Developmental Psychobiology*, 1974, *7*, 39–42.

Birren, J. Aging and psychological adjustment. *Review of Educational Research*, 1958, *28*, 475–490.

Bowlby, J. *Attachment and loss: Attachment* (Vol. 1). New York: Basic Books, 1969.

Bowlby, J. *Attachment and loss: Separation* (Vol. 2). New York: Basic Books, 1973.

Bronson, F. H., & Eleftheriou, B. E. Behavioral, pituitary and adrenal correlates of controlled fighting (defeat) in mice. *Physiological Zoology*, 1965, *38*, 406–411.

Coe, C. L., Mendoza, S. P., Smotherman, W. P., & Levine, S. Mother-infant attachment in the squirrel monkey: Adrenal response to separation. *Behavioral Biology*, 1978, *22*, 256–263.

Conner, R. L., Vernikos-Danellis, J., & Levine, S. Stress, fighting and neuroendocrine function. *Nature*, 1971, *234*, 564–566.

Coover, G. D., Goldman, L., & Levine, S. Plasma corticosterone levels during extinction of a lever-press response in hippocampectomized rats. *Physiology and Behavior*, 1971, *7*, 727–732.

Coover, G. D., Ursin, H., & Levine, S. Plasma corticosterone levels during active avoidance learning in rats. *Journal of Comparative and Physiological Psychology*, 1973, *82*, 170–174.

Davis, H., Memmott, J., MacFadden, L., & Levine, S. Pituitary-adrenal activity under different appetitive extinction procedures. *Physiology and Behavior*, 1976, *17*, 687–690.

Davis, J., Porter, J. W., Livingstone, J., Herrmann, T., MacFadden, L., & Levine, S. Pituitary-adrenal activity and lever-press shock escape behavior. *Physiological Psychology*, 1977, *5*, 280–284.

Dess-Beech, N., Linwick, D., Patterson, J., Overmier, J. B., & Levine, S. Shock predictability and controllability: Cortisol reactivity to subsequent aversive experience. Presented at the Annual Convention, American Psychological Association, Los Angeles, 1981.

Faranoff, A. A., Kennell, J. H., & Klaus, M. H. Follow-up of low birthweight infants: The predictive value of maternal visiting patterns. *Pediatrics*, 1972, *49*, 287–290.

Frankenhaeuser, M. Psychobiological aspects of life stress. In S. Levine, & H. Ursin (Eds.), *Coping and health*. New York: Plenum Press, 1980.

Friedman, S. B., & Ader, R. Adrenocortical response to novelty and noxious stimulation. *Neuroendocrinology*, 1967, *2*, 209–212.

Friedman, S. B., Mason, J. W., & Hamburg, D. A. Urinary 17-hydroxycorticosteroid levels in parents of children with neoplastic disease: A study of chronic psychological stress. *Psychosomatic Medicine*, 1963, *25*, 364–376.

Furedy, J. J., & Biederman, G. B. Preference for signaled shock phenomenon: Direct and indirect evidence for modifiability factors in the shuttlebox. *Animal Learning and Behavior*, 1976, *4*, 1–5.

Gann, D. C. Parameters of the stimulus initiating the adrenocortical response to hemorrhage. *Annals of the New York Academy of Sciences*, 1969, *156*, 740–755.

Ganong, W. F. The central nervous system and the synthesis and release of adrenocorticotropic hormone. In A. V. Nalbandov (Ed.), *Advances in neuroendocrinology*. Urbana: University of Illinois Press, 1963.

Glass, D. C. Stress, behavior patterns, and coronary disease. *American Scientist*, 1977, *65*, 177–187.

Gliner, J. A. Predictable vs. unpredictable shock: Preference behavior and stomach ulceration. *Physiology and Behavior*, 1972, *9*, 693–698.

Gould, R. The phases of adult life: A study in developmental psychology. *American Journal of Psychiatry*, 1972, *129*, 521–531.

Gunnar, M. R., Gonzalez, C. A., & Levine, S. The role of peers in modifying behavioral distress and pituitary-adrenal response to a novel environment in year-old rhesus monkeys. *Physiology and Behavior*, 1980, *25*, 795–798.

Hamburg, D. A., Hamburg, B., & DeGoza, S. Adaptive problems and mechanisms in severely burned patients. *Psychiatry*, 1953, *16*, 1–20.

Hanson, J. D., Larson, M. E., & Snowdon, C. T. The effects of control over high intensity noise on plasma cortisol levels in rhesus monkeys. *Behavioral Biology*, 1976, *16*, 333–340.

Harlow, H. F., & Zimmerman, R. R. Affectional responses in the infant monkey. *Science*, 1959, *130*, 421–432.

Hennessy, J. W., King, M. G., McClure, T. A., & Levine, S. Uncertainty, as defined by the contingency between environmental events, and the adrenocortical response of the rat to electric shock. *Journal of Comparative and Physiological Psychology* 1977, *91*, 1447–1460.

Hennessy, M. B., Kaplan, J. N., Mendoza, S. P., Lowe, E. L., & Levine, S. Separation distress and attachment in surrogate-reared squirrel monkeys. *Physiology and Behavior*, 1979, *23*, 1017–1023.

Kaufman, I. C. Mother-infant separation in monkeys. In J. P. Scott, & E. C. Sinay (Eds.), *Separation and anxiety: Clinical and research aspects*. Washington, D.C.: AAAS, 1973.

Klaus, M. H., Kennell, J. H., Plumb, N., & Zuehlke, S. Human maternal behavior at the first contact with her young. *Pediatrics*, 1970, *46*, 187–192.

Lefcourt, H. M. The function of the illusions of control and freedom. *American Psychologist*, 1973, *28*, 417–425.

Levine, S., Coe, C. L., Smotherman, W. P., & Kaplan, J. N. Prolonged cortisol elevation in the infant squirrel monkey after reunion with mother. *Physiology and Behavior*, 1978, *20*, 7–10.

Levine, S., Weinberg, J., & Brett, L. Inhibition of pituitary-adrenal activity as a consequence of consummatory behavior. *Psychoneuroendocrinology*, 1979, *4*, 275–286.

Lewis, M., & Goldberg, S. Perceptual-cognitive development in infancy: A generalized expectancy model as a function of the mother-infant interaction. *Merrill-Palmer Quarterly*, 1969, *15*, 81–100.

Lockard, J. S. Choice of a warning signal or no warning signal in an unavoidable shock situation. *Journal of Comparative and Physiological Psychology*, 1963, *56*, 526–530.

Lundberg, U., & Frankenhaeuser, M. Psychophysiological reactions to noise as modified by personal control over stimulus intensity. *Biological Psychology*, 1978, *6*, 51–59.

Mason, J. W. A re-evaluation of the concept of "non-specificity" in stress theory. *Journal of Psychiatric Research*, 1971, *8*, 323–333.

Mason, W. A. Social experience in primate cognitive development. In G. M. Burghardt, & M. Bekoff (Eds.), *The development of behavior: Comparative and evolutionary aspects*. New York: Garland STPM Press, 1978.

McMahon, A. W., & Rhudick, P. J. Reminiscing: Adaptational significance in the aged. *Archives of General Psychiatry*, 1964, *10*, 292–298.

Mendoza, S. P., Smotherman, W. P., Miner, M. T., Kaplan, J., & Levine, S. Pituitary-adrenal response to separation in mother and infant squirrel monkeys. *Developmental Psychobiology*, 1978, *11*, 169–175.

Miller, N. A perspective on the effects of stress and coping on disease and health. In S. Levine, & H. Ursin (Eds.), *Coping and health*. New York: Plenum Press, 1980.

Mineka, S., & Suomi, S. J. Social separation in monkeys. *Psychological Bulletin*, 1978, *85*, 1376–1400.

Murison, R. Experimentally induced gastric ulceration: A model disorder for psychosomatic research. In S. Levine, & H. Ursin (Eds.), *Coping and health*. New York: Plenum Press, 1980.

Noirot, E. Ultrasounds and maternal behavior in small rodents. *Developmental Psychobiology*, 1972, *5*, 371–387.

Overmier, J. B., Patterson, J., & Wielkiewicz, R. M. Environmental contingencies as sources of stress in animals. In S. Levine, & H. Ursin (Eds.), *Coping and health*. New York: Plenum Press, 1980.

Pribram, K. H., & Melges, F. T. Psychophysiological basis of emotion. In P. J. Vinken, & G. W. Bruyn (Eds.), *Handbook of clinical neurology* (Vol. 3). Amsterdam: North-Holland Publishing Company, 1969.

Reite, M., Short, R., & Seiler, C. Physiological correlates of maternal separation in surrogate-reared infants: A study in altered attachment bonds. *Developmental Psychobiology*, 1978, *11*, 427–435.

Rodin, J. Managing the stress of aging: The role of control and coping. In S. Levine, & H. Ursin (Eds.), *Coping and health*. New York: Plenum Press, 1980.

Rosenblum, L. A. Sex and age differences in response to infant squirrel monkeys. *Brain Behavior and Evolution*, 1972, *5*, 30–40.

Rosenblum, L. A., & Kaufman, I. C. Variations in infant development and response to maternal loss in monkeys. *American Journal of Orthopsychiatry*, 1968, *38*, 418–426.

Sackett, G. P. Exploratory behavior of rhesus monkeys as a function of rearing experiences and sex. *Developmental Psychology*, 1972, *6*, 260–270.

Sackett, G. P., & Ruppenthal, G. C. Some factors influencing the attraction of adult female macaque monkeys to neonates. In M. Lewis, & L. A. Rosenblum (Eds.), *The effect of the infant on its caregiver*. New York: John Wiley and Sons, 1974.

Seashore, M. J., Leifer, A. D., Barnett, C. R., & Leiderman, P. H. The effects of denial of early mother-infant interaction on maternal self-confidence. *Journal of Personality and Social Psychology*, 1973, *26*, 369–378.

Seay, B. M., & Harlow, H. F. Maternal separation in the rhesus monkey. *Journal of Nervous and Mental Diseases*, 1965, *140*, 434–441.

Seay, B., Hansen, E., & Harlow, H. F. Mother-infant separation in monkeys. *Journal of Child Psychology and Psychiatry*, 1962, *3*, 123–132.

Seligman, M. E. P. Chronic fear produced by unpredictable electric shock. *Journal of Comparative and Physiological Psychology*, 1968, *66*, 402–411.

Seligman, M. E. P. *Learned helplessness: On depression, development and death*. San Francisco: W. H. Freeman and Company, 1975.

Seligman, M. E. P., Maier, S. F., & Solomon, R. L. Unpredictable and uncontrollable aversive events. In F. R. Brush (Ed.), *Aversive conditioning and learning*. New York: Academic Press, 1971.

Selye, H. A syndrome produced by diverse nocuous agents. *Nature*, 1936, *138*, 32.

Selye, H. *Stress*. Montreal: Acta, 1950.

Smotherman, W. P., Bell, R. W., Starzec, J., Elias, J., & Zachman, T. Maternal responses to infant vocalizations and olfactory cues in rats and mice. *Behavioral Biology*, 1974, *12*, 55–66.

Smotherman, W. P., Hennessy, J. W., & Levine, S. Plasma corticosterone levels during recovery from LiCl produced taste aversions. *Behavioral Biology*, 1976, *16*, 401–412.

Smotherman, W. P., Hunt, L. E., McGinnis, L. M., & Levine, S. Mother-infant separation in group-living rhesus macaques: A hormonal analysis. *Developmental Psychobiology*, 1979, *12*, 211–217.

Smotherman, W. P., Margolis, A., & Levine, S. Flavor preexposures in a conditioned taste aversion situation: A dissociation of behavioral and endocrine effects in rats. *Journal of Comparative and Physiological Psychology*, 1980, *94*, 25–35.

Sokolov, E. N. Neuronal models and the orienting reflex. In M. A. B. Brazier (Ed.), *The central nervous system and behavior*. New York: Josiah Macy, Jr. Foundation, 1960.

Ursin, H., Baade, E., & Levine, S. (Eds.). *Psychobiology of stress: A study of coping men*. New York: Academic Press, 1978.

Vogt, J. L., & Levine, S. Response of mother and infant squirrel monkeys to separation and disturbance. *Physiology and Behavior*, 1980, *24*, 829–832.

Watson, J. B. Memory and "contingency analysis" in infant learning. *Merrill-Palmer Quarterly*, 1967, *17*, 139–152.

Weinberg, J., & Levine, S. Psychobiology of coping in animals: The effects of predictability. In S. Levine, & H. Ursin (Eds.), *Coping and health*. New York: Plenum Press, 1980.

Weinberg, J., Smotherman, W. P., & Levine, S. Early handling effects on neophobia and conditioned taste aversion. *Physiology and Behavior*, 1978, *20*, 589–596.

Weiss, J. M. Effects of coping responses on stress. *Journal of Comparative and Physiological Psychology*, 1968, *65*, 251–260.

Weiss, J. M. Effects of coping behavior in different warning signal conditions on stress pathology in rats. *Journal of Comparative and Physiological Psychology*, 1971a, *77*, 1–13.

Weiss, J. M. Effects of coping behavior with and without a feedback signal on stress pathology in rats. *Journal of Comparative and Physiological Psychology*, 1971b, *77*, 22–30.

Zigler, E. F., and Gordon, E. W. (Eds.). *Day-care: Scientific and social policy issues*. Boston, Mass: Auburn House Publishing Co., 1981.

CHAPTER 5

SOCIAL ECOLOGY AND CHILDBIRTH: The Newborn Nursery as Environmental Stressor

P. HERBERT LEIDERMAN, M.D.
PROFESSOR, DEPARTMENT OF PSYCHIATRY AND
BEHAVIORAL SCIENCES
STANFORD UNIVERSITY SCHOOL OF MEDICINE

PERSPECTIVE ON STRESS AND COPING PARADIGM

The stress and coping paradigm has been widely employed in the fields of adult social medicine (Antonovsky, 1980), psychiatry (Coelho, Hamburg, & Adams, 1974), behavioral sciences (Lazarus, 1966), and clinical psychology (Korchin, 1976) to account for an individual's reaction to threatening events, both internally and externally derived. The major stressors usually involve sudden alterations in the environment, though an unchanging environment itself may serve as a chronic stressor. An internal event might be a threatening alteration in the physiological and psychological equilibrium of the individual. A clinical example resembles the following: a nutritionally deprived woman—chronic physiological deprivation—living under poverty conditions in the inner-city—physical and social stressors—confronted with the desertion of her husband—a sudden event—forcing her to get a second job in order to support herself and her children—repeated stressor. Physiological, behavioral, psychological, and social adaptations must be made by the individual in this situation in order to cope with the stress factors in her life. Thus, the basic stress and coping paradigm consists of a person living in, and interacting within, an environment in which multiple, rather than single, factors are brought to bear. These factors, when seen collectively, are the crucial elements for predicting the relative success of an individual's adaptation.

In this chapter, I shall outline the basic components of the stress and coping paradigm and their uses in adult medicine, and then examine their applicability to child-development research. The greater part of this chapter will be devoted to illustrating how this paradigm is utilized in my own research, thereby delineating its limitations and its possible extension as a tool for developmental research.

Stress and Coping for the Adult—A Biological Perspective

The modern version of the concept of stress was introduced by Selye (1950) to account for the physical changes in the individual in response to stimulus events of severity sufficient to produce disequilibrium in the homeostatic physiological systems. These changes resulted from the organism's attempt to reestablish equilibrium after noxious stimulus agents acted directly on the tissues. Selye's major contribution was to show that tissue reactions were nonspecific with respect to the type of noxious agents. In other words, reaction was the same regardless of the agent's composition. He termed these reactions the General Adaptation Syndrome, and described its three phases: (1) the *stage of alarm*, in which the noxious stimuli produced disturbances in the tissue or in the physiological functions which were associated with specific signs of response, such as prolonged increases in body temperature, blood pressure, or endocrine functions; (2) the *stage of resistance*, in which the body's defenses would be called forth to mitigate or contain the noxious stimuli; and (3) the *stage of exhaustion*, ensuing when the body's defenses failed, and which could lead, potentially, to severe bodily damage or death. The degree to which the organism responded to the noxious stimuli in the alarm reaction phase depended upon the nature and effectiveness of the defenses. Whether the stage of exhaustion was reached depended on the severity of the onslaught of the noxious stimuli and on the biological resources available to the particular organism.

Stress and Coping for the Adult—Psychological and Social Perspectives

Selye's original conceptualization of stress was biological and individual in its orientation; that is, he conceived of stress as a physiological and biochemical response, specific to an individual with little concern for variations in the environmental or stimulus conditions. Selye placed little emphasis on the behavioral and psychological components of stress. Further, he did not delineate the nature of the stressor, and did not clearly differentiate it from the stress reaction itself.

In 1966, Lazarus introduced the psychological component which suggested that the individual's perception of threat might determine whether a given noxious stimulus could produce the stress reaction effects.[1] He suggested that varying psychological stimuli could lead to similar stress responses, thereby providing a psychological parallel to the physiological response schema postulated by Selye.

With the purely biological notion of stress developed by Selye, broadened by the psychological conceptualizations of Lazarus, the way was paved for the inclusion of social and cultural components in understanding stressors, stress reactions, and coping. On the stressor side of the paradigm, Smelser (1961) introduced the concept of social strain, thereby emphasizing the social forces that produce stress reactions in the individual. On the stress reaction and coping side of the paradigm, the psychological and social components were emphasized in chapters by Goldschmidt, White, and Mechanic, in the volume edited by Coelho et al. (1974). The adaptive process, as explored by these authors, was defined to include cognitively oriented social supports, problem solving, education, and culture, as well as the psychological defenses and physiological adaptations introduced by Lazarus and by Selye. Despite the historical background for the introduction of sociological concepts in stress and coping, their prominence in contemporary discussions of adult stress is quite recent. For an excellent summary of these issues, see Antonovsky (1980).

Stress and Coping—Environmental Perspectives

Because the stress and coping paradigm is a confluence of ideas from psychiatry, physiology, and psychology, the lack of precise delineation of elements of the paradigm is understandable (see Garmezy, Kagan, and Rutter, this volume). Selye was not precise about whether the stress reaction included the environmental events as well as the organisms's reaction to them, and, further, whether the coping and adaptive responses should be differentiated from the stress reaction itself. The fuzziness of definition was not due merely to a lack of scientific rigor. Rather, the concept of stress contained within it a problem of major proportions: the description and conceptualization of organism-environmental interaction without destruc-

[1] Clinically, the psychological conception of stress and coping had been suggested by Lindemann (1944) in his study of grief, following the Coconut Grove fire in Boston, and by Grinker and Spiegel in their studies of American pilots under the stress of combat (1945).

tion of the basic unity of this relationship. Nonetheless, the concept of stress was useful in linking environmental events to psychological and physiological responses (both normative and nonnormative), when describing the endeavors of the organism to reestablish a homeostatic equilibrium.

What has been absent from the stress and coping paradigm is detailed specification of the environment. Though Lewin, Lippitt, and White (1939) had introduced their psychological-field theory, there had been relatively little work carried out in the intervening period that precisely described the nature of specific environmental conditions (see Barker & Wright, 1949). This issue becomes extremely important since central to the concept of stressor is the implication that there has been an alteration in the environmental conditions. Any theory of stress must consider the nature of the environment, and, beyond that, the more complex ecological relationships which can involve more than one level of environmental complexity (see Bronfenbrenner, 1979, on the interrelationship of multiple levels of environment, in his advocacy of an ecological approach to developmental psychology).

What is the nature of "environment," in which change leads to stress reactions? Certainly it can be physical, though for a person it may more often involve changes in psychological and social circumstances, such as the loss of a close companion, loss of self-esteem, loss of a job or retirement, or loss of social status. Quantification of the physical and social environment, as it impinges on the individual, does not lend itself to simple physical measurements or even to assessment by outside observers. It depends upon an individual's appraisal of a particular situation, and is influenced both by current perceptions and prior experiences. The individual and his or her reactions to environmental conditions are inextricably linked. A quantitative determination of this relationship remains a basic problem for researchers in the area of stress and coping (see Moos, 1974).

Stressors and Stress Reactions in Child Development Research

Regardless of the heuristic value of the concept of stress and coping for understanding adult reactions to stressor events, its relative absence from the literature of child-development research is puzzling.[2] If the stress and coping paradigm has proven valuable in identifying relationships between complex biological, psychological, and social processes in adults, then why should these constructs not prove equally helpful in understanding the same reac-

---

[2] Exceptions are the work of Murphy and associates (1962) and Murphy and Moriarty (1976), which will be discussed later in this paper.

tions in the developing infant and child? An immediate issue is posed by these questions: What are the possible differences between adulthood and childhood? Do these differences necessitate modifications of the stress and coping model before it can be applied to developmental research? Examination of a child developmental handbook (see Carmichael, 1970) over the past decade reveals no references to stress and coping specifically, although similar ideas were expressed under the heading of emotion or emotional response. Lazarus (1966) mentioned developmental issues on only three pages. There are two chapters in Coelho et al. (1974) that deal with the developmental aspects of coping and adaptation. Perusal of child developmental abstracts for 1980 reveals only two references. Perhaps a brief examination of differences in adult and child developmental research might aid us in determining how these constructs might be utilized in the latter, and thereby contribute a markedly neglected environmental and biobehavioral component to developmental theory.[3]

Characteristically, stress and coping research, especially those studies employing experimental paradigms in adults, has been devoted to relatively short-term changes, which presupposes the relative psychological and physiological stability of the individuals under examination. Once stable baseline conditions are obtained, the internal or external perturbations can be measured. The research strategy for adults has frequently been cross-sectional, though relatively long-term longitudinal approaches have been used more recently. Examples of this life-span approach are reflected in the work of Baltes, Reese, and Nesselroade (1977), Lerner and Spanier (1978), Vaillant (1977), and Levinson, Darrow, Klein, Levinson, and McKee (1978), and are based in part on theoretical formulations of the life-span concept introduced by Erikson (1959).

The measurements made of stress and coping in adult research have been physiological, behavioral, and (far less frequently) social. In contrast to adults, children are in the midst of physical, psychological, and social growth. As a result, their environments are more varied and changing than are those of adults. Psychological growth and development is fairly rapid, and thus variability of reaction, even in brief time periods, is characteristic of children, as opposed to the comparative stability observed in adults. The effects of environmental and/or internal perturbations can be captured only by greater specification of environmental conditions, and by longitudinal strategies that take into account the greater variability in children, particularly during periods of early rapid development.

---

[3] This discussion of the use of the stress and coping paradigm in development refers to human research, since for many years developmental comparative psychologists have utilized the stress and coping paradigm successfully, especially for issues of prenatal and postnatal experience and subsequent development (see Levine, 1962).

Focusing further on the stressor side of the stress and coping paradigm, another difference between adults and children can be observed: children are less able than adults to ascertain whether or not environmental conditions and sudden dramatic events in their lives are relevant factors in their ability to cope; they are less able to discern which situations are potentially threatening. Lazarus characterized and defined this function in establishing the role of stressors in the stress and coping paradigm for adults. The absence of perceptual appraisal research in the field of child development has been a hindrance in furthering the general use of the paradigm as a research tool. The work of Kagan on novelty, discussed in this volume, indicates that the child is able to discriminate aspects of the environment that are discrepant and thereby potentially threatening. A verbal example of perceptual appraisal is given by the work of Wallerstein (this volume), exemplifying the fruitfulness of examining the verbal reports of children involved in divorce; their ability to assess the situation affecting them is certainly not unlike that of the adult's ability to assess the situation. Further, the child's appraisal of stress and the ability to cope are frequently reported in clinical research. The breadth of the schism between experimental and clinical research may lessen when both the child's individual perceptions and behavior are taken into account and used as components of an index to appraise the environment.

Turning to the stress reaction and coping side of the paradigm, one notes another difference between adult- and child-development research, namely the absence of physiological and biochemical parameters as indicators of children's reactions, unlike the characteristic studies of the 1950s and 1960s detailing stress and coping in adults. While undoubtedly there is greater difficulty in monitoring endocrinological and electrophysiological response in children relative to adults, such monitoring, if done noninvasively, falls within the accepted research guidelines imposed by human subjects committees. Promising leads in this area can be seen in the work of Kagan and Rosman (1964), Sroufe and Waters (1977) on cardiovascular response, and Maccoby, Doering, Jacklin, and Kraemer (1979) on androgens.

Coping and Adaptation in Child-development Research

Whatever the differences between adults and children in the appraisal of stressors and stress reactions, these are relatively minor when compared to those between adults and children on the coping and adaptation side of the schema. The immaturity of the child, and the attendant necessary dependence on adults for survival, constitutes one crucial feature. In contrast to the relatively autonomous adult, the infant or young child utilizes other people as part of the coping mechanism; thus, the child must use the social system as part of the effort at adaptation and survival. Coping and adaptation are not simply physiological or psychological reactions restoring equilibrium, rather they are responses which are embedded within the social matrix. Hence, the successful adaptation by the child includes the ability to demand of the immediate social environment those components, both social and physical, which will ensure survival.

When viewed in this way, the concept of coping for the developing organism is incomplete if the individual is considered as a completely autonomous entity. Adaptive and maladaptive responses are found in the relationship between the person and the social environment, rather than exclusively in the biology and psychology of the individual. In the case of children, successful coping includes not only psychological and psysiological adaptive responsiveness, but also the child's inherent ability to demand compensating care from the major caregivers. This perspective brings into focus the importance of evaluating family relationships, social and community supports, and, finally, the cultural values and habits of a given group in predicting the adaptive potential of the child.

The longitudinal investigations conducted by Murphy and associates (1962) and Murphy and Moriarty (1976) reflect a broad "ecological" viewpoint in the study of developmental factors in stress and coping, in its inclusion of familial, social, and cultural influences. Although heavily influenced by a psychoanalytic viewpoint, which placed less emphasis on current environmental conditions and more on personal historical aspects of development, these investigators nevertheless demonstrated how the ecological supports surrounding the children, in the form of teachers, counselors, and religious institutions could supplement family influences in strengthening the child's adaptive processes. Noteworthy in this research was the happy combination of clinical and research techniques which brought forth the subtle nuances of the environment that facilitated adaptation. However, as might well be expected of work begun in the late 1950s and continued through the 1960s—a matrifocal research era—these studies deemphasized the contributions of the father. This fact, evident in the seminal work of Murphy and her colleagues, indicates the difficulty of obtaining an encompassing ecological perspective.

STUDIES OF THE NEWBORN NURSERY AS AN ENVIRONMENTAL STRESSOR

I have attempted to discuss some of the reasons why the stress and coping paradigm has not been used extensively in developmental research. Further, I have emphasized how an ecological perspective provides a more complete picture of the adaptation of the child than does a simple individual psychological or physiological perspective. The remainder of this paper will attempt to illustrate how the paradigm might be utilized in research on the influence of institutional, social, and cultural forces on the child's ability to adapt. Some of the research conducted in my laboratory will provide evidence of the limitations of the stress and coping paradigm as a theoretical perspective, and how this perspective might be modified to include a broader definition of environment-organism interaction. This research will be used to illustrate some of the inherent pitfalls in a restricted view of coping, as opposed to a broader position that takes ecological circumstances into account. To do so, I will focus on the institutional arrangements within the newborn nursery—a cultural and environmental surround for childbirth in our technologically oriented society. Further, I will attempt to show how these arrangements impinge upon the mother-infant and father-infant relationships, and subsequently produce stress within the family unit that eventually affects the child. The outcome, as we shall see, will have a broader perspective when considered from the vantage point of the child and the family, rather than exclusively from the perspective either of the child or of the parents alone. This analysis will also emphasize the necessity of dealing with multiple types of stressors in accounting for stress responses and adaptation of the individual.

PREMATURITY AND THE NEWBORN NURSERY

Biological and Medical Considerations

One of the crowning achievements of American medicine in the second half of the twentieth century has been the improvement in the care of the preterm infant. While the mortality rates for preterm infants in the United States weighing between 1000 to 2500 grams was approximately 20% at mid-century (Eastman, 1950), mortality rates for this group are now approximately 5% when compared to full-term infants. Historically, infants below 1000 grams had little chance for survival; the survival rate has now increased to about 80% for infants born weighing between 750 to 1000 grams in university medical school hospitals (Sunshine, 1981). Clearly, modern technology and medicine have fostered remarkable advances in the care of the newborn-at-risk.

Biological advances in the care of the preterm infant began in earnest in the late 1940s with control of infection, better management of respiratory and nutritional problems, and more adequate monitoring of physiological processes by electronic means. Not all of these advances were without risk of morbidity for the preterm infant (e.g., excess of oxygen to aid respiration that led to later blindness). By the 1970s the technological advances included more sophisticated temperature and light control, and later, provision of water beds (Korner, Thoman, & Glick, 1974; Korner, Kraemer, Haffner, & Cosper, 1975), which simulate the uterine environment so as to ease the transition of preterm infants from intrauterine to extrauterine life. What was missing in the 1960s was a most important link in the chain of this technologically oriented process: the establishment of a viable relationship between the preterm infant and a responsible adult, after the infant was delivered in the socially isolated, biomedically advanced, technologically oriented infant care unit.

Social and Psychological Considerations

How did this separating of the mother from the care of her preterm infant come about? The history of premature care exemplifies some of the processes involved in the scientific progress made over the past 70 years which led to such a birthing arrangement. Before 1900 most preterm infants died. Near the turn of the century, Budin (1907) devised a simple arrangement for providing heat, cleanliness, and routine attention for the infant, revolutionizing care and markedly altering survival rates. Most importantly, he encouraged mothers to breast-feed, visit, and care for their infants. Cooney, in the United States, found these results so remarkable, he used preterm infants in incubators as part of the sideshow attractions of circuses and international exhibitions throughout the United States, though without mothers' participation in their care. One byproduct of this technology was a demonstration that infants could survive with only a minimum of human contact and without maternal interference, as long as they received proper physical care. However, there were some disquieting results. As reported by Klaus and Kennell (1976), mothers of premature infants would, on some occasions, refuse to take back their infants when the child achieved full birth weight and was ready to come home. The fact that the mother was a biological parent did not ensure that she was also the psychological and social parent of the infant.

The importance of the social-psychological components of care in the modern era began to be considered in the late 1960s. Until then, the caregiver entered the picture several days, or even several weeks, after the birth of the infant, depending upon the rate of weight gain and the health of the infant. The caregiver was prepared to "take delivery," as a six- to eight-week-old infant approached the requisite weight of 2500 grams. Despite the optimal physical and biological care provided in the hospital, growth and development of the preterm infant after discharge was found in many cases to present severe problems when compared to full-term infants. Furthermore, mothers of these infants often proved less equipped to care for their children once they were at home, than were mothers of full-term infants. This observation was especially true of infants from lower-class families; it was much less true for infants who were raised in middle-class families. Despite the optimal care provided by the nursery, some infants, in terms of subsequent growth and development, seemed to be at considerable risk once they were within the context of the biological family. What was the basis for these differences in growth and development for infants who were, at least biologically, quite similar to one another? Was it caused directly by the somewhat uncommon early relationship of the mother to the child? Was it caused by the sudden change in the environment once the child left the hospital? Or were there some other aspects of prematurity that resided either in the mother-infant relationship, or in specific environmental conditions that characterized the infant's nursery and/or postnatal world?

The preterm infant had long been thought to be at high risk for abnormal physical and behavioral development. This was attributed at various times to genetic, intrauterine, prenatal, and perinatal causes, as well as to the maternal attitudes and childrearing practices in the immediate postnatal period. Though biological factors were regarded as the most important, and were most readily observed, studies by Drillien (1959) in Scotland and by Broman, Nichols, and Kennedy (1975) in the United States indicated that infants from middle-class backgrounds, when they were evaluated as school children and at older ages, were not at higher risk for impaired cognitive development. These findings suggested the possibility that social factors, perhaps including the middle-class mother's psychological stance toward her child, played some part in fostering adequate cognitive development, previously assumed to be deficient in preterm children.

Among the psychosocial factors considered important in accounting for these manifest deficiencies when they were evidenced (and viewed here as potential stressor factors), was the institutional arrangement which traditionally surrounds the birthing process—the separation of the mother from the infant in the preterm nursery. This hypothesis received some support from experiments with animals which indicated there might be a critical, or sensitive, immediate postpartum period for the establishment of the mother-to-infant social bonding relationship. Some of those animal studies indicated that the absence of mother-infant contact in this period was found to lead to the mother's rejection of the newborn (Herscher, Richmond, & Moore, 1963). By analogy, these studies were thought to provide a mechanism accounting for some of the later dysfunctional mother-child relationships found previously with preterm human infants.

Clinical Considerations

The basic clinical problem facing those caring for the preterm infant and its mother was one reported by Budin: some mothers, after receiving a viable, reasonably well infant, did not seem to provide the enthusiastic care of their infants that one would anticipate. They had difficulty in "reading" their newborns. Further, some reported they felt incapable of caring for their infants, expressed uncertainty about their ability to deal with such a fragile creature, or were frankly depressed. Given the strong bias of clinicians and researchers in the developmental field (Rutter, 1972, 1979) to make maternal personality, feelings, and attitudes their central focus in accounting for dysfunctional child development, it is not surprising that the mothers of preterms were deemed to be the responsible agents, and were viewed as rejecting their maternal role much as they rejected the biological imperative of carrying their infants to full term (Kaplan & Mason, 1960). Thus, a new element introduced to account in part for some of the clinical phenomena, namely the environmental conditions that provided for separation of the neonate from the mother in the newborn nursery, was hypothesized to play a major role in producing the symptoms reported by mothers. It was reasoned these symptoms were manifestations of environmentally induced stress reactions produced not merely by the fact of a preterm birth, but also by a deprivational state generated by early caretaking being delegated to others, rather than being performed by the infant's mother.

Mother-Infant Separation in the Preterm Nursery: Psychological Reactions

Barnett, Leiderman, Grobstein, and Klaus (1970), working at Stanford University, began to study the possibility that these early environmental conditions of separation might serve as an institutional stressor which could set in motion a sequence of dysfunctional relationships, the first being the relationship of the mother to the child, and the second, other relationships important to the early development of the child. In an experimental study, the premature nursery was rearranged, permitting mothers to become involved, as early as they desired after giving birth, in the caretaking of their preterm infants. This nursery was modified for three month intervals, permitting mothers with infants in the nursery during those three months to become involved in early caretaking. During the alternative period, mothers with infants in the nursery experienced the routine arrangements of separation until the infant achieved a weight of 2000 grams, approximately one week before discharge. Both the separated and contact mothers could be in contact with their infants in the week immediately preceding the infant's discharge from the hospital. Twenty-three mothers and infants comprised the contact group; 22 mothers and infants comprised the separated group; 23 mothers and infants comprised the full-term control group, who experienced the routine neonatal arrangements of 12- to 24-hour separation after childbirth, with hospital discharge in 2 to 4 days. The usual period of a mother's separation from her infant after birth was several hours to 1 to 2 days for the contact group, compared to periods of 3 to 12 weeks for mothers in the separated group. Caretaking by the mothers consisted of physical contact with their infants as long as they wished, and included assisting the nurse in feeding their infants when the infants were able to manage oral feeding.

The basic hypothesis was that the modification of the physical arrangements, in the immediate postnatal period to reduce separation, would influence the psychological reactions and expectations of the mothers, making them feel more competent, less guilty, and more effective in caring for their infant. In essence, their presence and their activity could serve to reduce the stress provided by the environmental surround while adding to the mother's sense of efficacy in caring for her child. The increment in self-esteem would eventuate in an improved mother-infant relationship that would in turn enhance the infant's growth and development in a manner commensurate with that of a full-term infant. In these studies conducted with middle-class families (Leifer, Leiderman, Barnett, & Williams, 1972; Seashore, Leifer, Barnett, & Leiderman, 1973), it was found that during the immediate postpartum period, and continuing throughout the period of separation and for several months after the infant was taken home, the separated group of mothers was less close physically to their infants, had a reduced sense of confidence with regard to their maternal role, and reported a sense of lowered personal efficacy and self-esteem; this contrasted markedly with the contact mother group and with the control group comprised of mothers of full-term infants. Many of the separated mothers felt guilty and incompetent over the handling of their infants. Reports such as "I don't feel like I am a mother," or "I am frightened by her crying," were not uncommon. Even their manner of holding their infants differed from that of full-term mothers and preterm contact mothers. Theirs was less close and more rigid, as if they were carrying an inanimate object.

These feelings and behaviors continued throughout a major portion of the infant's first year for some of the noncontact mothers, but were gradually reduced as the mothers became more experienced and gained confidence in handling their infants. One year after discharge, most separated mothers appeared to have regained their sense of self-esteem and efficacy and could not be differentiated from either the groups of mothers of full-term infants or the preterm infant-contact mothers. These improvements in attitude and self-esteem were paralleled by an increase in the physical expressions of affection, such as smiling, looking at and holding their infants close, behaviors which had been demonstrably less common in the separated group during the first several months after discharge.

Leiderman, Leifer, Seashore, Barnett, and Grobstein (1973) and Leiderman and Seashore (1975) continued to follow these infants into their second year. By the middle of the second year, they found differences in caretaking behavior of mothers of both preterm and full-term neonates were influenced by the gender and birth order of the infant as well. Further, mothers of preterm first-born children seemed to be more negatively influenced by the separation than were mothers of second-born children. Furthermore, mothers of male infants handled them more cautiously and talked to them less than did mothers of female infants. However, these differences gradually diminished by the end of the second year.

The obvious conclusion was that by the end of the infant's second year the evident signs of maternal stress effects following birth of a preterm infant, and subsequent separation, had essentially disappeared. Cognitive studies at two years also revealed no differences between preterm separated infants, the full-term controls, and the preterm contact infants. It should be noted, of course, that these mothers were predominately of middle-class status and from intact families in which, when the study began, both mother and father were living together in the home. In addition to the possible differences in value orientation and maternal caretaking skills that may differentiate socio-economic groups, many of the families participating in the study had community and family support networks available to mitigate against some of the deleterious effects of separation. Thus, these findings were consistent with the earlier observations of Drillien (1959) and parallel studies by Broman et al. (1975), in which the deleterious effects of preterm birth were less obvious in families with middle-class backgrounds.

Mother-Infant Separation and Social Class

Klaus and Kennell subsequently, at Case-Western Reserve University, joined in a series of studies that were performed in Guatemala and in Cleveland, Ohio (Kennell, Trause, & Klaus, 1975; Klaus, Jerauld, Kreger, McAlpine, Steffa, & Kennell, 1972; Klaus & Kennell, 1976). They initially studied preterm infants, and, subsequently, the consequences of very early contact of mothers and their full-term infants following birth. An additional and particularly important aspect of their research was the fact that they employed a sample of black, relatively economically deprived mothers. Further, they were interested in the effects of contact between mother and infant within one hour after birth, compared to the several hours delay in contact between mothers and infants that had marked the Leiderman study.

Allowing some mothers to have such very early contact, they found differences between the caretaking habits of this group in comparison with mothers who had been deprived of contact opportunities; contact mothers were found to be more comfortable with and concerned about their infants when evaluated one year later during a visit to the physician's office. Further, Klaus and Kennell found these effects were maintained into the second year of the child's life. Follow-up studies, performed when the child was four years old, revealed cognitive differences between the groups of children that favored those born to mothers who had been allowed early contact with their infants. Furthermore, these mothers maintained their relationships with their children throughout their participation in the study. Particularly noteworthy in their study were the positive effects of early contact observed in a group experiencing many non-specific stressors such as minority status, poverty, and ghetto residence, in addition to more specific effects of inexperience with newborn infants, and an unmarried marital status. However, for Klaus et al. (1977), the importance of maternal contact within an hour after birth was considered by them to be the salient factor in accounting for their striking results.

Both of these early studies demonstrated that conditions of the institutional environment did affect, for a time, the mother-infant and mother-child relationships. They diverged, however, in that the Leiderman study conducted with middle-class families found that the negative effects of lack of perinatal contact disappeared by the infant's second year of life, whereas in the Klaus and Kennell studies there continued to be measurable deficits in the lower-class population group for as long as four years after hospital discharge.

Further tests of the effects of the social class variable, apart from the effects of very early contact, are reflected in studies reported by O'Connor, Vietze, Sherrod, Sandler, and Altemeier (1980). They dealt with the effects of a hospital rooming-in situation in comparison with routine postnatal care for 291 mothers and infants in an urban public hospital in the southern United States. The sample consisted of both white and black mothers, only one-third of whom had an employed member in the household. Approximately 40% of the mothers were married, their median age was 18 years, and their median education level achieved was two years of high school. Except for the presence of racial variations, this sample was quite similar to the one studied by Klaus and Kennell. In this study, mothers were randomly assigned to one of two conditions: (1) rooming-in, beginning some 7 hours after delivery, or (2) routine care, beginning some 12 hours after delivery. The mothers in the rooming-in situation had approximately 10 hours of additional contact with their infants compared with the routine hospital group.

At 17 months following discharge, 10 of the 145 mothers who had belonged to the routine care group were found to be inadequate parents, as measured by several standards: (1) hospitalization of their infants for inadequate care; (2) referral for protective services; and (3) placement of the child outside the home by the courts or the parents. By contrast, there were only two such cases of the 146 mothers in the rooming-in group. These findings, applicable to lower-class families, supported the previously reported observations of positive consequences for a considerable portion of the infant's first year if mother-infant contact had occurred within hours after birth. It should be noted that contact between mothers and infants in the O'Connor et al. study came 7 hours after birth, an interval that would have been deemed inappropriate in terms of the need for early contact, i.e., within an hour after birth. What is particularly important is that these observations affirmed the generality of the variable contact findings, at least during the first year, in a white and black lower-class group, which differed demographically from the predominately white middle-class sample observed at Stanford, and the predominately black lower-class urban sample observed at Case-Western Reserve University in Cleveland.

Klaus et al. (1977) extended their studies of early contact to a lower middle-class and lower-class sample in Guatemala where they permitted very early contact, within the first hour after birth, between mothers and infants. Follow-up of these cases one year later indicated greater amounts of breast-feeding and greater weight gain in the group of very early contact infants compared to the group deprived of this advantage. Although the two groups were not truly comparable, these data too suggest that merely minutes of contact within the first hour following birth can enhance later caretaking functions of participant mothers. The diverse cultural and racial aspects of these studies provide an important perspective on the significance of the contact variable. The most important aspect of this later study was that it extended the earlier studies to a nonindustrialized urban society, with a markedly different cultural orientation and childcare practices.

Replication of the Klaus and Kennell studies with a Swedish middle-class population (deChateau, 1976) has been reported, revealing that very early contact influenced the frequency and duration of breast-feeding three months later. However, the effects of early contact were not prominent in other aspects of behavior, including reports of maternal self-esteem and self-confidence. This study, however, provided additional evidence of the buffering effects of middle-class background and middle-class social environments which appeared to mitigate the deleterious effects of early postnatal separation of mother from infant.

In a well-controlled, well-designed test of the very early contact hypothesis, Svejda, Campos, and Emde (1980), in Denver, studied 30 lower-middle-class mothers from intact families. One group of 15 mothers and infants had contact for 15 minutes immediately after birth. Within approximately one-half hour, a further five minutes of contact were allowed the mothers and infants in the privacy of the mother's room. At this time, the mother was gowned with the nude infant lying at her side. By contrast, the control group received routine care. The contact mothers had an additional 10 hours of baby contact during the first 36 hours. The authors reported that at 36 hours there was no difference in maternal behavior between the two groups. The only major difference was gender-based; early contact mothers talked to their female infants more, and routine contact mothers touched their female infants more and looked at their male infants more, than did the contrasting group.

In comparing these discrepant findings with the results obtained in the studies conducted by Klaus and Kennell, it should be noted that in the Denver study the fathers were present at the birth of the 13 control infants and 13 of 15 experimental infants. It may be that the differences in the results of the studies can be explained by the fact that these mothers had the manifest physical presence and social support of their husbands at the time of childbirth, and that the husband presumably would be more likely to be involved in the future care of the child.[4] This study, too, raises the issue of the importance of considering education, social class, and marital status as possible modifier variables on the effects of early separation.

The Denver study, while not supportive of Klaus and Kennell's basic findings on the effects of early contact, does not address the question of whether there are delayed effects later, especially during the first two years of the infant's life. Nonetheless, the favorable social and economic circumstances of this study's sample may have minimized the more dramatic benefits of early contact that have been observed in economically and socially disadvantaged samples.

Another cross-national study reported by Grossmann, Thane, and Grossmann (1981), with a middle-class West German sample, was designed to examine the effects of very early contact within one hour after birth versus extended contact for several hours after birth. This study divided 54 mothers and their infants into four groups: (1) very early contact; (2) 5 hours of extended contact; (3) neither early nor extended contact; and (4) both early and extended contact. They evaluated the mothers' behavior while still in the hospital 8 to 10 days postpartum. They reported that for the first 5 days after birth, early contact, but not extended contact, was found to have a significant positive effect on mothers' caressing behaviors but not on their caretaking functions. The major effect of early contact on tenderness behavior of mothers was associated with those who *planned* their pregnancies. By 8 to 10 days, mothers without early contact touched their infants as often as

---

[4] See Sosa, Kennell, Klaus, Robertson, and Urrutia (1980) for the effects on the mother, related to the presence of a supportive companion at childbirth.

did mothers under the early contact condition. These findings, again characteristic of a middle-class sample, point to the possible cross-national role of social and economic supports, and planfulness, in reducing the negative effects of separation (see Lamb & Hwang, 1982, for a critical review of the issue of separation, and early and extended contact in the neonatal period).

Prematurity as Stressor

Having considered the event of separation in the neonatal period as a possible stressor for both preterm and full-term infants and mothers, we must now question whether prematurity itself may account for some of the maternal reactions reported in the various studies.[5] In this formulation, the infant is also seen as a potential source of stress for the family. A series of studies (Field, 1980; Goldberg, Brachfeld, & Divetto, 1980) have demonstrated that prematurity affects the mother-child relationships and creates other deficiencies in parental caretaking.

Evidence of inadequate parenting can be seen in reports on abused and neglected children. Investigators (Elmer & Gregg, 1967; Klein & Stern, 1971) have reported a greater incidence of prematurity in abused and neglected children, in samples collected in Pittsburgh and in Montreal. These studies did not report birthing conditions of the infants, but, based upon the period during which the research was conducted, it is likely that the mothers did not have early contact with their infants. Despite the suggested evidence that prematurity does contribute to inadequate parenting, Minde (1980) has pointed to a confounding factor—many of the children reported by these investigators were not only born prematurely but also had other medical abnormalities and deficiencies. Thus it might not be prematurity alone which could account for these findings, but other aspects of deviancy in these children. Nonetheless, despite this note of warning, the joint effect of an unexpected premature birth and/or the presence of other anomalies did appear to be related to a greater subsequent incidence of deficient parenting.

A more direct approach to examining the effects of prematurity on childcare can be seen in the study of Egeland and Vaughan (1981). They studied the childcare practices of a group of lower-class welfare mothers. The group which provided the least amount of care and showed abuse and neglect of their offspring, did not include a greater number of mothers of preterm infants when compared with a group that provided optimal infant care. They concluded that early separation in the neonatal period, as de-

---

[5] The possibility exists, of course, that it is not prematurity itself which accounts for these reactions but unanticipated prematurity and subsequent separation which leads to the deficiencies in childrearing. This issue will not be examined in this paper.

duced from prematurity of the infant, did not distinguish the two groups through a period extending as long as nine months after delivery.

Rode, Chang, Fisch, and Sroufe (1981) examined the infant-mother relationship by studying the effects of separation at birth on subsequent attachment behavior of the infants to their mothers after 12 months of age. These investigators followed a group of 24 middle-class infants (20 preterms and 4 seriously ill full-term infants) who had been separated from their mothers for approximately 27 days. These infants were tested at 12 to 19 months of age in the Ainsworth Strange Situation (Ainsworth, Blehar, Waters, & Wall, 1978). The patterns of attachment response of this group of infants proved to be no different when compared with a group of normal infants. The results suggest that the resiliency of the mother-infant social bond, despite early separation, was sufficient to ameliorate the effects reported by Kennell and Klaus.

Goldberg, Brachfeld, and Divetto (1980), however, did examine the question of inadequate parental care in their study of mothers with preterm infants. They evaluated maternal caretaking by selecting four groups of infants: (1) full-term; (2) healthy preterm; (3) ill preterm; and (4) post-mature infants. These infants were studied over their first year of life in a series of mother-infant interactions conducted both at home and in the laboratory. The results suggest that the preterm infant is not as well adapted to normal caregiving as is the full-term infant. Such infants are less alert, less responsive to their caregivers, and unable to give clear distress signals by crying when the attention of another is needed. The researchers conclude that the parents of preterms are denied the gratification of the signs of growth and development for a considerable period of time. The birth of a preterm infant appears to confront the caregiver with a poorly adapted social partner; the parents must put forth a great deal of effort during the first year with relatively little return in positive responsiveness from their offspring. It would appear that the infant plays a major part in shaping the behavior of the mother, an inference that is consistent with the recognition of the influencing role of the infant on the caregiver (Bell, 1968).

Apart from the contribution of the infant's behavioral repertoire to the mother's behavior, recent studies focus on the effects of preterm infants on mothers' expectations of their infants' ability to achieve developmental milestones (Smith, Leiderman, Selz, MacPherson, & Bingham, 1981). In this study, mothers of infants born preterm, when their offspring were 18 months old, were asked to record their expectations for social, psychomotor, and cognitive development for the age range of six months to nine years. Mothers were asked to rate the developmental milestones both for their own child as well as those that they would expect for a typical child. The mothers of pretermers did not differ from mothers of normal children in judging the achievement of these developmental milestones for typical children. However, in rating their own children, they predicted substantial lags for their own child until approximately two years of age. At that time, they tended to advance their expectations so that these exceeded the typical levels reported by the mothers of full-term infants. This expected precocity held for the areas of social, psychomotor, and cognitive development. Assuming successful replication of the results, the study suggests that the mothers of preterm infants may harbor unrealistic expectations for their young children, thereby creating some of the conditions that presage later dysfunctional parent-child relationships.

Somewhat compensatory for the unrealistic expectations of mothers for preterm infants are the scattered reports that fathers play a greater role in the caretaking of preterm infants, complementing and, in some instances, substituting for the deficiencies in maternal caregiving. This result has been reported by Minde (1980) and Goldberg (1979) and is supported by clinical observations made in our earlier studies. The infant's potential for adaptive behavior lies not only in his or her own inherent abilities, nor even, in this instance, in the relationship to the mother, but may well extend to other social resources, such as the father as an object of attachment who can compensate for a lack of maternal infant caretaking.

Mother-Infant Separation: Coping and Adaptation

The longer-term follow-up of the Case-Western Reserve and Stanford research programs may shed some light on the coping and adaptation side of the stress and coping paradigm. A follow-up study is still underway for the Cleveland sample, and has been completed through eight years of age for some children in the Stanford sample (Leiderman, 1978, 1981). In the latter study, the most important finding was the relationship of prematurity to marital stability. Those families with preterm infants had a much higher rate of divorce than did the parents of full-term control infants. The effects of early mother-infant separation on parental divorce failed to differentiate the preterm contact and separated groups. Whatever the effects of prematurity, they involved not only the mother-child relationship, but had ramifications that extended to the marital relationship. The longer-term effects influenced the entire family system rather than individual members of the family exclusively.

Another unanticipated effect of the study of early mother-infant separation was the by-product that followed upon the conduct of the research. Many nurseries throughout the United States changed their practices shortly after these studies were underway, despite the absence of concrete findings and the lack of a thorough understanding of the basic underlying processes. Thus, whatever the social forces involved in society at that time—greater independence of women in choosing their birthing procedures, the general climate of the 1960s and early 1970s of a more "democratic" participation in decision-making affecting one's self—the heretofore closed doors of the nurseries were thrown open to parents. Mothers, rather than being excluded, were actually encouraged to participate in caretaking of their infants while still in the hospital. Subsequent research findings buttressed what proved pragmatically to be a better arrangement. Adaptation to the stress of the premature birth of an infant led to the rearrangement of institutional practices which had, up until this time, been considered to be the best, the most effective, and the most convenient setting for all parties involved.

CONCLUSION

Three major points are worth making about this cautionary recital of studies that concern both the family, and the hospital as an institutional stressor. The first point is that the major stressors themselves are built into institutionalized arrangements which in turn are derived from the dominant cultural values of the society. These institutional forms are built upon, and then justified as part of, the contemporary ideology of experts. Despite the lack of supporting or contradictory evidence, these arrangements persist, even though they may hold great stress-related costs to the individual. When these stresses become sufficiently powerful, or real damage becomes a probable outcome, there is a press for change to reduce these stressors. The nature of these critical events that must occur for the individual, and/or the system that allows for change, is essentially unknown. Stresses stemming from these institutionally induced arrangements inspire adaptive responses by bringing scientists and physicians who, by virtue of their professional responsibility, are able to help to modify them. Individual adaptation is enhanced by the coping behaviors which are instituted by others. Subsequently, the adaptation takes place at the level of the system rather than the individual.

The second point to be made about these studies is that a single stressor does not seem sufficient to account for the maintenance of maladaptive behaviors, though the stress experience may be sufficient (and perhaps necessary) to initiate such reactions. A preterm birth in conjunction with a parents' minority status and relative poverty, combined with a lack of adequate social supports, can generate a complex of stressors that lowers the adaptive threshold of individuals, and hence fosters dysfunctional relationships within the family. In contrast, the better "buffered" middle-class families seem to have access to compensatory institutions and to social supports that are not easily or readily available to families buffeted by poverty. These might include information resources, neighbors, friends, and, of course, family members able and willing to assist in the crisis. These ameliorative forces and their effects are more usual, and hence less dramatic, in the lives of middle-class families. However, in the case of the economically deprived groups, the ameliorative action of institutions, including very early contact and supportive physicians seems to exercise a more powerful effect on the mother-infant relationship. Stated in another way, the remedial measures are much more likely to affect individuals and families with multiple stressors while the same measures may not be as necessary for individuals exposed to relatively few or to less severe stressors.

The third point to be made about these studies is more specific to the stress and coping paradigm. The adaptive or maladaptive responses are not necessarily viewed as residing within the individual. The normal infant and young child can call forth, from the family, physical safety, adequate nutrition, and stable arrangements within the household. These essentials are provided by parents and by society. Where the family and social systems are inadequate, the presence of a preterm infant exacerbates stress within the family, and increases the risk for marital dissolution. The condition of prematurity, when introduced into a family, affects the social system and ultimately the child.

The coping and adaptive arrangements of the family include not only the attitudes of the mother and father toward the preterm infant, which surely affects their behavior to the newborn, but also the arrangements they might provide for subsequent caretaking of the infant.

There is a reciprocal element to the mother-infant relationship. Despite the fact that the mothers of premature infants are particularly hard-working, they often derive little reward for this, at least during the infant's earliest years. The mother's attempt to achieve gratification from her infant may lead to her neglect of the marital relationship, and can accentuate marital discord. The situation, however, is not inevitably bleak. When an infant is born prematurely, there is also an increased likelihood for some families to develop greater shared parental responsibility for the infant in order to provide for adequate caretaking. Adaptation and coping, therefore, go beyond the responsibility of any single member of the family, including the mother. It can occur through shifts within the family, and, beyond it, to changes in the social world, where ideally there will be available adequate physical and social support systems for preterm (or at-risk) infants and their families.

A CONCLUDING COMMENT ON STRESS, COPING, AND ADAPTATION

I have attempted to examine the possible usefulness of the stress and coping paradigm as it might apply to developmental processes in infancy and early childhood. The differences between the adult and child versions of the paradigm exemplify the importance of longitudinal and ecological factors, when considering the adaptation of children. This is necessary because of the immaturity of the cognitive system of the developing child, the relatively long period of dependency, and the role of familial and social systems as significant components of the coping process. In examining the environmental and stressor components, I have attempted to illustrate how culturally and socially derived stressors (separation of mother and infant in "high-risk" nurseries in Western technologically oriented societies) influence mothers in caring for their infants. These experiences of mothers, especially under circumstances when other chronic, deleterious environmental factors (poverty, prematurity, single parenthood) obtain, exercise a negative effect, at least in the short run, on the infant's caretaking, with possible extensions into a longer term future that will influence the lives of both parent and child. Further, I have indicated how the expectations of mothers regarding the child may partially explain subsequent maladaptive responses to her offspring. For the longer term, I have attempted to show that the stress reaction and coping responses do not reside exclusively in the infant and young child but are entwined in the social system of the family and the larger society beyond. These components may exercise a positive influence on social and medical institutions, modifying these arrangements which, in turn, can accentuate or attenuate stress factors in the child's life.

In presenting the stress and coping paradigm, I have indicated that the perceptual appraisal system of the child may be somewhat less complex and more limited than that of the adult. This is particularly critical when considering the child's appraisal of possible threats within the environment. However, children are not dependent solely on their own perceptual appraisal system but have available to them the perceptual appraisal system of their caregivers and other household members who are responsible for their well-being. The mother initially, and, very soon thereafter, the father and other caregivers, can serve as the immediate filterers of environmental stimuli that impinge on the infant and young child. These caregivers serve as a modulating interface between the child and the world; their task is to assess and respond to the infant's requirements and demands, and to react to and shape his or her responses in a manner consonant with their own expectations and with the goals they set for their infant. In a successful system, environmentally derived stressors, as well as the needs of the infant, are appropriately assessed by the caregivers to ensure exposure to a variety of experiences, sufficient in amount and moderate in intensity, designed to promote the growth and development of the young child. The pace of development of the young child can become the crucial element in determining the rate of and exposure to environmental vicissitudes by the caregivers. The assessment of the child's perceptual capacities must necessarily take into account the dynamic interplay between the developing infant and the patterned environment of the family and the community.

Turning to the coping and adaptation side of the stress and coping paradigm, I have provided examples which indicate that this paradigm should be applied not only to the child but broadened to include the wider domain of familial, community, and cultural systems. Coping and adaptation are more than functions of an individual's efforts and talents. Some actions by family or society, in the short term, may be harmful to the individual child (i.e., not committing all of the family resources to a child with a reduced likelihood for survival), though such action may be beneficial to the larger social group. The gain for the group through the removal of the least viable organism is presumed to be a strengthened potential for adaptation to a variety of environments, though this may come at the expense of the vulnerable individual. The adaptive potential is retained at the group level and not at the level of the individual, though in most instances it would include appropriate concern and care for the individual child.

I have emphasized the ecological viewpoint as the basis for a more appropriate developmentally based stress and coping paradigm. Given the potential of the young organism to become established in a variety of environmental niches, and given the ambiguity of future projections for any developing individual, predictions of adaptive success or failure could be aided by knowledge of the child's experience in diverse ecological situations, especially as these are modulated by concerned and trusted caregivers. The basic unit of adaptation is the individual-environmental fit, and it is this complex which should serve as the unit of analysis and the basis for determining the long-term potential for adaptive success.

The final word, if any is possible, on stress reaction and coping in developmental research clearly cannot be provided in this chapter. Stress and coping have had little utility in developmental research in the past because the ecological conditions, over time, have not been an essential element in the analysis of child behavior, nor have we had adequate assessment methods for the perceptual appraisal of threat by the child. Stress and coping research with adults has included many more of these aspects. But, particularly in developmental research, the lack of ecological concerns is clearly not suitable for a developmental stress and coping model in which the child is viewed as undergoing relatively rapid change within a continually changing social matrix.[6] While a nonecologically oriented stress and coping paradigm possibly may have been heuristically valuable in the past for

---

[6] See Harmon and Emde (1978), Lipsitt (1981), and Parke and Tinsley (1982) for further discussion of this point.

adult stress research, it is unlikely to be so in the future. In any case, for the developing organism, we need to consider all of the components of the social and physical world which impinge upon, shape, or respond to the developing child. In this way we can understand children's requirements for a variety of social and physical resources that can assure their continued survival and attainment of maturity in a complex social system. For the child-development researcher and the clinician, there is no alternative but to get on with the difficult task of the search for understanding of the broadened picture of a child's environment, together with an appreciation of the child's individualized, ever-changing patterns of behavior.

REFERENCES

Ainsworth, M., Blehar, M. C., Waters, E., & Wall, S. *Patterns of attachment*. Hillsdale, N.J.: Lawrence Erlbaum Associates, 1978.

Antonovsky, A. *Health, stress, and coping*. San Francisco: Jossey-Bass, 1980.

Baltes, P. B., Reese, H. W., & Nesselroade, J. R. *Life span developmental psychology: Introduction to research methods*. Monterey, Calif.: Brooks/Cole, 1977.

Barker, R. G., & Wright, H. F. Psychological ecology and the problem of psychosocial development. *Child Development*, 1949, *20*, 131–143.

Barnett, C., Leiderman, P. H., Grobstein, R., & Klaus, M. Neonatal separation: The maternal side of interactional deprivation. *Pediatrics*, 1970, *45*, 197–205.

Bell, R. A reinterpretation of the direction of effects in studies of socialization. *Psychological Review*, 1968, *75*, 81–93.

Broman, S. H., Nichols, P. L., & Kennedy, W. A. *Preschool IQ: Preschool and early developmental correlates*. Hillsdale, N.J.: Lawrence Erlbaum, 1975.

Bronfenbrenner, U. *The ecology of human development*. Cambridge, Massachusetts: Harvard University Press, 1979.

Budin, P. *The nursling*. London: Laxton Publishing Company, 1907.

Carmichael, L. *Manual of child psychology* (3rd Edition). New York: John Wiley & Sons, 1970.

Coelho, G. V., Hamburg, D. A., & Adams, J. (Eds.). *Coping and adaptation*. New York: Basic Books, Inc., 1974.

deChateau, P. *Neonatal care routines: Influences on maternal and infant behavior and on breast feeding*. Thesis, Umea University Medical Dissertations, New Series #20. Umea, Sweden, 1976.

Drillien, C. M. A longitudinal study of growth and development of prematurely and maturely born children (III. Mental development). *Archives of Diseases in Children*, 1959, *34*, 37–45.

Eastman, J. J. *Williams obstetrics* (10th Edition). New York: Appleton-Century-Crofts, Inc., 1950.

Egeland, B., & Vaughan, B. Failure of "bond formation" as a cause of abuse, neglect and maltreatment. *American Journal of Orthopsychiatry*, 1981, *51*, 78–84.

Elmer, E., & Gregg, G. S. Developmental characteristics of abused children. *Pediatrics*, 1967, *40*, 596–602.

Erikson, E. Identity and the life cycle. *Psychological Issues*, *1*, 1959.

Field, T. Interactions of pre-term and term infants with their lower- and middle-class teenage and adult mothers. In T. Field (Ed.), *High-risk infants and children*. New York: Academic Press, 1980.

Goldberg, S. *Adaptation to stress in parent-infant dyad.* Paper presented at Keystone Conference on parenting. Keystone, Colorado, 1979.

Goldberg, S., Brachfeld, S., & Divetto, B. Feeding, fussing and play: Parent-infant interaction in the first year as a function of prematurity and perinatal medical problems. In T. Field (Ed.), *High-risk infants and children. Adult and peer interactions.* New York: Academic Press, 1980.

Goldschmidt, W. Ethology, ecology and ethnological realities. In G. V. Coelho, D. A. Hamburg, & J. E. Adams (Eds.), *Coping and adaptation.* New York: Basic Books, Inc., 1974.

Grinker, R. R., & Spiegel, J. P. *Men under stress.* Philadelphia: Blakiston, 1945.

Grossmann, K., Thane, K., & Grossman, K. E. Maternal tactile contact of the newborn after various postpartum conditions of mother-infant contact. *Developmental Psychology,* 1981, *17,* 158–169.

Harmon, R. J., & Emde, R. N. *Clinical and research perspectives on perinatal influences in the family.* Presented at the Annual Convention, American Academy of Child Psychiatry, October, 1978.

Hersher, L., Richmond, J. B., & Moore, A. U. Modifiability of critical period for the development of maternal behavior in sheep and goats. *Behavior,* 1963, *20,* 311–319.

Kagan, J., & Rosman, B. L. Cardiac and respiratory correlates of attention and an analytic attitude. *Journal of Experimental Child Psychology,* 1964, *1,* 50–63.

Kaplan, D. M., & Mason, E. A. Maternal reactions to premature birth viewed as an acute emotional disorder. *American Journal of Orthopsychiatry,* 1960, *30,* 539–552.

Kennell, J. H., Trause, M. A., & Klaus, M. H. Evidence for a sensitive period in the human mother in parent-infant interaction. In *Parent-infant interaction.* CIBA Foundation Symposium (Vol. 33) (N.S.). New York: Elsevier, 1975.

Klaus, M. H., Jerauld, R., Kreger, N. C., McAlpine, W., Steffa, M., & Kennell, J. H. Maternal attachment: Importance of first postpartum days. *New England Journal of Medicine,* 1972, *286,* 460–463.

Klaus, M. H., & Kennell, J. H. *Maternal-infant bonding.* St. Louis: C. V. Mosby Company, 1976.

Klein, M., & Stern, L. Low birth weight and the battered child syndrome. *American Journal of Diseases in Children,* 1971, *122,* 15–18.

Korchin, S. J. *Modern clinical psychology: Principles of intervention in the clinic and community.* New York: Basic Books, Inc., 1976.

Korner, A. F., Thoman, E. B., & Glick, J. H. A system for monitoring crying and noncrying, large, medium and small neonatal movements. *Child Development,* 1974, *45,* 946–952.

Korner, A., Kraemer, H. C., Haffner, M. E., & Cosper, R. N. Effects of waterbed flotation on premature infants: A pilot study. *Pediatrics,* 1975, *56,* 361–367.

Lamb, M. E., & Hwang, C. Maternal attachment and mother-infant bonding: A critical review. In M. E. Lamb, & A. L. Brown (Eds.), *Advances in developmental psychology* (Vol. 2). Hillsdale, N.J.: Lawrence Erlbaum Associates, 1982.

Lazarus, R. S. *Psychological stress and the coping process.* New York: McGraw-Hill Book Company, 1966.

Leiderman, P. H. The critical period hypothesis revisited: Mother to infant social bonding in the neonatal period. In F. D. Horowitz (Ed.), *Early developmental hazards: Predictors and precautions.* Boulder, Colo.: Westview Press, 1978.

Leiderman, P. H. Human mother to infant social bonding: Is there a sensitive phase? In K. Immelmann, G. Barlow, L. Petrinovich, & M. Main (Eds.), *Behavioral development.* The Bielefeld Interdisciplinary Project. New York: Cambridge University Press, 1981.

Leiderman, P. H., Leifer, A. D., Seashore, M. D., Barnett, C. R., & Grobstein, R. Mother-infant interaction: Effects of early deprivation, prior experience, and sex of child. In J. I. Nurnberger (Ed.), *Biological and environmental determinants of early development.* Association for Research in Nervous and Mental Disease (Vol. 51). Baltimore, Maryland: Williams & Wilkins Press, 1973.

Leiderman, P. H., & Seashore, M. J. Mother-infant separation: Some delayed consequences. In *Parent-infant interaction*. CIBA Foundation Symposium (Vol. 33) (N.S.). New York: Elsevier, 1975.

Leifer, A. D., Leiderman, P. H., Barnett, C. R., & Williams, J. A. Effects of mother-infant separation on maternal attachment behavior. *Child Development*, 1972, *43*, 1203–1218.

Lerner, R. M., & Spanier, G. B. *Child influences on marital and family interaction: A life span perspective*. New York: Academic Press, 1978.

Levine, S. Psychophysiological effects of infantile stimulation. In E. L. Bliss (Ed.), *Roots of behavior*. New York: Harper & Row, 1962.

Levinson, D. J., Darrow, C. N., Klein, E. B., Levinson, M. H., & McKee, B. *The seasons of a man's life*. New York: Alfred A. Knopf, 1978.

Lewin, K., Lippitt, R., & White, R. K. Patterns of aggressive behavior in experimentally created social climates. *Journal of Social Psychology*, 1939, *10*, 271–299.

Lindemann, E. Symptomology and management of acute grief. *American Journal of Psychiatry*, 1944, *101*, 141–148.

Lipsitt, L. P. Importance of collaboration and developmental follow-up in the study of perinatal risk. In V. Smeriglio (Ed.), *Newborns and parents: Parent-infant contact and newborn sensory stimulation*. Hillsdale, N.J.: Lawrence Erlbaum, 1981.

Maccoby, E., Doering, C. H., Jacklin, C. N., & Kraemer, H. C. Concentration of sex hormones in umbilical-cord blood: Their relation to sex and birth order of infants. *Child Development*, 1979, *50*, 632–642.

Mechanic, D. Social structure and personal adaptation: Some neglected dimensions. In G. V. Coelho, D. A. Hamburg, & J. E. Adams (Eds.), *Coping and adaptation*. New York: Basic Books, 1974.

Minde, K. Bonding of parents to premature infants: Theory and practice. In P. M. Taylor (Ed.), *Parent-infant relationships*. New York: Grune and Stratton, Inc., 1980.

Moos, R. H. *Evaluating treatment environments*. New York: John Wiley and Sons, 1974.

Murphy, L. B., & Associates. *The widening world of childhood: Paths toward mastery*. New York: Basic Books, 1962.

Murphy, L. B., & Moriarty, A. E. *Vulnerability, coping and growth: From infancy to adolescence*. New Haven: Yale University Press, 1976.

Mussen, P. H. (Ed.) *Carmichael's manual of child psychology* (3rd Edition). New York: John Wiley & Sons, 1970.

O'Connor, S., Vietze, P. M., Sherrod, K. B., Sandler, H. M., & Altemeier, W. A. Reduced incidence of parenting inadequacy following rooming-in. *Pediatrics*, 1980, *66*, 176–182.

Parke, R. D., & Tinsley, B. R. The early environment of the high risk infant: Expanding the social context. In D. Bricker (Ed.), *Application of research findings to intervention with at-risk and handicapped infants*, 1982.

Rode, S. S., Chang, P. N., Fisch, R. O., & Sroufe, L. A. Attachment patterns of infants separated at birth. *Developmental Psychology*, 1981, *17*, 188–191.

Rutter, M. *Maternal deprivation reassessed*. Harmondsworth: Penguin Books, Inc., 1972.

Rutter, M. Maternal deprivation 1972–1978: New findings, new concepts, new approaches. *Child Development*, 1979, *50*, 238–305.

Selye, H. *The physiology and pathology of exposure to stress*. Montreal: ACTA, 1950.

Seashore, M. D., Leifer, A. D., Barnett, C. R., & Leiderman, P. H. The effects of denial of mother-infant interaction on maternal self confidence. *Journal of Personality and Social Psychology*, 1973, *26*, 369–378.

Smelser, N. J. *Social sources of stress*. Paper presented at APA meetings. New York, 1961.

Sosa, R., Kennell, J. H., Klaus, M. H., Robertson, S., & Urrutia, J. The effect of a supportive companion on perinatal problems, length of labor, and mother-infant interaction. *New England Journal of Medicine*, 1980, *303*, 597–600.

Smith, C., Leiderman, P. H., Selz, L., MacPherson, L., & Bingham, E. *Maternal expectations and developmental milestones in physically handicapped infants*. Paper read at Biennial Meetings of the Society for Research in Child Development. Boston: 1981.

Sroufe, L. A., & Waters, E. Heart rate as a convergent measure in clinical and developmental research. *Merrill-Palmer Quarterly*, 1977, 23, 3–27.

Sunshine, Philip. Personal communication. Director, Stanford Neonatal Nurseries, 1981.

Svejda, M., Campos, J. J., & Emde, R. N. Mother-infant "bonding": Failure to generalize. *Child Development*, 1980, 51, 775–779.

Vaillant, G. E. *Adaptation to life*. Boston: Little, Brown, & Co., 1977.

White, R. W. Strategies of adaptation: An attempt at systematic description. In G. V. Coelho, D. A. Hamburg, & J. E. Adams (Eds.), *Coping and adaptation*. New York: Basic Books, Inc., 1974.

CHAPTER 6

STRESS IN INFANCY: Toward Understanding the Origins of Coping Behavior

LEWIS P. LIPSITT
PROFESSOR OF PSYCHOLOGY AND MEDICAL SCIENCE
DIRECTOR, CHILD STUDY CENTER
BROWN UNIVERSITY

INTRODUCTION

In this chapter, stress is used to refer to the introduction, imposition, or intrusion of a perturbation of a kind that usually results in the organism taking some kind of corrective or stabilizing action which then serves to eliminate or reduce the intensity of the perturbation. Such actions, of which there is a great diversity, may be termed coping behaviors or tactics. The available repertoire of coping behaviors depends upon many factors: the species of the organism, developmental maturity, the learning experiences by which the organism has diversified or become constrained in its strategies, and various intercurrent events. In brief, a stress is a perturbing event; the specific reaction to the stress mediated by an organismic response is coping; and the termination of the stress marks the success of the coping process.

This essentially Cannonian view (1925) of stress and coping is too simple, of course, but it suffices as a model for approaching an understanding of much of infant behavior. In actuality, multiple perturbations often occur simultaneously and the rules by which infants respond are confounded by the relative intensities of the multiple perturbations and the comparative strengths of the available responses.

What has just been said refers principally, of course, to perturbations of the organism which are essentially noxious, disturbing, or unsettling. This account honors the hedonic basis of perturbation, but acknowledges only the sort of perturbation which we would regard as annoying. However, not all perturbations are exclusively aversive. On the one hand, some pleasant stimulus conditions may be so overwhelming as to have negative overtones or consequences. On the other hand, perturbations imposed by stressful events are often offset by the pleasures of sensation which typically accompany successful coping with noxious stresses. Some pleasures of sensation indeed require for their occurrence the prior presence of negative perturbation, as in the anxiety that precedes a successful mountain climb or debate. The infant's satisfaction that accompanies feeding when hungry is an example of this sort. The rewarding experience of the baby's successful struggle to free its respiratory passages for breathing when threatened with occlusion is another. Pleasure and annoyance are twin issues of the overarching hedonic cloak that envelops most of the infant's response systems, and they virtually dictate that ambivalence (or approach-avoidance conflict) will shadow practically all of the infant's behavior.

More will be said later about the hedonic character of infancy. Suffice it to note now that learning processes, perhaps particularly those that occur early (and, we think, lastingly) in infancy, are heavily dependent upon the pleasures of sensation that generally accompany successful coping behaviors. In learning-theory parlance, these pleasures are called reinforcing events. Although the specific conceptualization of the response-reinforcement sequence and the learning process that ensues therefrom is that of Thorndike (1911), the principle is not unfriendly to the supposition of how response accretion occurs in human development as espoused by Freud, Piaget, Erikson, or Skinner: Those responses that are followed by a satisfying state of affairs for the behaving organism will tend to be repeated in the future when a similar occasion presents itself, and those that are followed by unsatisfying or hurtful consequences will tend later to be avoided.

An appreciation of the reinforcing or hedonic consequences of effective coping behavior goes a long way toward understanding the role of stress in development, and understanding particularly the ontogeny of coping strategies under stressful circumstances in the first year of life.

STRESS IN DEVELOPMENT DURING THE FIRST YEAR

There is much that occurs in the normal life of the newborn, and in the child developing throughout the first year, that is quite patently stressful.

The human signal of distress is the response of crying, an adaptive mechanism that has the typical function and consequence of attracting attention, aid, solace, and the technical expertise of nearby persons who are adept in diminishing the aversive conditions that instigated the cry. Crying is one of the first mechanisms that the infant has in its repertoire of responses, initially as a gift of the species, for coping with distress. Like many of the newborn's coping mechanisms, the cry is also a rudimentary, biologically rooted social behavior in that the infant enlists through this tactic the reciprocating coping behaviors of other persons. Other infantile defensive responses instigated by adverse stimulation, which often provoke caretaker response, particularly during feeding, include respiratory occlusion reflexes. The nature of these response patterns bears a closer look, particularly in the context of other aspects of biological development which evoke concern and fascination from responsible adults centering their attention upon the child.

Neonatal behavior and subsequent development

The human baby doubles in weight during the first three months of postnatal life and triples within the first year. From birth to six months of age, babies increase in weight about two grams every 24 hours. From six months to three years, the daily increase averages about .35 grams, and from three to six years about .15 grams per day. Growth rate is thus faster in the first six months of life than it will ever again be, but already it is slowing down. Scholars concerned with the morphology of infancy and with the nutritional implementation of growth and sustenance (e.g., Dobbing, 1974; Dobbing & Sands, 1979) have conjectured, with good empirical support, that this is, if not a critical period of development, a *vulnerable* period in which failures of nutritional inputs can produce marked deficits of growth and development. Some of these may be of long duration, and perhaps even have cross-generational influences.

The behavioral advances in infancy are equally astounding. From birth to one year of age, the infant emerges from a condition of largely subcortical functioning to one of cortical behavioral mediation (McGraw, 1943); from a responsive but unthoughtful being to a contemplative, wary, striving person with a special yearning to be in physical, visual, and auditory contact with certain specific people (Ainsworth, 1973). Not surprisingly, the persons specially selected for this privilege are those who have been most frequently attentive, and most concerned with the delivery of pleasure and the cessation of pain. Such special persons will be rewarded with the smile of the baby by about two months of age. This psychological achievement is clearly under the control of specific stimulation and cortical mediation, although the facial musculature has been capable since birth of executing the smile maneuver.

Clear recognition of specific other persons, and discriminative responses to them, are apparent by six months of age, with obvious attachment to the most evident caretakers by about eight months. The first step, the eventual utterance of meaningful sounds, and the capacity of the child to engage in reciprocating exchanges by the end of the first year, are all, of course, exceptionally rewarding events for the infant's caretakers. The pleasures and annoyances of the caretakers themselves, moreover, are instrumental in generating, promoting, sustaining, and reinforcing the infant's own burgeoning behavioral repertoire (Emde, Gaensbauer, & Harmon, 1976; Lipsitt & Werner, 1981).

That most people do not remember the first year of life does not obviate the effectiveness of early experiences in setting the stage for later aspects of development. The human infant is capable of only minimal reflection on the past and future, and in this respect has much in common with lower animals. Infants do not guffaw reflectively (they have no sense of humor) and, although they cry, they do not weep. Contemplating one's destiny and understanding one's personal history are characteristics only of cognitive organisms. Humans do not seem capable of such activities requiring long-term memory and long-term anticipation until (1) they have experienced simpler events requiring the association of stimuli with responses, and responses with response-consequents, both of these processes involving short-term memory of stimulus events, and until (2) a significant shift of brain function from subcortical to cortical mediation has taken place.

Interestingly, and perhaps importantly, these two maturational processes move rapidly and together in the first year of life. It is not an absurd hypothesis that the rudimentary short-term associative experiences must occur for optimal development, just when (in the first year) dendrite proliferation and myelination are, like the rest of the infant's body, in their peak growth periods. Under this supposition, infancy may be regarded as a period of instigation and rehearsal of later cognitive and emotional functioning. Infantile attachment behavior may be considered, in this view, as a mechanism for coping with the cessation of caretaking attentions, the threat of abandonment, and the loss of (by now) needed social stimulation. As such, rudimentary attachment processes are rehearsals of adaptive behaviors to be deployed defensively in the future against stressful occurrences.

Attachment Behavior as Stress Reduction

Attachment processes have biological roots (Bowlby, 1969), probably antedating the history of mankind. Attachment or bonding may be regarded as part of the evolutionary history that prepares human infants for defense against hostile interpersonal encounters long before they will be in need of such talent, and before they will be motorically capable of capitalizing upon their early-acquired appreciation of the need for self-defense. Says Bowlby (1969): "We may conclude . . . that . . . the way in which attachment behavior develops in the human infant and becomes focused on a discriminated figure is sufficiently like the way in which it develops in other mammals, and in birds, for it to be included legitimately, under the heading of imprinting—so long as that term is used in its current generic sense" (p. 223).

Infancy can be seen in this respect to be a period of rehearsal or practice for later defense against noxious stimulation and territorial intrusion. Attachment behavior bears a similarity in this regard with the much earlier manifested startle-response to loud sounds, and head-shaking or hand-face activity in response to respiratory threats. This characterization of infancy as survival training suggests a psychobiological basis for the presence very early in development, even in the neonatal period, of other effective systems of self-defense, such as are manifest in infantile responses to gravity loss, pressure on the palms, and rustling noises. While all of these stimulating events elicit explicitly defense-related behaviors (the Moro reflex, the Babkin reflex, and vigorous arousal, respectively), other aspects of the response repertoire commonly conceived as appetitive (or approach as opposed to avoidance) systems can be characterized as defense processes. Even the rooting reflex and the smile can be seen as positive components of a larger hedonic network biologically adapted to enhance the probability of proximity with protective adults. Whatever the larger conceptualization, stress seems a salient instigator of the complete sequence of events. Moreover, contrary to a simple picture of homeostasis-seeking in the human infant, the psychobiologically adaptive experience often appears to be one in which the organism practices *departures* from a steady-state into various conditions of threat and arousal. The familiar infant games of pat-a-cake and peek-a-boo may be seen, in this view, as promoting disequilibrium, and increasing tension and stress—with, of course, an eventual behavioral and emotional resolution. Not surprisingly, these games are typically accepted by infants, like tickling in adults, only if played with familiar attachment figures.

The interplay of emotional and cognitive development in the formation of infantile attachment has been explicated by Bowlby (1969) in terms of three critical stages; he believes these to be crucial as precursors of the adult affectional system. These parts of the attachment cycle, which will ultimately lead to a cementing of attachment and love only when an adequate stage of cognitive reflection is reached at about three years of age, take place long before the child is able to remember. During the first period, at around two to three months, nondiscriminative social responsiveness will be acquired. The baby recognizes persons as persons, i.e., can distinguish them from inanimate objects. In the second phase, between the ages of two and six months, infants continue to manifest a special interest in other humans, but now discriminate among diverse familiar figures, responding differently, for example, to mother than to father or to siblings. The third phase of the cycle accompanies the advent of a neuromuscular capacity for reaching out, or for using distance receptors to seek proximity. With the achievement of the third phase, the baby acquires instrumentality with respect to the instigation and sustaining of the pleasures of interpersonal (as opposed to autistic) contact. This period coincides with Piaget's characterization of the infant as having a conception of object permanence. The ontogenetic basis for such behavior must surely depend upon repetitive experiences, on previous disappointments following anticipations of expected events, and on the pleasures associated (as in the peek-a-boo game) with the requiting of the child's intentions and bids for accustomed events to occur again.

Nonetheless, it is not, according to Bowlby, until the child is about three years of age that the fourth and essentially final stage of early attachment is reached when the child really understands and can reflect on the true nature of his or her relationships with attachment figures. At this point, the child understands that the mother has goals in her interactions with the child, revealed in her anticipations, her promises, and her regrets when expectations are not fulfilled. The child, in turn, adjusts his or her behavior accordingly, to maximize the pleasures derived from executing the mother's wishes. Alas, the child also can, by now, gain some pleasure from thwarting the mother's diminution of his or her autonomy.

The ontogeny of attachment is a *stressful* process, involving a perpetual tug between the infant's egoistic claims on the environment and the burgeoning insistence of the caretakers on the reciprocities of the infant. We are more accustomed to thinking of the *Sturm und Drang* of adolescence, not of infancy, in these terms.

THE HEDONIC INFANT

In this section, some salient aspects of sucking behavior and avoidance responses in the human infant will be considered as adjustive responses to endogenous and exogenous perturbations. Patterns of sucking behavior appear to be under control of factors relating to the condition of the organism, such as whether the infant was premature, asphyxiated at birth, or malnourished. On the other hand, incentive-motivational environmental variables, such as the quality and quantity of fluid delivered into the infant's mouth contingent upon its own rate of sucking or the strength of its suck, also are relevant.

The human newborn carries on a transaction with the environment, right from the start, involving behavioral self-regulation of caloric intake and of the pleasures of sensation. In fact, a case may be made that this begins in utero, as the fetus is known to ingest as much as 500 ml of amniotic fluid per day toward the end of gestation (Bradley & Mistretta, 1973; Mistretta & Bradley, 1977). This reciprocating interaction between infant and environment (or infant and caretaking conditions) manifests itself early and develops; this is to say that the character of the interaction accrues, or undergoes alterations (some of them of a learned nature), dependent upon the association between the responses and the response-consequents. More will be said of this subsequently. For now it need only be added that what holds for appetitive behavior holds, as well, for aversive responding. Those responses, followed by unsatisfying or annoying conditions, elicit objection and escape, and they tend not to be repeated. Pleasantness and unpleasantness of response-consequents will, in this view, affect the perpetuation or cessation of behavior. These response-consequents, as determinants of behavior, are as critical for understanding the flow of behavior as are the instigators that elicited the behavior in the first place. The newborn infant will suck upon practically any object placed in its mouth, but the facility with which it attains a pressure seal around the nipple, the delight with which the sucking will continue, and the perpetuation of the instigated behavior will depend, to an extent, upon the context within which all of these take place. For example, if the infant receives a bitter substance in response to its suck, or if respiratory occlusion accompanies the latching on to the nipple, then, it should be apparent, the sucking behavior will be interrupted or aborted entirely. The infant sometimes expresses its discontent quite profoundly, and to the great consternation of its mother who (sometimes) is fretful that her infant dislikes her. The hedonic features of the infant's behavior, and the signal value that these have for those caring for the infant, can be of great importance in eliciting immediate response from caretakers, as well as in producing more prolonged affective reactions.

Theoretical Considerations

The hedonic aspects of the infant's demeanor were of great interest to Darwin (1877). He was captivated by the intrinsic fascination of his son's face, particularly the child's hedonically mediated changes in facial expression. He made copious notes of his observations and eventually proposed that there is evolutionary significance to these physiognomic features of development. Thus, as Lipsitt and Werner (1981) have noted, the study of "hedonics" in infancy has an honorable tradition dating at least to the mid-nineteenth century. Similarly, in his attributions of psychosexuality to infants, Freud (1927) supposed that movement through the various stages involved progressive shifts in the anatomical loci of pleasure reception. The perioral region, in this view, is the earliest bodily area through which the infant presumably receives its greatest comfort and delight, and this region gradually yields to others as normal psychosexual maturation ensues. The "pleasure principle," which Freud postulated as the impetus for and perpetuation of behavior, would yield eventually to the "reality principle," as the infant learns through the imposition of social controls and differentiable contexts that sometimes the pleasures of sensation are denied or postponed. The environmental thwarting of behaviors which are biologically based in, or driven by, the infant's quest for pleasures of sensation is itself, of course, a perturbation to which the coping tactics of the infant must be addressed. The annoyance occasioned by the frustration entailed in reward denial or postponement is also a perturbation which calls forth a variety of coping maneuvers, some of them perhaps more successful than others, but all of them adjustments to a series of stressful circumstances (e.g., crying, screaming, regurgitation, head-banging, and the like). An important point in this regard is that perturbation in the midst of psychobiological needs characteristically activates a succession of adaptive mechanisms. Some of these may be requited by allaying the noxious perturbation and causing cessation of the condition of deprivation that set off the cycle of events in the first place.

Perturbation, its consequences, and its adaptive significance have been dealt with in the context of such diverse and divergent theoretical orientations that one might suppose it virtually impossible to construct a promising theory of human development without an acknowledgment of a role for hedonic factors. Although Piaget's theory (1932, 1952) could not be easily characterized as a reinforcement or incentive-motivational theory, Piaget (1952) did not overlook the child's pleasure of successful experiences in his search for the conditions that perpetuate searching and problem-solving behavior. Some of Piaget's more apt descriptions of the changing panorama of behavior with successive experience relate to the surprise and glee which infants in the sensorimotor period manifest when they eventually find a hidden object, or when they finally grab at a pendulum at just the propitious moment to enable its grasp. The perturbation created by the presence of an object just out of reach or a suddenly receding item in the visual field impels—in the child that can appreciate the frustration or loss—search and discovery activity clearly directed toward diminishing the perturbation or stress. Indeed, Piaget's theory supposes that increasing age (or cognitive maturation) involves enhanced appreciation of differences between how things are and how they might be. Cognitively generated perturbations proliferate with increasing age and with greater understanding of less complicated features of the natural environment.

Perturbation, and its resolution, has a place also in theories about the development of attention, particularly visual attention (e.g., Kagan, 1970; Uzgiris & Hunt, 1970), where the burden is to predict and understand what adjustive processes will occur (visual fixation, vocalization, quieting, thrashing, or smiling) and to what features of the stimulus events they will occur. Studies of the deployment of attention by infants to a continuum of visual stimuli differing from a familiarized stimulus often result in an inverted-U function, indicating that greater visual attention is invested in (or the infant is most fascinated with) stimuli of intermediate distinctiveness relative to the familiarization stimulus, with neither very similar nor very different stimuli attracting as much attention. It can be presumed that the stimuli which attract greater attention are those which are moderately dissonant and thus perturbing with respect to the familiarization stimulus. As Kagan (1970) put it: "events . . . moderately discrepant from established schemata, and that activated hypotheses in the service of assimilation had the greatest power to recruit and maintain attention in the young child." Activating hypotheses in the service of assimilation must surely be preceded by cognitive unrest or perturbation. These in turn impel coping processes that may dispel the apparent dissonance. The pleasures inherent in the diminution of dissonance imposed by discrepant experiences are, of course, obvious in persons of all ages.

Even in Watsonian behaviorism, the hedonic basis of behavioral change during development is assumed. Life begins with three major response mechanisms or unconditioned patterns of behavior, each of them having affective concomitants: fear, rage, and love (Watson, 1928). In this view, any neutral stimuli which are paired sufficiently often with any of the three congenital responses will themselves acquire the capacity to evoke the relevant response-pattern, e.g., outraged crying or a satisfied appearance of quietude. The monolithic adoption of the classical conditioning model of Pavlov apparently was honored more in theory than in practice by Watson. His major demonstrations of learning, including that of Albert (Watson & Rayner, 1920), who was conditioned to fear furry objects through use of a loud noise which initially called forth crying and other fear-induced behavior, were in actuality instances of paradigms later to be characterized as operant learning (Church, 1972). Nonetheless, the reliance on the hedonic features of infant behavior and learning processes is what is important here, and there is no question about the pertinence in this work of Thorndike's (1913) pronouncement that those behaviors followed by satisfying states of affairs will tend to be repeated in the future, whereas those followed by unsatisfying states would not. During the early history of behaviorism, paradoxically, there was little research activity investigating the hedonic processes per se that presumably facilitated the cumulative effects of experience. There was enough carried out principally by Young (1936), however, to keep the hedonic vocabulary current, and to supply a modicum of reputable evidential support for the "satisfying affairs" required by Thorndike's dictum.

Sucking Behavior Controlled by the Pleasures of Sensation

The "pleasures of sensation," to borrow Pfaffmann's (1960) phrase, are the building blocks of Thorndike's "satisfying states of affairs." What we call incentives for perpetuating instrumental behavior, and for determining the style of that behavior once it has begun, are essentially opportunities for experiencing the pleasures of sensation. This is apparent even in the human newborn. Research on the effects of the sweet taste on infants' sucking behavior and associated autonomic nervous system functions provides the opportunity to explore the mechanisms through which pleasures of sensation serve to reduce psychobiological perturbations (i.e., provide pacification in the presence of threats or stress). Such research also illuminates the processes by which certain response-contingent events may come to act as reinforcers for learning.

Numerous recent studies have led to the inexorable conclusion that human infants are keenly sensitive, shortly after birth, to small changes in gustatory stimulation, and that profound preferences exist in the normal newborn for sweeter fluids (Crook, 1979; Lipsitt, 1976, 1977; Steiner, 1979). The human newborn is capable of acting on its differentiations among taste substances, and may engage in appropriate behaviors to either terminate or perpetuate the taste. This is done through modulation of sucking behaviors. The human newborn effectively controls, through behavioral self-regulation, the gustatory and caloric substances that are visited upon the tongue and stomach—up to a point. The oral-ingestive system, and the behavioral regulatory mechanisms which are such an important feature of it, is dependent, to a large extent, upon hedonic mediation in carrying out its basic functions, which are to reduce the stress of hunger and assure the assimilation of nutritious substances. The autonomic accompaniments of pleasant and unpleasant stimulation, such as are indexed by heart-rate changes, represent some of the earliest responses of infants to stress and stress reduction. The hedonic mediation of infantile behavior is perhaps never clearer than when an infant quickly grows quiet, after a period of distressed crying, when it is lifted, rocked, or offered sweet fluid. On the other hand, heart-rate increases may follow when a sweeter (more savory) substance is introduced into the infant's mouth, and even in the presence of the slower sucking rates which sweeter fluids promote. A large number of studies yielding such findings as these has been conducted by the author and his students and colleagues (see references).

In our neonatal laboratory at Women and Infants Hospital of Rhode Island, babies are placed in a special crib in which various psychomotor and autonomic responses can be recorded under diverse conditions of stimulation. Breathing is monitored by an infant pneumobelt around the abdomen, and electrodes are placed on the chest and on one leg. These sensing units permit the polygraphic monitoring of the primary electrocardiogram and respiration. A cardiotachometer provides a momentary reading of heart rate which is recorded on one of the polygraph channels. Another channel is used for recording sucking behavior, which is accomplished by means of a specially constructed device consisting of a stainless steel housing with a pressure transducer, over which a commercial nipple is pulled. Polyethylene tubes run into the nipple from pump sources which deliver fluids which can be selected at any time from three different wells simply by means of a switch. The drops of fluid which the infant receives, however, are on demand of the subject. When the baby engages in a criterion suck, which requires a preset sucking amplitude, a small drop of fluid (usually .02 ml) is delivered by the pump from the appropriate well and into the baby's mouth. Very small amounts of fluid are delivered to the baby, in order to minimize the cumulative effects of ingestion and to maximize the control of the infant's behavior by the sweetness, or incentive value, of the fluid received.

The infant may receive no fluid for sucking, or might receive a fluid such as plain distilled water, or 5% or 15% sucrose. A polygraph event marker records delivery of each fluid drop, or of each criterion suck during no-fluid conditions.

As our studies reveal, normal newborns typically suck in bursts of response separated by rests. The parameters of burst length and rest length constitute individual difference variables which are of interest in and of themselves, especially because they are subject to variations due to perinatal risk factors. These two response characteristics (burst length and interburst interval) are joined by other parameters—such as the sucking rate within bursts and number of sucks per larger unit time—in being significantly influenced by the fluids received by the baby, contingent upon its own behavior. If the infant is switched from a no-fluid condition to water, or from a 5% sucrose solution to a sweeter solution, several behavioral consequences typically ensue. Sucking bursts characteristically become longer. The interburst intervals tend to become shorter, and intersuck intervals become larger. Because sucking rate within bursts slows down with the increasing sweetness of the fluid, and simultaneously with the infant taking fewer and shorter rest periods, more responses are typically emitted over a two-minute period for the sweeter, or hedonically more positive, fluids. These effects are often compromised in high-risk infants. The greater the severity of risk requiring intensive care, the less avid will be the infant's sucking behavior generally, and the less will be the effect of an incentive shift, such as from 5% to 15% sucrose (Cowett, Lipsitt, & Vohr, 1978).

We have investigated the interrelationships among these various sucking-response parameters and the effects of different incentive conditions not only on the sucking behavior, but on heart rate as well. Moreover, we have been able to document the effects of brief experiences that the infant has had with one fluid condition upon sucking behavior to a subsequent, differently tasting substance.

To study the effects of previous experience on subsequent sucking behavior, five groups of newborns were treated differentially with respect to the successive experiences that they had in sucking upon the automatic nipple (Kobre & Lipsitt, 1972). These infants, all of them three days old, received one of five reinforcement regimens for the 20-minute period, after passing a screening test that resulted in rejecting those few infants for this study who had a mean sucking rate lower than 30 sucks per minute during the initial 2-minute testing period. A total of 20 minutes of responding was recorded for each subject, in four successive 5-minute periods. One group received only sucrose, a second group received water throughout, and a third received sucrose and water, alternated twice, in 5-minute units. A fourth group received no fluid throughout the four 5-minute periods and was compared with the group that received sucrose alternated with no fluid. Between each period, the nipple was removed for one minute to allow the tube to be flushed with water and the child to be picked up.

Comparison of the first three groups revealed that sucking rate within bursts slows down for a fluid-sucking condition relative to a no-fluid-sucking condition, and that sucking rate within bursts is slower still for sweet-fluid sucking, relative to sucking for plain water. There is an orderly progression, then, from no fluid to plain water to 15% sucrose sucking, with the sucking response becoming slower as the sweetness of the fluid increases. Moreover, under the sucrose condition, infants invest a larger number of sucks during a comparable period of time than under either the water or no-fluid condition. This effect, a consequence of the infants taking fewer rest periods under the sweet-fluid condition, also occurred in the comparison of the water with the no-fluid condition.

Infants sucking for sucrose throughout the 20-minute period produced more sucks than the groups receiving water throughout. Both groups, moreover, had stable response rates for their respective fluids throughout the four 5-minute blocks. All of the foregoing effects lead to consideration now of the most interesting finding, which concerned subjects who were alternated from one 5-minute period to another between sucrose and water, or between sucrose and no fluid. These groups showed marked effects attributable to the alternating experience. When sucking for sucrose, for example, the group which received sucrose and water in alternating periods was comparable to that group which sucked only for sucrose throughout the 20-minute period. When the alternating sucrose and water group was switched to water, however, response rate during each of those 5-minute water periods was reliably less than in the counterpart controls in the water-throughout group. It must therefore be concluded that when newborns have experience in sucking for sucrose, an immediately subsequent experience with water "shuts them off." Infants, under these conditions, displayed their apparent aversion for the water by markedly reducing the instrumental sucking behavior that would put that fluid in their mouths. When they were switched from water to sucrose, response rate went back to the normative level.

Infants thus optimize their taste experiences by modulating oral behavior that determines the rate at which drops of fluid enter their mouths. This type of effect occurred also in the group that was alternated between sucrose and no fluid; the alternated group showed lower response rates when sucking for no fluid after experience in sucking for sucrose. Such negative contrast effects suggest that incentive conditions control immediate response rates, but that also the pleasures of sensation have effects, as well, upon subsequent occasions in which the same response is paired with other incentive conditions. The negative contrast effect demonstrated here must be one of the most rudimentary sorts of behavioral control due to prior experiential circumstances. Previous studies of habituation in the newborn have suggested (e.g., Engen & Lipsitt, 1965) that infants subjected to a regimen of successive presentations of a stimulus may habituate to that stimulus and show recovery of response to a novel or dishabituation stimulus. The suggestion from such studies is that memory processes are already working in the newborn such that there is a lasting impression made, admittedly of unknown duration, of the experience endured. The negative contrast effects obtained here with respect to sucking behavior support that at least short-lived memory mechanisms are present. Thus any adaptations or adjustments that the infant may adopt for coping with stress have the potential for transferring to subsequent periods of time in which the previous experience can have an effect upon subsequent responding.

Thus far we have concentrated on the changes which occur in neonatal sucking behavior dependent upon the incentive conditions available, such as the sweetness of fluid which the infant's sucking behavior is instrumental in obtaining. A succession of studies from this laboratory has demonstrated that when infants suck for sweeter fluid their response rates within bursts of sucking slow down as if to facilitate savoring of the sweet fluid (Lipsitt & Werner, 1981). Additional data, now involving the heart-rate response, further substantiate our supposition that a hedonic or savoring mechanism is operative in the earliest days of life. An interesting interplay occurs between sucking behavior and heart rate. With increases in sweetness of the fluid, and even as sucking rate within bursts diminishes as is typical for sweeter fluids, heart rate increases. This is so even in the first burst after the switch to the sweeter fluid. The heart-rate enhancement takes place within only a few sucks, thus obviating the conclusion that the higher heart rate results from the increased number of sucks per burst which is also characteristic of the sweet-fluid conditions. Crook and Lipsitt (1976) showed that the enhanced heart-rate effect under sweet-sucking conditions occurs even when the length of sucking burst is controlled statistically, and when heart rates are measured only during actual sucking and not during interburst intervals. Detailed analyses by Crook and Lipsitt of the synchronously varying heart rate and sucking were made possible by tape recording each interbeat interval and each intersuck interval for subsequent computer processing.

An alternative interpretation of the increased heart rate during sucrose sucking, relative to water sucking, is that there is greater energy expenditure during the high-incentive condition. In this view, higher heart rates are secondary to this energizing phenomenon, a supposition compatible with the observation that when sucking under the high-incentive conditions, more sucks are emitted and fewer rest periods occur even though within-burst sucking is slower. However, the appropriate study has been conducted to rule out the possibility that the higher heart rates under the sweeter fluid conditions are artifacts of increased sucking amplitudes. The enhanced heart rate is almost always seen within a few sucks of the switch from no fluid to sucrose, or from water to sucrose. Within a few seconds, or a few sucks, the effect of the sweet taste on the tongue is reflected in a higher heart rate. The possibility that the heart rate effect is an artifact of differential sucking amplitudes has, through this observation and by statistical controls, been ruled out (Ashmead, Reilly, & Lipsitt, 1980).

Finally, Crook (1976) has studied the effects of the quantity of the response-contingent fluid upon sucking rhythm and heart rate, complementing the extensive findings now available on sweetness. Temporal organization of neonatal nutritive sucking and heart rate were studied in consecutive periods to analyze the effects of two quantities of response-contingent fluids. Crook found that cumulative pausing time and intersuck intervals are affected by the amount of fluid delivered for each sucking response, just as with sweetness variations. Heart rate accelerates quickly to a stable level at the start of sucking bursts, and within-burst heart rates are higher with the larger drops of fluid (.03 ml per suck versus .01 ml). Sweetness and amount of fluid thus operate in comparable ways. They are collapsible incentive-motivational variables. It is not unreasonable to suppose that in these situations it is the "pleasures of sensation" (Pfaffmann, 1960) that control important features of the newborn's motor and autonomic responses. If coping behavior is regarded as responses to perturbative conditions of sensory stimulation, then it is apparent that the human infant in the first days of life has the capacity to modulate its behavior to accommodate to stressful conditions.

Aversive Responses in the Infant

Aversive or avoidance behavior is also noted within the first few days of life, even in the first few minutes when the baby expresses itself with a loud cry. Defensive and angry behaviors of this sort unquestionably have adaptive significance and may be considered as psychobiological adjustments to stress.

Newborn infants have well-organized constellations of defensive behaviors that are readily elicited in response to aversive stimulation. When such noxious intrusions become quite intolerable, the baby moves into a very vigorous mode of objection which can be best described as an angry pattern of behavior involving crying. Aversive behavior occurs in human infants under conditions in which biological threat or stress exists. In its milder forms, such behavior is manifested in the autonomic and withdrawal responses to moderately intense stimulation, such as bright lights; annoyances of touch, such as pin-pricks; unpleasant odorants and tastes; and loud noises. The amount of response to such stimulation is directly proportional to the intensity of the stimulus. The type of response pattern which occurs to specific stimuli reveals the biological adaptiveness of the young nervous system, in that the responses are often instrumental in helping to divert threats to the infant's safety. A sudden increase in illumination near the infant's open eyes, for example, causes the lids to close. If the skin surface is touched with great pressure, or is pricked with a pin, the infant withdraws the offended part of its anatomy from the stimulus. If a noxious trigeminal stimulant, such as ammonia, is presented near the nostrils, the baby turns its head from the locus of stimulation, and signals through vocalization and facial expressions of annoyance that the experience is disturbing. If the tongue is stimulated with a bitter taste, withdrawal of the tongue occurs and the lips purse and remain tightly closed. The different facial expressions of the newborn in response to differential hedonic stimulation have been described in detail by Steiner (1979), who has found species-specific patterns for human infants, and who has documented that these facial expressions tend to remain even in infants who have suffered severe neurological damage or cranio-facial anomalies. Each of the sensory modalities, it seems, can be excessively stimulated to produce its own aversive style of response, usually culminating in crying when less vigorous aversive responses fail to enable escape from the noxious condition.

Threats to the blockage of the infant's respiratory passages elicit particularly vigorous responses from the normal newborn. The response to the threat of respiratory occlusion has been incorporated as a test item in both the Graham (1956) and Brazelton (1973) neonatal behavior scales, and is assessed by placing a gauze pad or a piece of cellophane for a brief time over the infant's face. The response tested is apparently to the threat of respiratory occlusion rather than actual oxygen deprivation, for the typical pattern of coping behavior exercised by the normal newborn occurs even when the mouth or nose is left free for air exchange. Stimulation that threatens or supports respiratory occlusion produces a response pattern consisting of five components. These are executed in such an orderly fashion as to suggest that they constitute a fixed action pattern that begins with milder responses and proceeds toward extreme arousal if the initiating stimulus situation is not reduced by earlier modes of coping, in the serial progression of response adaptation (Lipsitt, 1979). The five components of the behavior pattern are, in the usual order expressed: (1) side-to-side head waving, (2) head withdrawal, with backward jerks and grimacing, (3) facial vasodilation, (4) arm jabbing directed toward the face area, and (5) crying. The continuum of response involves escalating vigor. The pattern is interrupted when the noxious or threatening stimulation is reduced or removed.

The angry behavior just described can occur in the natural course of infant feeding. When anger in the newborn results from respiratory occlusion during feeding, the action pattern results, and becomes effective in freeing the respiratory passages by displacing the offending object, or by impelling the mother to adjust her feeding style. Such reciprocating behavior on the part of the mother might involve manipulation of her breast to free the infant's nostrils, or holding her infant differently. British pediatrician Mavis Gunther (1955, 1961) reported on her own careful observations of the ways in which the nursing mother and her infant reciprocate one another's behavior, even immediately after birth, and, quite possibly, with lasting effects. When suckling at the breast, according to Gunther, the baby's nostrils periodically and fortuitously become occluded. This generates aversive reactions from the infant, who begins to withdraw from the nipple and breast, and might be returned to it only with great difficulty, especially after a bout of prolonged occlusion. Because the newborn ordinarily sucks by creating a secure pressure seal between its lips and the nipple, unlatching from the breast is not accomplished easily, especially by a hungry infant. Moreover, mere brief intervals of respiratory occlusion elicit only minor coping strategies as opposed to the vigorous objections which are called forth by prolonged threats. The baby first engages in minor head movements, swaying the head from side to side and pulling the head backwards. If these actions succeed in freeing the nasal passages for breathing, the progression of the behavior pattern is aborted. If these minor maneuvers do not succeed, however, the normal infant may execute more vigorous patterns of behavior, such as arm waving, pushing against the mother's breast, and crying, all of this accompanied by increasing facial vasodilation. If none of these coping strategies succeeds in wresting the infant free of the offending object, the fail-safe crying response occurs, thrusting the nipple from the mouth and freeing the respiratory passages for air exchange.

The interactions and adaptations just described suggest that components of the action patterns of newborns may be selectively reinforced, resulting in these behaviors becoming learned and perpetuated through periodic practice, with reinforcement renewed on subsequent occasions. Thus, under some circumstances, the baby might be reinforced for retreating from the breast rather than remaining at it. Gunther has described some instances in which the infant was clearly reluctant when put to the breast after a single apparently aversive experience. Although she does not render the sequence of activities described in these terms, it seems clear that the setting conditions, the behavior of the baby in that setting, and the subsequent aversion to the feeding situation can be understood as operant learning. When the response of uncoupling from the breast is reinforced by a satisfying state of affairs (freedom from occlusion or the threat of it), the baby will adaptively decline that position, or otherwise resist it, when put to the breast again. The negative consequences of being at the breast now override the positive features which, at the outset, were strong.

More will be said in the next section concerning the possible long-term consequences of this sort of reciprocating interaction, or mutual coping behavior, of the mother and infant. For now it needs only to be added that the type of behavior described, involving aversion on the part of the infant to threats to its respiration, can occur also in the bottle-feeding situation. The newborn's lips are thick and close to the nostrils; some commercial nipples are especially constructed with a shield that can produce the same kind of threats to respiration as were described for breast-feeding babies.

CRISES AS FAILURES OF THE HEDONIC SYSTEM

In this section, we consider the possibility that some aberrations of development in the first year of life, even those that may have life-threatening implications, might result from failures of the hedonic system to reinforce adaptive behavior adequately. Behavior which is adaptive is taken here, as at the outset of this chapter, to mean those action patterns or maneuvers of the organism which tend to reduce stress or annoying perturbations and maximize the pleasures of sensation. When a normal infant is respiratorily occluded, for example, the adaptive maneuver is (for the baby or the mother) to shift or move in such a way as to reduce the irritant and gain safe space for air exchange.

Learning Processes Based upon Hedonic Adjustments

One may note, first, that hedonic mediation enables learning to occur, by rewarding adaptive or corrective behavior. Those behaviors are perpetuated which are followed by satisfying states of affairs. It has also been observed, almost routinely in neonatal intensive care units, but also in a systematic way in studies of sucking avidity in high-risk newborns (see, e.g., Cowett, Lipsitt, Vohr, & Oh, 1978), that in the premature child the greater the severity of perinatal risk, the less affected is the infant—at 40 weeks conceptional age—by differences in the incentive-motivational or rewarding properties (sweetness) of the fluid for which the infant sucks. While much too little is known of the possible developmental consequences of such behavioral limitations, the inference seems justified that the typical lags found in early development of premature and other high-risk infants (see, e.g., Field, Sostek, Goldberg, & Shuman, 1979; Sameroff, 1978), are due, at least in part, to the impediments to learning occasioned by failures of the hedonic system. It is quite plausible that the behavioral lethargy of some infants can be attributed to an accumulation of adverse conditions, including both congenital and experiential hazards. The absence or reduced strength of basic unconditioned responses or reflexes automatically places the child's learning processes at risk, for there must be suitable responses in the behavioral repertoire for learning to occur, whether of the classical or operant variety. Any compromises in the capacity of the infant to adjust to stressful stimulation, or to take actions which perpetuate available incentive conditions, must almost certainly result in diminished learning potential. Indeed, failure to *experience* stress, and to be subjected to conditions in which behaviors will be executed which are differentially rewarding, would seem to constitute a learning hazard in itself. Such a state of affairs could come about because the organism (1) lacks the hedonic mediating mechanisms which inform and reinforce appropriate behavior, (2) has not been presented with challenges or perturbations from the reduction of which learning could occur, or (3) does not have in its response repertoire the appropriate motoric behaviors to enable the variety of actions from which some will be rewarded more than others. In all events, there is failure of the hedonic system to be effectively paired with patterns of behavior that reduce stress and enhance reward. Let us see how such failures might have implications for developmental hazards in the post-neonatal first year of life.

Crib Death: A Stress Hypothesis

About 8,000 babies each year in the United States alone die of a poorly defined condition known as sudden infant death syndrome (SIDS) or crib death. This number is in addition to those infants (about 14 in 1000 births) who succumb in the first few days of life due to quite well understood perinatal hazards such as birth asphyxia. The incidence of SIDS is 2 to 3 deaths per 1000 live births and most of these occur during the age period from two to five months after birth. The term SIDS is applied to the death when thorough investigation of the circumstances surrounding the death, usually including an autopsy, have led to no clear answer as to the cause of death. Paradoxically, the SIDS diagnosis is applied as a residual; it is a diagnosis of no-diagnosis. Several authoritative reviews and definitive analyses of the data concerning crib death and the hypotheses generated to explain the pathology of it (see, e.g., Valdes-Dapena, 1967, 1978) reveal the current failure to gain a scientific understanding of the phenomenon. Obscure anatomical and physiological factors might well be involved in the final pathway to crib death. Indeed some researchers (e.g., Anderson & Rosenblith, 1971; Carpenter & Emery, 1974; Lipsitt, 1976; Steinschneider, 1972; Swift & Emery, 1973) have found specific disposing characteristics (e.g., respiratory distress, apnea, or apparent inability of the infant to divert threats to its own respiratory passages) which might, in ways not yet well understood, jeopardize the infant's ability to defend itself with appropriate behavioral adjustments when respiratorily stressed.

Lipsitt, Sturner, and Burke (1979) began with the extensive perinatal and pediatric records of 15 crib death cases, then composed two control groups, one consisting of the very next births of the same sex and the other of the very next births of the same sex and race. The deceased group proved to vary from the controls in several ways, all of them in a direction connoting greater perinatal stress and biological hazard in that group. There were reliable differences in Apgar scores in the first few minutes of life. (The Apgar test is a quickly administered scale for assessing vital signs, such as adequacy of respiration, heart rate, pallor, and muscle tone.) The deceased group did more poorly than either control. Infants in the deceased group were identified significantly more often, moreover, as having respiratory anomalies. More of the deceased group had mothers with anemia during pregnancy. More had required intensive care than the controls. The deceased infants were hospitalized longer. The infants that ultimately died required more resuscitative measures during the neonatal period. Infants who succumbed were already showing, in general, that they were beginning life with some fragility or deficiency in coping with stress, perhaps particularly stresses relating to breathing. One might be tempted to conclude, in fact, that there are frank physiological deficiencies in these infants, and that the deaths can hardly be mysterious. However, these infants are babies who do survive the neonatal period and seem well at the time of their deaths. Moreover, many infants with the same or comparable symptoms and constellations of symptoms do not succumb. So many more survive who appear this way than do not makes prediction of which infants are truly in jeopardy, at least at the present state of knowledge, seem quite impossible. Only retrospective actuarial statistics reveal the seeming order in the characteristics of the SIDS cases. Any attempt to predict, on the basis of the epidemiological statistics currently available, would lead to an intolerably large number of false predictions.

The supposition has to be entertained that the disposing characteristics of infants who ultimately die of crib death may conspire with critical experiential conditions to cause some small number of the physiologically predisposed infants to become especially vulnerable. One line of research relating to this supposition has suggested that a basic learning disability may be implicated (Lipsitt, 1976, 1979). Noting that crib deaths usually occur within the 2- to 4-month age period, it may be observed that this is a critical time period during development, when many of the basic reflexes with which the baby is born are becoming transformed rapidly. Like the grasp reflex, many of the responses of the infant are very strong at birth but begin to weaken soon after. Turning the head to touches near the mouth, and other response patterns—including those that are involved in the so-called swimming reflex—change drastically within the 2- to 4-month age period. In her careful documentation of the ontogeny of reflexes in the first year of life, Myrtle McGraw (1943) showed that the "obligatory" character of these reflexes diminishes over the first six months, to be eventually superseded by a slower (more "voluntary") pattern of behavior seemingly in synchrony with the maturation of cortical tissue (myelination and dendrite proliferation) and function. Of great interest from the point of view espoused here, that there may be implications for crib death in this transition, is the fact that McGraw documented a particular kind of transitional behavior for practically every reflex studied, and she regarded that transitional period, between the reflexive and the voluntary, as decidedly stressful. She referred to these transitional phases as characterized by "disorganized behavior" and "struggling activity" (McGraw, 1943, pp. 34–36).

Of additional interest is the fact that the disorganized transitional period to which McGraw drew attention tended to occur, for most response systems, at around 100–150 days of age, just the age period in which infants are most at risk for crib death. Although McGraw was not concerned with crib death in her studies, the inference might be drawn (to promote further study) that there is a link between the two phenomena. The relevance of the link might occur in the following ways. First, the respiratory occlusion reflex which was detailed earlier in this chapter has a course like those that McGraw described, beginning as a reflex found in the repertoire of normal newborns. There are, of course, individual differences in its elicitability and strength, with some expectable compromise in the capacity of infants born at risk, probably proportional to the degree of risk. This respiratory defense system, available at birth, will be gradually supplanted by a slower, more deliberate, cortically mediated response pattern. If the reflex component subsides well before the later pattern appears, the infant may be in the critical "disorganized" period for an unusually long period of time, and in jeopardy as a result. By the same token, if the reflex subsides rapidly, this may compromise the opportunities available to the child to experience respiratory threat, and thus learn the appropriate hedonically mediated maneuvers required for the full development of the normal to-be-acquired "voluntary" behaviors. Inadequate opportunity to acquire the required defensive behaviors could be occasioned, then, by too rapid diminution of the reflex component, by too slow acquisition of the mature coping maneuvers characteristic of the older normal child, or by too debilitating a period of "disorganization" appearing between the two. Little is known about the origins of an adequate repertoire of defensive behaviors in the developing human. It is not unlikely, however, that after the first weeks of life, during which the infant is protected by inborn reflexes from most threats to respiration, much of this type of behavior is importantly dependent upon learning.

INFANTILE STRESS AND CONTINUITY: AN EVOLUTIONARY PERSPECTIVE

In their observations and conceptualizations, developmental theorists emphasize the positive features of development, by which is meant those experiences which tend to promote development to a higher, more mature, or more adaptive mode of functioning. Among the processes to which special attention is paid are the beginnings of antigravitational postural controls, such as turning over, pulling to standing, climbing, and holding objects or transferring them from hand to hand. In the social sphere, we study the onset of smiling, the beginnings of attachment, the discrimination of family members from others, and the ritualization of eating and other bodily functions.

The study of infancy has been mostly the study of positive/appetitive/approach behavioral processes. We do not often deal with the processes underlying events when things do not go right. Information about the dire consequences of the untoward experience or misadventure has come largely from clinical observers who have been called on to examine afflicted cases, to determine the etiology in specific instances, and to implement remedial measures. Occasionally attention has been directed as well to the salubrious effects that the experience of stress may have. René Spitz (1965), for example, accepted the importance of displeasure in the following way: "It follows that to deprive the infant of the affect of unpleasure during the course of the first year of life is as harmful as to deprive him of pleasure. Pleasure and unpleasure have an equally important role in the shaping of the psychic apparatus and the personality. To inactivate either affect will upset the developmental balance. . . . The importance of frustration for developmental progress cannot be overestimated—after all, nature itself imposes it" (p. 147).

One of the most compelling issues in the field of developmental psychology, regardless of one's stand on the relative importance of pleasant and annoying experiences, relates to the supposition of enduring influences of early experience. Human and animal developmentalists have been concerned with continuity for many years. The idea was promoted in psychology, especially by Sigmund Freud and John B. Watson. The assumption that the cumulation of early life experiences, *beginning* in infancy, is critical for and determinative of later development and behavior has been almost universally embraced by human development scholars.

Freud presumed that trauma during the earliest stages of human maturation could cause fixation at that level, thus precluding psychosexual development to the next stages, and that life-long personality attributes, temperamental characteristics, and behavior patterns would be forever affected by those early experiences (Freud, 1949). Similarly, Watson believed that infants subjected to conditioning experiences would carry with them lasting residual effects, phobic or affectional, depending upon the circumstances (Watson, 1928). Interestingly, both Freud and Watson also assumed that reversibility is possible under very special circumstances. For Freud, this could occur through later psychoanalysis involving free association and dream dissection designed to search for and understand the earliest origins of the disturbance; and for Watson, through empirically established counterconditioning techniques. The *reversibility of*, or *constraints on*, the *possible* consequences of profound early experience is as fascinating and important a topic as the enduring influences of early experience.

Does infancy make a difference, or is infantile experience a waste of time? That is the impertinent question, somewhat facetiously put. Connectivity between events is sometimes illusory, and putative causal associations between earlier conditions and later apparent consequences often turn out, on careful examination, to have been happenstance.

Retrospective reconstructions of events and their possible connections pose a special problem for developmental scientists. If we know, for example, that a child was abused or deprived as an infant, and the child is now found to be seriously antisocial, delinquent, or violent, it is a plausible conclusion that the history of infantile abuse and deprivation was the cause. From a yearning to understand, we might embrace such an apparent confirmation of the connection, and thus affirm our predilection. Moreover, such an "explanation" would honor the essentially linear human development models of both Watson and Freud which have prevailed in the twentieth century. Fortunately, increasing attention is paid now to the subtly interacting conditions which work in combination, either to attenuate the effects of otherwise powerful antecedents, or to turn a minor developmental crisis into a life catastrophe (see, e.g., Sameroff, 1975).

There is another aspect to this. The science of human development is not a conclusively foretelling science. Prediction and understanding of human developmental regularities is not (do I dare say?) as easy as forecasting in astronomy. Our astronomer colleagues can tell us, within an infinitesimal error of measurement, where Saturn and Jupiter will be on the first day of the year 2082, at 10:02 A.M. EST. The essentially closed system of the heavenly bodies allows the inferring of future states and fates from past regularities. In human development, on the other hand, destiny is subject to unknown, unanticipated intrusion of events and conditions that greatly attenuate knowledge of continuities and prediction of outcomes in individual instances. As actuarial experts in the service of insurance companies know, it is much easier to make correct probabilistic statements about the future (e.g., the death dates) of groups of persons (say, white males aged 45) than it is to correctly forecast the same event for individuals.

Another example may be found in the study of human development in relation to adverse perinatal factors. Although cerebral palsied and mentally retarded infants are more likely than normal infants to have been subjected to a variety of adverse perinatal conditions (e.g., asphyxia, twinhood, prolonged forceps use, malnutrition), anticipation from those specific precursors to the outcome in specific individuals is extremely tenuous indeed. There are many, many more infants subjected to these conditions who do *not* become cerebral palsied or mentally retarded than do. It appears that intervening or interceding conditions can be powerfully important in disrupting anticipated effects.

This need not mean that there is little or no continuity between earlier conditions or experiences and later events. There are two caveats to be honored in this connection. The first is that the overpowering or reversing effect of later experiences on a seemingly preset condition does not diminish the importance of the earlier condition. This is, in fact, what we *attempt* to do in successful remediation of any kind, educational or psychotherapeutic. If I get a headache whenever I have a certain experience A, but not when I take aspirin immediately after A, prediction from the experience to the headache will be poor at best. Nonetheless, A was a powerful determinant of the sequence. The aspirin merely aborted the initial antecedent-consequent relationship. Were A not importantly associated with headaches, I would not have taken the aspirin. Thus A *and* the aspirin were joint causes of my no-headache condition. Apparent non-continuities may be instances of continuities not yet fully revealed, or continuities that have been interfered with.

The second caveat is not unrelated to the first. The structure of behavior, like morphological structures, is sometimes deceptive, disguising underlying commonalities in parentage or experience. Two brothers may look very dissimilar and only a chromosomal analysis will reveal common parentage. By the same token, a frog and a tadpole hardly look like the same species, yet the frog had identical early experiences to those of at least one tadpole—itself at an earlier stage. Again, apparent non-continuities can be examples of continuities not yet sufficiently investigated. There are laws of behavioral development that describe verifiable regularities in antecedent-consequent relationships. In time, research is likely to reveal other regularities involving multiple, interactive variables that will also be precursors of outcomes. It would not be surprising were some of these factors to include those that we now regard as merely fortuitous circumstances or events.

Contextual factors play an important role in seeming discontinuities. Thus an early tendency toward anxiety might be abated if the individual's life circumstances are critically altered; there might then appear to be no connection between earlier stress index and later behavior. By the same token, if individual differences in an attribute like temperament flourish and are markedly affected by intercurrent or transient events, then the impression of discontinuity may be given of an otherwise fairly stable characteristic. Continuity of attributes is probably manifested most strongly when some powerfully controlling condition appears in the life of the individual, and persists.

Persisting contextual circumstances conduce to persisting personal characteristics, or continuity. If the tasks required of the person should shift markedly, however, as when a significant stress is introduced, then the stable coping techniques of the person suddenly *seem* unstable. Indeed they will *be* unstable in a highly variable set of contextual circumstances.

Life stress seems to disrupt and diminish continuity, as shown in the study of attachment behavior of infants (Waters, 1978). When Waters examined the stability of specific attachment behaviors at 12 and 18 months of age, along with the persistence of rated behavior categories and behavior patterns, he found no evidence of stability of discrete attachment indices in a time-sampling procedure. However, when classifications were used based upon patterns of interactive behaviors, the components of which could vary from one age to another, substantial stability was revealed. Forty-eight of 50 children retained the same classification from 12 to 18 months of age. Further evidence of such stability was obtained by Vaughn, Egeland, Sroufe, and Waters (1979) when life stress of the sample was considered. Families under high stress have children who show less persistence or apparent continuity of attachment behaviors (38% of the infants changed classification) relative to the children from lower-stress homes (4% changed classification). Thus contextual factors which produce resounding intercurrent changes in behavior may becloud the manifestation of stability in presumably endogenous attributes. It appears that continuities in human behavior may be attenuated by drastic conditions of life or intercurrent disruptions.

An interesting argument presented recently by Woodson (in press) concerns the evolutionary process through which infants arrive at mechanisms for surviving and thriving in the face of biological and environmental threats. The proposition has implications for the continuity issue. Woodson asserts that behaviors, like biological characteristics, are the product of an evolutionary process. The need to cope with the task of surviving hazards, in his view, had to have been among the strongest of selective pressures shaping infant behavior. The infant's *behavior* helps to resolve the consequences of perinatal complications which threaten transition of the newborn to extrauterine life and, by extension, other transitions as well.

One consequence of this supposition is that behavioral compensatory mechanisms, evolved as strategies for coping with threats, may obviate *apparent* continuities between early life events and later conditions of the organism. Woodson likens the situation to the invention and use of shock absorbers in cars, which effectively reduce the correlation between the state of the road and the smoothness of the ride. Similarly, early behavior may help to resolve perinatal complications which would otherwise have caused a subsequent deficit. The resolution of earlier-manifested developmental conditions, such as mild spastic diplegia resulting from neonatal asphyxia, is not uncommon (Solomons, Holden, & Denhoff, 1963). Modern technological procedures for assaying such damage have led to the finding that a large proportion of infants are born with intraventricular hemorrhage which eventuates in no apparent deficit on later assessment (Volpe, 1977). The apparent discontinuity may be due, in part, to experiential events instigated as adaptive mechanisms to stress.

Let us look more closely at an example of such behavioral compensation or coping in the presence of stress. The example is also from Woodson and neatly provides an instance in which the behavior of the baby is important for correcting a biological perturbation. Equally important, however, is the environmental support system in the form of the primary caretaker. Woodson notes that in a thermo-neutral environment the baby is typically quiescent, resting in a semiflexed posture. As the temperature drops, increased flexion takes place, helping to reduce heat loss by decreasing skin surface area. The behavioral response to cold contributes directly to maintenance of body temperature, along with increased metabolic activity and decreased subcutaneous blood flow. The feeling of cold resulting from ambient temperature drop produces other changes in behavior as well. The infant becomes active and it cries. The activity probably has consequences similar to that of shivering in adults, but crying has an effect on the caretaker, who usually responds with close and sustained physical contact resulting in heat-loss retardation for the baby.

These are clear illustrations in which the defensive behaviors of infants can facilitate recovery from a stress condition and promote physiological integrity. The newborn's response to respiratory occlusion, as shown earlier, follows a similar pattern. Oxygen depletion, or the threat thereof, serves as the stimulus, in normal infants, of defensive behaviors involving head-jerking, arm-thrashing, and crying (Gunther, 1961; Lipsitt, 1977). All of these responses serve to deflect the obtrusive stimulus and to regain the respiratory pathways for breathing. Success in gaining recovery from the insult is rewarded by stress reduction and the achievement of autonomic equanimity, a series of events accompanied by positive hedonic tone, and which can be learned. Thus facility in the execution of such beneficial psychobiological sequences is itself rewarding, and generates its own perpetuation through fundamental learning processes. Infantile learning processes have evolved, apparently, in ways conducive to the perpetuation of the livelihood of the baby. Moreover, these early manifested reflexes undergo a shift from essentially subcortical mediation to essentially cortical functioning with the passage of time. The result is that the child is then able to anticipate respiratory hazards and take evasive action before real threats to respiratory integrity occur.

CONCLUDING STATEMENT

> During the first six months, the baby has the rudiments of a love language available. . . . There is the language of the embrace, the language of the eyes, the language of the smile, vocal communications of pleasure and distress. It is the essential vocabulary of love before we can speak of love. Eighteen years later, when this baby is full grown and "falls in love" for the first time, he will woo his partner through the language of the eyes, the language of the smile, through the utterance of endearments, and the joy of the embrace. In his declarations of love, he will use such phrases as "When I first looked into your eyes," "When you smiled at me," "When I held you in my arms." And naturally, in his exalted state, he will believe that he invented this love song.
>
> Selma Fraiberg
> *Every Child's Birthright*, 1977

Few observers of infancy and the enduring echoes of infantile experience have captured as well as the late Selma Fraiberg the importance of the early months and years of life as a period of rehearsal, a time for the practice and fine tuning of responses essential to survival, socialization, and the preservation of self-esteem. Even so, one has to scrutinize the passage carefully to find that she has honored both sides of the hedonic coin by a tip of the hat to "distress." The developmental stresses of human infancy, and the durability of the young child in the presence of those stresses, have never been widely celebrated. Indeed, there has not been as much research attention to the earliest stages of life that one might expect, given the position of prominence that the infantile stages have in the major theories of human development, such as those of Freud, Erickson, and Piaget. No major theorist, on the other hand, has suggested that infancy is a waste of time. Quite the contrary, each has formulated specific propositions about the life-span relevance of the earliest periods of life. Why, one must therefore ask, do we not know more about stress and its effects upon the infant, and about the resiliency of the stressed infant?

The answer may be found in our own tastes as developmental investigators. Our emphasis, in our observations and studies of infancy, has been, as in the touching passage from Fraiberg, on "approach" behaviors of the infant. We have found more appealing the study of infants consuming coveted substances, obtaining objects with which to have pleasure, and achieving proximity to persons to whom they are, or are becoming, attached. The eating, touching, and looking behaviors of infants are more attractive to adults, even to presumably impartial investigators, than crying or tantrum behavior, or response patterns suggestive of distress, detachment, and despair.

In the first year of life a great deal of aversive behavior occurs. The human newborn is, in fact, a defensive creature, capable of rage and withdrawal when threats occur. For example, the greatest amount of crying occurs in the earliest months of life. Although, as with other aspects of growth and development, the rate decelerates virtually from the beginning of life, crying is the best index of human suffering that we have. We must study aversive and defensive coping behaviors, and their antecedents and developmental consequences, as carefully as we have studied sucking, swallowing, reaching, touching, attaching, and clinging.

One of the essences of human development is the capacity for defense. Biological defensiveness, well suited for protection against tissue damage, constitutes a rehearsal model for the infant who, in time, must be able also to deploy psychological defenses in the presence of a variety of stressful stimuli. The transformation of early adaptation styles, through practice into adequate psychological coping styles later, is one of the tasks of development.

The closer study of such transitions should be one of the tasks of developmental investigators. Future research needs to honor, more than previously, the infant fighter coping with perinatal risks and with hazardous stresses of which there are so many.

REFERENCES

Ainsworth, M. D. S. The development of infant-mother attachment. In B. Caldwell, & H. Ricciuti (Eds.), *Review of child development research* (Vol. 3). Chicago: University of Chicago Press, 1973.

Anderson, R. B., & Rosenblith, J. F. Sudden unexpected death syndrome: Early indicators. *Biologia Neonatorum*, 1971, *18*, 395–406.

Ashmead, D. H., Reilly, B. M., & Lipsitt, L. P. Neonates' heart rate, sucking rhythm, and sucking amplitude as a function of the sweet taste. *Journal of Experimental Child Psychology*, 1980, 29, 264–281.

Bowlby, J. *Attachment and loss: Attachment* (Vol. 1). New York: Basic Books, 1969.

Bradley, R. M., & Mistretta, C. M. The sense of taste and swallowing activity in fetal sheep. In R. S. Comline, K. W. Cross, G. S. Dawes, & T. W. Nathanielsz (Eds.), *Foetal and neonatal physiology. Proceedings of the Sir Joseph Barcroft Centenary Symposium*. Cambridge, England: Cambridge University Press, 1973.

Brazelton, T. B. *Neonatal behavioral assessment scale*. Philadelphia, Pa.: Lippincott, 1973.

Cannon, W. D. *The wisdom of the body*. New York: Norton, 1932.

Carpenter, R. G., & Emery, J. L. Identification and follow-up of infants at risk of sudden death in infancy. *Nature*, 1974, *250*, 729.

Church, R. M. The role of fear in punishment. In R. H. Walters, J. A. Cheyne, & R. K. Banks (Eds.), *Punishment*. Baltimore: Penguin Books, 1972, pp. 107–118.

Cowett, R. M., Lipsitt, L. P., Vohr, B., & Oh, W. Aberrations in sucking behavior of low-birthweight infants. *Developmental Medicine and Child Neurology*, 1978, *20*, 701–709.

Crook, C. K. Neonatal sucking: Effects of quantity of the response-contingent fluid upon sucking rhythm and heart rate. *Journal of Experimental Child Psychology*, 1976, *21*, 539–548.

Crook, C. K. Taste and the temporal organization of neonatal sucking In J. M. Weiffenbach (Ed.), *Taste and development: The genesis of sweet preference*. Bethesda, Md.: U.S. Department of Health, Education, and Welfare, 1977.

Crook, C. K., & Lipsitt, L. P. Neonatal nutritive sucking: Effects of taste stimulation upon sucking rhythm and heart rate. *Child Development*, 1976, *47*, 518–522.

Darwin, C. A biographical sketch of an infant. *Mind*, 1877, 2, 285—294.

Dobbing, J. Later development of the brain and its vulnerability. In J. A. Davis, & J. Dobbing (Eds.), *Scientific foundations of pediatrics*, Philadelphia, Pa.: W. B. Saunders Co., 1974.

Dobbing, J., & Sands, J. Comparative aspects of the brain growth spurt. *Early human development*, 1979, 3, 79–83.

Emde, R. N., Gaensbauer, T. J., & Harmon, R. J. *Emotional expression in infancy: A biobehavioral study*. New York: International Universities Press, 1976.

Engen, T., & Lipsitt, L. P. Decrement and recovery of responses to olfactory stimuli in the human neonate. *Journal of Comparative and Physiological Psychology*, 1965, 59, 312–316.

Field, T. M., Sostek, A. M., Goldberg, S., & Shuman, H. H. (Eds.), *Infants born at risk: Behavior and development*. New York: Spectrum Publications, 1979.

Fraiberg, S. *Every child's birthright: In defense of mothering*. New York: Basic Books, 1977.

Freud, S. *Beyond the pleasure principle*. New York: Boni & Liveright, 1927.

Freud, S. *An outline of psychoanalysis*. New York: Norton, 1949.

Graham, F. K. Behavioral differences between normal and traumatized newborns. I. The test procedures. *Psychological Monographs*, 1956, *70*(20, Whole No. 427).

Gunther, M. Instinct and the nursing couple. *Lancet*, 1955, *1*, 575.

Gunther, M. Infant behavior at the breast. In D. M. Foss (Ed.), *Determinants of infant behavior*. New York: Wiley, 1961.

Kagan, J. The determinants of attention in the infant. *American Scientist*, 1970, *58*, 298–306.

Kobre, K. R., & Lipsitt, L. P. A negative contrast effect in newborns. *Journal of Experimental Child Psychology*, 1972, *14*, 81–91.

Lipsitt, L. P. Developmental psychobiology comes of age: A discussion. In L. P. Lipsitt (Ed.), *Developmental psychobiology: The significance of infancy*. Hillsdale, N.J.: Lawrence Erlbaum Associates, 1976.

Lipsitt, L. P. The study of sensory and learning processes of the newborn. In J. Volpe (Ed.), *Clinics in perinatology* (Vol. 4, no. 1). Philadelphia, Pa.: Saunders, 1977.

Lipsitt, L. P. The newborn as informant. In R. B. Kearsley, & I. Sigel (Eds.), *Infants at risk: Assessment of cognitive functioning*. Hillsdale, N.J.: Lawrence Erlbaum Associates, 1979.

Lipsitt, L. P., & Werner, J. S. The infancy of human learning processes. In E. S. Gollin (Ed.), *Developmental plasticity*. New York: Academic Press, 1981.

Lipsitt, L. P., Sturner, W. Q., & Burke, P. Perinatal indicators and subsequent crib death. *Infant Behavior and Development*, 1979, *2*, 325–328.

McGraw, M. *The neuromuscular maturation of the human infant*. New York: Columbia University Press, 1943.

Mistretta, C. M., & Bradley, R. M. Taste in utero: Theoretical considerations. In J. M. Weiffenbach (Ed.), *Taste and development: The genesis of sweet preference*. Bethesda, Md.: U.S. Department of Health, Education, and Welfare, 1977.

Pfaffmann, C. The pleasures of sensation. *Psychological Review*, 1960, *67*, 253–268.

Piaget, J. *The moral judgment of the child*. New York: Collier Books, 1932.

Piaget, J. *The origins of intelligence in children* (Margaret Cook, trans.). New York: International Universities Press, 1952.

Sameroff, A. J. Transactional models in early social relations. *Human Development*, 1975, *18*, 65–79.

Sameroff, A. J. Caregiving or reproductive casualty? Determinants in developmental deviancy. In F. D. Horowitz (Ed.), *Early developmental hazards: Predictors and precautions*. Boulder, Colo.: Westview Press, 1978.

Solomons, G., Holden, R. H., & Denhoff, E. The changing picture of cerebral dysfunction in early childhood. *Journal of Pediatrics*, 1963, *63*, 113–120.

Spitz, R. *The first year of life: A psychoanalytic study of normal and deviant object relations*. New York: International Universities Press, 1965.

Steiner, J. E. Human facial expressions in response to taste and smell stimulation. In H. W. Reese, & L. P. Lipsitt (Eds.), *Advances in child development and behavior* (Vol. 13). New York: Academic Press, 1979.

Steinschneider, A. Prolonged apnea and the sudden infant death syndrome: Clinical and laboratory observations. *Pediatrics*, 1972, *50*, 646–654.

Swift, P. G. F., & Emery, J. L. Clinical observation on response to nasal occlusion in infancy. *Archives of Diseases in Childhood*, 1973, *48*, 947–951.

Thorndike, E. L. *Animal intelligence*. New York: Macmillan, 1911.

Uzgiris, I., & Hunt, J. McV. Attentional preference and experience: II. An exploratory longitudinal study of the effect of visual familiarity and responsiveness. *Journal of Genetic Psychology*, 1970, *117*, 109–121.

Vaughn, B., Egeland, B., Sroufe, L. A., & Waters, E. Individual differences in the infant-mother attachment at 12 and 18 months: Stability and change in families under stress. *Child Development*, 1979, *50*, 971–975.

Valdes-Dapena, M. A. Sudden and unexpected death in infancy: A review of the literature, 1954–66. *Pediatrics*, 1967, *39*, 123–138.

Valdes-Dapena, M. A. *Sudden unexpected infant death 1970 through 1975: An evolution in understanding*. (Publication number HSA 78-5255) Bethesda, Md.: U.S. Department of Health, Education, and Welfare, 1978.

Volpe, J. (Ed.), *Clinics in perinatology* (Vol. 4, number 1). Philadelphia, Pa.: W. B. Saunders, 1977.

Waters, E. The reliability and stability of individual differences in infant-mother attachment. *Child Development*, 1978, *49*, 483–494.

Watson, J. B. *Psychological care of infant and child*. New York: Norton, 1928.

Watson, J. B., & Rayner, R. Conditioned emotional reactions. *Journal of Experimental Psychology*, 1920, *3*, 1–14.

Woodson, R. Newborn behavior and the transition to extrauterine life. *Infant Behavior and Development*, in press.

Young, P. T. *Emotion in man and animal: Its nature and relation to attitude and motive*. New York: Wiley, 1943.

CHAPTER 7

STRESS AND COPING IN EARLY DEVELOPMENT

JEROME KAGAN
PROFESSOR OF HUMAN DEVELOPMENT
DEPARTMENT OF PSYCHOLOGY
HARVARD UNIVERSITY

STRESS, COPING, AND DEVELOPMENT IN THE OPENING YEARS OF LIFE

Introduction

One of the significant generalizations wrenched from laboratory work in biology and psychology during the last three decades is that the organism's biological or psychological reactions to an event depend upon its preparedness, which often means its stage of development. This principle rests on many functional relations that have survived replication, from modification of future sexual behavior following administration of sex hormones during a critical phase in development (Phoenix, Goy, & Resko, 1968), to the probability of crying following encounter with an unfamiliar person (Décarie, 1974). In both of the above examples, if the organism's structure is such that it can either ignore or resist the intruding event, no untoward consequences occur. Although departure of the mother has little observable effect on the behavior of 3-month-old infants, that same event produces clear distress in 12-month-olds. As a result, infants placed in day-care centers prior to six months do not show the distress often seen in children placed in surrogate care around the first birthday (Kagan, Kearsley, & Zelazo, 1978). Similarly, the modeling of an act which is on the threshold of comprehension and mastery has no effect on a 10-month-old but produces inhibition, protest, and even crying in a 2-year-old.

These robust phenomena are psychological examples of one of the great insights of experimental embryology. Prior to the critical phase of tissue organization, transfer of a few cells from one locus to another has no untoward consequences. After the period of organization has passed, however, that transfer leads to morphological anomaly. We begin, therefore, with a major principle: *the consequences of an event are dependent upon the structural readiness of the organism.*

This principle is vital to any discussion of stress and coping. A hard-headed attitude toward the use of exotic language in psychology would insist that stress and coping do not have any meaning not captured by the simpler words "incentive event," and "reaction." It is possible to defend such a seemingly tough position and to suggest that the current popularity of the concept of stressor reflects a profound shift in the community's mood regarding the causes of human unhappiness. During the latter part of the nineteenth century, and the opening few decades of this century, the efficient cause of psychological symptoms was internal conflict between standards and desires, between one's competence and the demands of reality, or between inconsistent beliefs. In each of these classes of conflict, the source of the disequilibrium was located inside the person in psychic processes. Even the neobehaviorists' attempts thirty years ago to use the simple language of learning theory to demystify psychoanalytic propositions posited approach-approach and approach-avoidance conflicts (Dollard & Miller, 1950). Animals were in conflict over their motivation for food and an equally strong motive to avoid electric shock. John Dollard and Neal Miller did not describe the animals' vacillation as caused by the stress created by past electric shock. But by the mid-1960s, the external events that had been viewed as only the potential beginning of a sequence that might generate dysphoric affect and disorganized behavior had become the primary causal agents. A mother's death, not the child's subsequent affective reaction, was awarded primary incentive force.

An extratheoretical reason for the change lies with the fact that sociologists and epidemiologists began to study the same phenomena that psychiatrists and psychologists had been pursuing. The latter are disposed to name and quantify internal mechanisms; the former code life events. Scientists usually ascribe special potency to the events they are able to measure, and, in the hands of epidemiologists and sociologists, maternal death assumed agentic power.

But there is a more important reason why the cause of distress moved outside. Commentators on modern society began to rewrite the traditional explanations of the psychological profile of its poor and minority citizens, and philosophical essays on the contemporary American scene began to concentrate on the helplessness of adults in the face of external forces that seemed resistant to benevolent management. As impersonal forces assumed more salience, the important transduction of an external event by belief became subordinate to the traumatic event.

Nevertheless, most investigators who indicated external events as malevolent, when pressed, would acknowledge that its consequences were not uniform, but dependent upon the beliefs, temperament, and past history of the victim. Theoretically, therefore, stressors remained simply arousing events, and coping reactions were still responses that individuals made to those events.

What is a Stressor?

Scholars have considerable freedom in selecting events for stressor status; hence, the concerns of a society have a subtle, but nonetheless, real effect on that choice. Compared with essays written a half century ago, the most recent surveys of research reveal a preoccupation with events that threaten the child's attachment to its parents and the adult's love relationship with spouse or sweetheart, rather than guilt over hostility and sexuality, or frustration born of disappointed desires for enhanced power. I suggest that the increased interest in intimacy and bonding is due, in part, to the social fact that the average contemporary adult is concerned with his or her lack of trusting relationships with others, worried over the high frequency of divorce and interpersonal anger that permeate the society, and troubled by the number of working mothers who leave their biological children in surrogate care. A reasonable reaction to this violation of traditional norms is to point to fragile or broken love relationships as the major villain in adult misery. If adults believe that their angst is due to unsatisfying love relations—either now or in the past—then, from the person's perspective, that conclusion has validity. The anthropologist's distinction between "emic" and "etic" frames is important in this discussion. The emic explanation, what Rorty (1979) calls consensual belief, is the community's modal interpretation of a regular phenomenon; a village's belief in the power of sorcery to cause illness is an obvious example. The etic explanation uses concepts selected by an observer outside the community. Although scientific explanations are more than an etic perspective, because they involve empirical tests of the validity of an explanation, one of their characteristics is that they frame explanations of behavior in terms different from those used by the person or community whose behavior is under study.

Even though many American adults believe that disruption of the child's early attachment to the parents is a cause of future problems, from the perspective of empirical fact, it is not clear that these disruptions are as formative as the community assumes. Citizens of fifth-century Athens believed that young children became undisciplined and uncontrollable if their mothers were too protective. If Socrates had used the word "stressor" as we do today, he might have regarded a close attachment between mother and infant as stressful because it bred fearfulness, cowardice, and a resistance to being socialized (Golden, 1981). Thus the definition of a stressor depends on the adult's ego ideal and the experiences that are presumed to divert the child from the desired psychological course. But let us be generous and assume that the words "stress" and "coping" have a special meaning not contained in the simpler words "event" and "response," and ask what those meanings might be.

Definitions of Stress

Stress can be defined in three different ways, only one of which seems satisfactory. The most popular strategy declares that certain conditions are stressful because they are correlated with particular socially undesirable outcomes; intuition implies that these conditions create anxiety, anger, and frustration in the recipient. Harsh punishment, frequent change of residence, divorce, poverty, indifferent parents, and a host of other events which can be objectively tallied are classified as stressful because the scholar believes that they create a special internal state in the recipient that is regarded as inimical to psychological health, and because these conditions are predictive (at levels far less than 1.0) of outcome reactions that the investigator believes are unwanted by the recipient. The problem with this definition of stress is that it ignores interaction between the event and the psychological and biological properties of the recipient, some of which are related to its stage of development, some to its biologically based temperamental qualities and prior history. Sackett, Ruppenthal, Fahrenbruch, Holm, and Greenough (1981) have reported that different macaque species do not react similarly to the same stressor; in this case, identical conditions of isolated rearing for the first six months of life. Rhesus show much more deviant behavior than pigtails following this experience. Surprisingly, crab-eaters (M. *fasicularis*) show almost normal profiles of social behavior despite the six months of prior isolation. If the objective events we call stressful, a priori, do not always provoke inimical reactions in the recipient (and we think this is true), this is not the best way to define stress, although it may be extremely useful in preliminary phases of investigation. But the scientist should try continually to replace it. The metaphor for this definition of stress is a hammer blow of fixed force creating a uniform deformation in the homogeneous surface it strikes. But psychological systems do not work this way. The effect of a mother's slapping of her child's face will depend on the child's age, prior history, and his or her interpretation of the maternal act. We must have information about the target before we can make inferences about consequences.

A second, even less satisfactory, approach is to define what is stressful in terms of outcome only. The investigator lists a set of outcomes which are presumed to be produced by stressful events, finds individuals who display these outcomes and then, after examining the history of the subject, decides that parts of that history must have been stressful, even though the history may not contain conditions theorists would regard as stressful. This deduction is an example of the logical fallacy of asserting the consequent. The presence of B in the syllogism, if A then B, does not imply A. This strategy makes the unwarranted assumption that a particular outcome (a criminal record, for example) has one major etiological history, and that the outcome has the same psychological meaning across all members of the category.

A third strategy, which I favor, defines a stressor conjunctively as a class of events and a specific reaction to exemplars of that class. This is also a useful approach to the definition of affective states. Guilt, for example, is an internal reaction that follows the violation of a standard for which the person believes he or she had a choice. Guilt is neither a particular autonomic, facial, or cognitive reaction, nor the state that always accompanies violation of a standard. Thus I shall assume that events that belong to the class "stressful" are typically accompanied by internal changes that have an undesirable affective component. I suspect that a majority of psychologists and psychiatrists would agree that the undesirable affects include the states that have been given names like anxiety, fear, anger, sadness, depression, hatred, hopelessness, shame, and guilt. Thus, I shall use the word "stressor" in this paper to refer to an event and an accompanying affective reaction, and shall use the phrase "incentive event" to refer only to a stimulus complex which might or might not provoke an affective reaction and, therefore, might or might not be a stressor.

Spring and Coons (1982), as well as others, adopt a slightly different approach to the definition of stress. They suggest that stress might be defined as a disruption or alteration in physiological, emotional, or behavioral functioning. But they reject that decision because there are always alterations in function and, therefore, everyone will always be under stress. A second strategy is to define stress in relation to the characteristics of the individual and his or her life context. "A situation or an event is deemed to be a stress if it is perceived as such by the individual, or, from the judgment of a rater, it outstrips the available resources for coping."

This rule prevents an observer from ever calling an event a stressor unless he can know the internal reaction. Because available methods do not permit this inference, Spring and Coons reject this approach. But they argue that stress might be defined in terms of events whose properties are objectively specifiable, and whose probability of occurrence is independent of the reactions or characteristics of the targets. They are willing to name some events stressful, regardless of how they are perceived.

Coping

Coping, as a descriptor or construct, refers to a special class of individual reactions to stressors. Once again, the investigator has three definitional choices. He or she can decide, a priori, that certain reactions are examples of coping, and ignore interaction, or declare that certain outcomes must imply a coping reaction. These strategies are subject to the same criticism raised in the discussion of the definition of stress.

A more useful definition of coping treats it as a reaction to a stressor that resolves, reduces, or replaces the affect state classified as stressful. If anger is the affective reaction of a 10-year-old to parental divorce, and disobedience to the parental requests resolves the anger and does not bring on a new stressor, it is a coping reaction. If anxiety is the reaction to the same stressful event, withdrawal from social interaction into academic studies might be a coping response. The coping reaction chosen to deal with a specific stressor will vary with the affect generated, as well as with the child's history and temperament. There is extraordinary variation among children in the selection of a coping response.

The stressful affect and coping reactions generated will depend in a special way on the child's level of development. Young children are likely to become fearful of stressors, while older children are likely to become angry. Dianne Lusk (1978) reported that four-year-olds appreciate this developmental principle. To an oral description of pictures illustrating varied stressful events occurring to targets of different ages (a person in a puddle, someone being victimized by another), 4-year-olds claim that infants would become frightened while older children and adults would become angry.

The reaction to an event that is a candidate for a stressor is due, in part, to the degree to which the child believes he understands the incentive. Once the period of infancy is over, an important pair of factors that determines the potential of an event to generate inimical affect is the child's ability to understand the event and his or her opportunity to act in a way that either permits avoidance of the incentive or protects the child from the cognitive consequences of the incentive. If a child is subject to unjust peer torment because of his ethnic membership, less anger will be generated if the child believes the hostility reflects the aggressor's irrational prejudice and not the child's properties. The anger will also be less intense if the child can physically avoid his tormenters, or find an activity that is so involving he has little time to dwell on the prejudice. Obviously, this is easier if the stressor is acute than if it is chronic.

Stressors in Early Development

I now describe some stressful conditions that occur during the first three years of life which last a relatively short time—one to six months at most—in the hope that an analysis of these phenomena might inform the effects of stressors in older children which have a much longer duration. Each of these stressors appears to involve the affect psychologists usually call anxiety. During the opening years of life, events differ in their potential to create a state of uncertainty, and in the dominant profile of reaction each provokes. During the first three months, pain and physical discomfort are primary sources of stress, leading to irritability and disturbances in feeding and sleeping. During the period four to twelve months, unassimilable discrepancy and unpredictable events are frequent stressors, leading to behavioral inhibition, withdrawal, and crying. During the second year, parental restriction, punishment, and prolonged separation are stressful events that provoke inhibition, protest, depression, and occasionally apathy. Let us consider in some detail two universal stressors that appear during the first year—encounter with an unfamiliar adult, and departure of a target of attachment.

Anxiety to Strangers and to Separation

The most effective incentive for stranger-anxiety is the approach of an unfamiliar adult who behaves in an unusual manner, usually by being unresponsive or overly reactive. Below 5 or 6 months of age this event usually does not lead to any behavior that might be regarded as indicative of fear. (It is of interest that Izard [personal communication] reports that the pattern of facial expression normally called fear [retraction of the mouth, widening of the eyes, raising of eyebrows] to the incentive of an injection does not appear until 6 or 7 months of age.) But between 6 and 15 months, the unfamiliar adult is likely to produce a stereotyped reaction (the probability is far less than 1.0). The child becomes motorically inhibited, stops playing, his or her facial expression changes in a special way, and, on occasion, the child will cry. But as suddenly as this correlated set of reactions appears, it vanishes during the second year. We now ask how does the child cope with this event?

During the period of vulnerability, the behavioral signs of fear can be avoided completely if the stranger's behavior is predictable. Indeed, when Rheingold and Eckerman (1973) had strangers approach the infants gradually, and talk to them softly, they observed no signs of fear, and suggested that stranger-anxiety might not exist. Or if the stranger allows the child to control the adult's behavior in a playful context, the signs of anxiety do not occur. If one-year-olds can act in a way to control an unexpected reaction of a toy, the signs of anxiety are not manifested (Gunnar, 1980). Thus, if the child can assimilate or control the incentive event, it need not be stressful. Further, if the child has toys, or can run to the mother when the stranger approaches—that is, if the child has a response she can issue to the stressor, even though she may not assimilate the event—the stressful consequences are far less striking, at least in their overt manifestation.

Similar phenomena occur when separation from the mother is the incentive. The behavioral signs of fear to the incentive of maternal departure appear around 8 months of age, peak at about 15 months in children growing up in many different cultural settings, and are infrequent by 30 months (see Figure 7-1).

The growth function for separation distress, that is, the tendency to cry and/or show serious inhibition of play following departure of the primary caretaker, is similar among children being raised in the United States, in barrios in urban Guatemala, in subsistence farming Indian villages in the Guatemalan highlands, in Israeli kibbutzim, in Kung San bands in the Kalahari desert (Kagan, 1976), and among infants diagnosed as suffering from failure to thrive (Jameson & Gordon, 1977). Moreover, the developmental course of distress in blind children, in reaction to unfamiliar adults or to

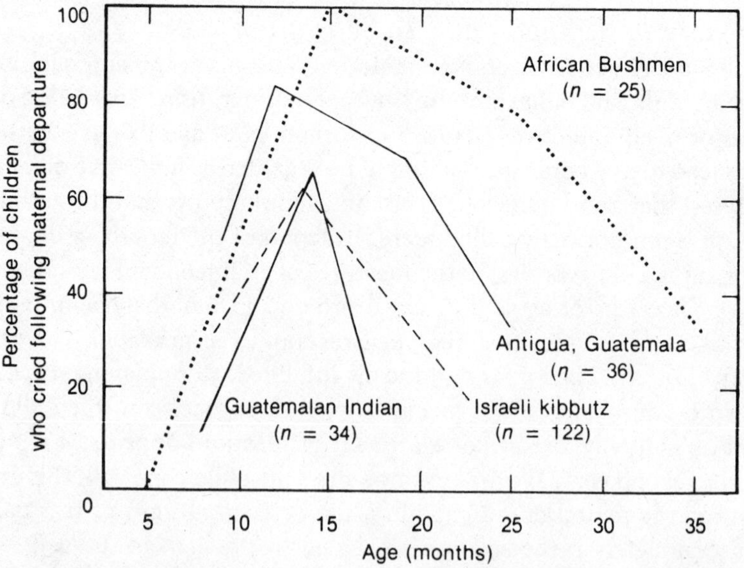

Figure 7-1. Proportion of children showing separation protest in various cultures.

maternal separation, is not much different from the function noted in those with sight.

Selma Fraiberg gathered detailed longitudinal observations on 10 blind infants observed bimonthly in their homes (Fraiberg, 1975; Adelson & Fraiberg, 1974). Not only did smiling and responsiveness to the voice of the mother or other familiar persons occur at about the same age for blind as for sighted children (at about 3 months), but apprehension and distress at being held by an unfamiliar adult emerged between 7 and 15 months. Separation distress was only a few months delayed in the blind children, emerging between 10 and 15 months. This is remarkable, considering the fact that the child cannot see that the parent is gone. The incentive for the blind child's display of separation distress is the sudden absence of the mother's voice or absence of the sounds that accompany her bodily movements. Fraiberg (1975) describes the case of Karen, who showed her first sign of separation distress at about eleven months.

> Mother remarked that she can't leave Karen with anyone anymore, which has not been the case until very recently. Karen cries and is unhappy even with her grandmother, whom she has known since birth. Added to Karen's behavior today is her need to always be in contact with mother. . . . Observer's report at 11 months 13 days. "Karen let herself down to the floor and started to creep to the box, which was about two feet away from her. She was somewhat hesitant or cautious, but she was curious. At this moment, mother got up to go to Debbie (the younger baby sister) to give her the pacifier because she was fussing. Karen immediately started to whimper, reversed direction, and went back to cling to the mother's chair, and when mother sat down again, reached to touch mother's arm. Mother then reached down and touched Karen's hair. (p. 330)

As with stranger-anxiety, if the child can play with someone while the mother is absent, behavioral signs of distress are less likely to occur. Or if the mother departs in a familiar room from an exit that she normally uses, distress is far less likely than if the mother takes an exit she rarely uses, or leaves the child in an unfamiliar place. Again, if the stressor can be assimilated, affective consequences are muted.

Anxiety to an Unfamiliar Peer

Less well documented, but following similar dynamics, is the occurrence of signs of anxiety to an unfamiliar child of the same age and sex. Inhibition of play, clinging, and remaining proximal to the mother, when in the presence of an unfamiliar child, peak during the second year, usually before the second birthday. Chinese and Caucasian children reared at home or in a day-care center were allowed to play with an unfamiliar child at 13,

20, and 29 months of age. The majority of children showed their peak signs of distress (inhibition of play and vocalization, and increased proximity to the mother) at 20 months of age. The incentive for the anxiety is the unfamiliar child, for pairs of children who are familiar with each other are less inhibited than pairs who are unfamiliar. Jacobson (1980) observed pairs of children 3 times, when they were 10, 12 and 14½ months. The children displayed much less play, more staring at each other, and more time proximal to the mother when the other child was unfamiliar than when the partner was familiar.

The appearance of inhibition to an unfamiliar child also occurs in children from other cultures, including children growing up on kibbutzim. Zaslow (1977) replicated the original finding summarized earlier in a cross-sectional study of 96 Israeli infants who were seen at 14, 20, and 29 months of age. Half the subjects lived in nuclear family households in Jerusalem. The other half lived in infant houses on kibbutzim and visited the parents' homes for only a few hours in the late afternoon and early evening. Each child's behavior was coded first while he played in an unfamiliar setting alone where his mother was reading a magazine or book, and after an unfamiliar peer and the peer's mother were introduced into the room. Both the kibbutz- and family-reared Israeli children showed their greatest inhibition of play at 20 months of age. However, group rearing exerted an effect. The kibbutz-reared 29-month-olds were still showing apprehension, although less frequently than the 20-month-olds.

In a final longitudinal study, children played with the same child monthly from 13 to 22 months of age. Most of the children did not show apprehension to the peer until they approached 20 months of age, even though each had been with the same child in the same setting on 3 or 4 prior occasions. The apprehension was not due to the fact that the child had forgotten his friend, for mothers reported that their children asserted on the trip to the laboratory that they were going to see a particular child. Thus, both developmental stage, as well as prior experience with peers, influence the degree of initial apprehension with other children. The maturation of cognitive competences determines the basic developmental function for the apprehension, and guarantees that it will begin at or soon after the first year, peak during the second year, and decline during the third year. Extensive experience with peers can influence the age of emergence of the apprehension, the age of decline, and perhaps its intensity during the period of its display.

Distress following Modeling

We have recently discovered a new incentive for distress which seems to involve the child's evaluation of his or her competence. The phenomenon emerges during the period 18 to 24 months of age when children become seriously inhibited, cry, and seek proximity to the mother, immediately after watching an adult woman model some acts that are moderately difficult to remember and to implement. The setting is quite simple. A child is playing happily with some toys while the mother sits nearby. A female examiner comes to the child and models three acts (e.g., the examiner picks up two plates and two dolls and makes the mother doll cook supper; she has a doll talk on a toy telephone; she picks up some animals and makes them go for a walk). The examiner then says, "Now it's your turn to play," and returns to the couch, while coders behind a one-way vision screen note the occurrence of the signs of uncertainty listed above. The procedure has been administered to 2 longitudinal and 2 cross-sectional samples of children. The first longitudinal sample consisted of 14 children seen monthly from 13 to 22 months and 16 children seen monthly from 20 to 26 months (15 of these children were seen from 20 to 29 months and again at 30, 32 and 34 months). All 30 children were Caucasian and middle class. The second sample, also longitudinal, Caucasian, and middle class, consisted of 3 boys and 3 girls who were between 17 and 19½ months when the longitudinal observations began. All were seen every 3 weeks in their homes for 13 to 14 visits until they had passed their second birthday. The third sample consisted of 12 Caucasian children seen only once in the laboratory at 23 months of age. The final sample consisted of 48 children between 13 and 36 months of age living in small villages of about 100 people on small islands in the Fiji group.

Figure 7-2 shows the growth function for the occurrence of signs of distress—clinging, crying, inhibition of play, protests, and requests to go

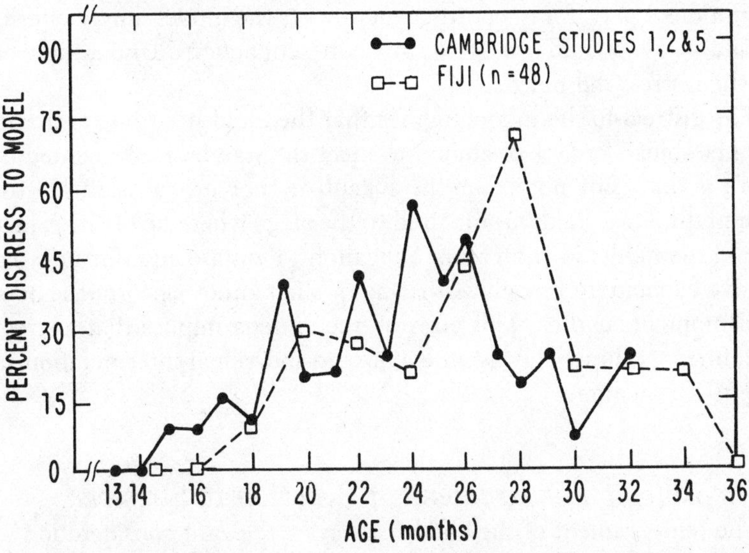

Figure 7-2. Proportion of children showing distress to the model.

home—that occurred within one minute after the modeling of the acts. In general, distress first occurred after 17 to 18 months, and reached a peak just before the second birthday in the American sample, and just after the second birthday in the Fiji group.

Unpublished data gathered by Gellerman (1981) as part of her doctoral research affirm the lawfulness of this growth function for a group of 7 Vietnamese children who had recently arrived in the United States. Gellerman visited the homes of the 7 children every 2 to 3 weeks from 15 to 26 months of age and administered the modeling procedure. No child showed distress to the model prior to 17 months of age; the incidence of distress peaked at 24 months, and then declined. Thus, similar growth functions for distress to the model occurred for 5 different samples differing in ethnicity and, presumably, prior history.

We interpret this developmental function as reflecting the emergence of at least two processes. One process involves the child's feeling of obligation to implement the acts of a model. The second involves the child's awareness of his or her inability to implement the modeled actions, either because the children forgot what the model did, or because they were unsure of their ability to do so. As a result, the child becomes uncertain, and may begin to cry or cling to the parent. We can eliminate the possibility of complete memory failure for the modeled acts because in many cases of distress, after the child had left the mother's side and begun to play again, he or she would display an exact or fragmented version of one of the model's prior actions. There may have been a temporary forgetting of the model's behavior, but it was not permanent.

We can also rule out the possibility that the child's distress was due to the interruption of play, for in control experiments the model simply interrupted the child's play, but did not display any coherent actions. Under these conditions the distress did not occur.

The distress to the model implies that the child has some awareness of his or her ability, or lack of ability, to meet the standard represented by the model's action. But note that the incentive that provokes the distress is impotent until the child has matured to the stage where he or she is ready to interpret the model's action as an obligation to imitate and, further, has the cognitive capacity to recognize that he or she cannot perform the acts witnessed moments earlier. This class of phenomena implies that a stressor is best defined conjunctively as an event-cum-individual interpretation rather than either one alone.

The Role of Temperament in Reaction to Stressors

The temperament of the child is always a relevant consideration in the study of stress (Thomas & Chess, 1972, 1977). In all of the studies described above there were moderately persistent individual differences in degree of dysphoric affect and behavior. Some children react with signs of fear to almost all discrepant situations; others rarely do; still others show signs of mild uncertainty (Garcia-Coll, 1981; Kagan, Kearsley, & Zelazo, 1978). This variation in vulnerability to distress is associated with ethnicity as well as with a higher and less variable heart rate while processing visual and auditory information.

One source of evidence for a relation between a disposition toward behavioral inhibition to unfamiliar incentives and heart rate while processing discrepant information came from a longitudinal study of children, half Caucasian, half Chinese, who were assessed 8 times over the period from 3½ to 29 months of age. Detailed descriptions of the procedures and major results appear elsewhere (Kagan, Kearsley, & Zelazo, 1978). Continuous heart rate data were gathered on these children during the habituation phase of visual and auditory episodes. We evaluated the variability of each child's heart rate during each stimulus presentation by coding heart rate range. Range was defined as the difference between the highest and lowest heart rates on those trials during the familiarization period when the child was highly attentive and not irritable. Trials during which the child's fixation time was less than 80% of the stimulus exposure period, or when more than one second of fretting occurred, were eliminated from all analyses. The child's absolute heart rate levels were far from their upper limit. Behavioral evaluations of inhibition were made in situations when the child was with an unfamiliar peer; with the mother, a familiar caretaker and a stranger; following separation; and as part of a visit to an unfamiliar day-care center. In all of these situations, the Chinese children, as a group, were more inhibited than the Caucasians. For example, during an episode administered at 20 months of age, the child was placed with the child's mother, an unfamiliar woman, and (for the day-care children) the primary caretaker from a day-care center, or (for the home controls) a female friend of the mother. The Chinese children spent twice as much time proximal to the mother as did the Caucasian children over the 45-minute session ($F = 9.61$, $1/64$, $p < .01$).

A standard maternal separation procedure was administered on each of the 8 sessions. Every one of the children cried on at least 1 of the 6 occasions, and most cried on 2. Although the occurrence of separation protest displayed a regular growth function for both ethnic groups, the Chinese children protested earlier and more often than the Caucasians. Of the 59 children tested 6 times from 5 to 20 months, almost 25% of the Chinese protested in 5 or all 6 of the sessions, while only 6% of the Caucasians protested as often. Moreover, the Chinese showed separation distress at an earlier age than the Caucasians (the age when more than 50% of the children fretted was 9 months for the Chinese and 11 months for the Caucasians). In a third situation, the child played with an unfamiliar peer at 13, 20, and 29 months of age. Again, the Chinese were significantly more inhibited than the Caucasians at all 3 ages. They stayed closer to their mothers, played and vocalized less, were more fretful, and made significantly fewer initiations, either cooperative or aggressive, toward the other child.

Finally, each child was taken to an unfamiliar day-care center with his or her mother and a female observer for a 30-minute observational period, when the child was 29 months old. As in the other episodes, the Chinese were significantly more inhibited than the Caucasians. They stayed closer to their mothers for a longer time, played less, and were less likely to initiate overtures to the unfamiliar children. When the children were 29 months of age, their mothers ranked a set of 16 qualities with respect to how characteristic each quality was for their child. The Chinese mothers were more likely than the Caucasians to report that the child's tendency to "stay close to the mother" was highly characteristic of their children. By contrast, the Caucasian mothers reported that laughter, talkativeness, and activity were most characteristic of their children.

Additionally, the Chinese children had more stable heart rates than the Caucasians on most trials of all episodes, and especially from 7 to 29 months of age. The consistent difference in range between Chinese and Caucasian infants was not solely a function of larger or more frequent cardiac decelerations or accelerations among the Caucasians. In a separate analysis, we compared the heart rate ranges of the two groups for those trials in which neither an acceleration nor deceleration occurred. The Chinese continued to show smaller average heart rate range values than Caucasians at most ages and on most episodes. In addition, the Chinese children had smaller heart rate ranges under conditions when they were not attending to an event, a time when the child was seated on the mother's lap, but the child's attention was not directed at any particular stimulus.

Despite the ethnic differences in both behavioral inhibition and heart rate range, there was no relation between heart rate range and apprehension or inhibition within each ethnic group. However, when we selected pairs of children who were matched on care, ethnicity, and sex, but who varied on behavioral signs of anxiety, there was the expected relation to heart rate range. Of 7 pairs of children matched on form of care, ethnicity, and sex, the 6 children with consistently low heart rate ranges showed separation distress more frequently than their matched counterparts who displayed high heart rate ranges ($p < .05$).

In the longitudinal sample of older children followed from 20 to 29 months (described earlier), we also coded heart rate and range to a series of visual episodes. Both heart rate and range were negatively correlated (the correlation averaged $-.56$), and both were moderately stable across age (coefficients in the fifties). Further, the children with higher and more stable heart rates showed distress to the model on more occasions, than did those with lower and more variable heart rates. Two-thirds of the children with higher and less variable heart rates showed distress to the model on 5 or more of 17 occasions, in contrast to only 20% of the children with low and variable heart rates.

Additionally, on each monthly visit to the laboratory, the same pair of children played together in a room familiar to them, while the mothers sat on a couch nearby. The children with the most stable heart rates were least likely to imitate the other child during the period 23 to 26 months of age, when imitation begins to appear with some frequency ($r = -.78$, $p < .01$). Thus, for this sample of two-year-olds, those with consistently high heart rates and low heart rate ranges were more likely to show behavioral signs of inhibition to uncertain incentives.

In the most recent and most extensive study of this functional relation, the reactions of 21-month-old children to 6 uncertain incentives were filmed (play warm-up, encounter with a stranger, the display of actions by a model, exposure to a robot, and separation from the mother). The coding of discrete behavioral signs of inhibition (withdrawal, clinging to the mother, proximity to the mother, crying, failure to play) from the videotape records of 117 children across 6 incentives permitted us to select the 28 most- and 30 least-inhibited children. These 58 children returned to the laboratory one month later and were retested in the same 6 situations. There was reasonable stability of the frequency of inhibited behaviors across the month separating the 2 sessions. The children who clung to their mothers, showed distress vocalizations, minimal play, and withdrawal on the first session, also did so on the second session ($r = .63$ for the group; $p < .05$).

After each behavioral session, the experimenter, mother, and infant moved into another laboratory setting where heart rate and respiration were recorded continually during a 20-minute presentation of 6 separate episodes involving classes of visual and auditory information. The visual episodes contained 2 series of familiar objects (women and dogs) and 2 of unfamiliar objects (abstract patterns and scrambled figures). Each set of chromatic slides consisted of 8 different exemplars of the same category, each exposed for 10 seconds. The auditory series consisted of a voice, without visual support, speaking meaningful phrases, and 8 unusual environmental sounds. The apparent source of the auditory stimulus was a sketch of a smiling face in the center of the child's visual field.

There was a significant negative relation between heart rate and a more sophisticated index of heart rate variability, the average standard deviation of the inter-beat interval for each of the 6 episodes. Further, the extremely inhibited children showed higher and less variable heart rates than the extremely uninhibited children. When the analysis was restricted to each of the

6 episodes, the episode which we believe was among the most difficult to assimilate produced the best association between high heart rate and low variability on the one hand, and behavioral inhibition on the other. During the fifth episode the children heard a series of short, recorded phrases spoken by a human voice, but without any visual sign of a person. This episode followed one in which the child saw slides of dogs, a category of events familiar to all the children. The rise in heart rate and the decreased variability of heart rate to this episode provided the best single predictor of behavioral inhibition (Garcia-Coll, 1981).

Eleven of the extremely inhibited and 11 of the extremely noninhibited children were brought back 10 months later (when they were 31 months old) for an assessment of behavior with an unfamiliar peer, as well as for a reevaluation of their autonomic reaction to visual information. After the session in which an inhibited and uninhibited child played together, each child participated in a laboratory session, during which heart rate was gathered while the child was listening to a narrated story consisting of 26 chromatic slides, each 10 seconds in duration. There was a significant positive relation between heart rate stability at 21 and 31 months. More important, the 5 children who had the most stable heart rates on both occasions—21 and 31 months—were behaviorally inhibited at both 21 and 31 months. The 3 children classified as behaviorally inhibited at 21 months, but who had variable heart rates at that age, were the least inhibited with the peer and with an observer who visited them in their homes when they were 31 months old. Thus, at 21 months of age, the behaviorally inhibited children who had more variable heart rates turned out to be less inhibited 10 months later than the inhibited 21-month-olds with stable heart rates, suggesting that variability of heart rate at 21 months was able to differentiate the inhibited children who remained behaviorally inhibited from those whose behavior changed over the 10-month period.

We suggest that the individual differences in heart rate and heart rate variability are due, in part, to differences in the degree to which the child actively attempts to assimilate unfamiliar and discrepant events. We call this state active vigilance. Children do not have a general disposition to have a stable or a variable heart rate; all children are capable of both variable and stable patterns. An important determinant of heart rate variability is the child's psychological state, and we suggest that children and adults differ in their proneness to the state we call active vigilance when they encounter discrepant, deviant, or unexpected events. The children who were more vigilant to the visual and auditory information (and had higher and more stable heart rates) apparently were also more vigilant with the adult model and with the peer and, as a result, were more likely to become anxious when they could not understand or perform the model's actions, or deal with the behavior of the other child.

As children gain information they gain mastery of the situation, and the vigilance subsides. The relations between a higher and less variable heart rate and behavioral signs of apprehension is in accord with current physiological theory. Under resting conditions, the heart rate is typically under parasympathetic influence and vagal tone tends to keep the heart rate low and variable because the heart cycle is yoked to the inspiration-expiration respiratory cycle (Fitzgerald, 1976). This phenomenon is called sinus arrythmia. Katona and Jih (1975) suggest that heart rate variability is a sensitive index of the degree of parasympathetic control of the heart. But when sympathetic tone is increased, the vagal influence on the heart is inhibited, respiratory control of the cardiac cycle is diminished, and heart rate tends to rise a little and become much less variable. There are a great many studies indicating that heart rate rises and becomes more stable when adults are attempting to cope with difficult problems (Martin, 1961; Light, 1981).

Our suggestion that infants differ in their proneness to vigilance, wariness, and anxiety is in accord with the work of others. Tennes, Downey, and Vernadakis (1977) found that individual variation in cortisol production among infants was correlated with vulnerability to distress following maternal departure. Bronson (1972) has reported that infants who were wary at four months were fearful at nine months, and the vulnerability to fear was independent of the number of caretakers to which the infant had been exposed. Additionally, the tendency to show inhibition with unfamiliar adults apparently has a significant degree of heritability in 22-month-old children (Plomin & Rowe, 1979). Comparisons of identical and fraternal twins revealed that indices of the tendency to approach or to avoid a stranger showed intraclass correlations in the neighborhood of 0.5 for identical twins, compared to correlations that hovered near zero for fraternal twins. By contrast, interactive behavior with the mother showed no evidence of heritability (Plomin & Rowe, 1979). Finally, Suomi, Kraemar, Baysinger, and DeLizio (1981) have found that individual differences in *fearfulness* among one- to two-year-old macaques, which tend to be significantly stable over time and smaller between siblings than between unrelated animals, were associated with the degree of heart rate reactivity to a series of conditioned stimuli administered to infants when they were one month old. Specifically, the one-month-old monkeys who showed large changes in heart rate to auditory conditioned stimuli were more likely to become fearful two years later than infants with minimal heart rate changes to the conditioned signals. It is possible that the tendency, in infants, to show a large change in heart rate to a brief conditioned stimulus is mediated by the same or similar mechanisms that lead two-year-old children to show stable heart rates while they are attempting to assimilate discrepant symbolic information.

In addition to the possibility of a genetic component, we believe that maternal stress during the period when the autonomic nervous system is differentiating, during the fourth through the sixth week postconception, may affect this disposition. Patterson, Potter, and Furshpan (1978) suggest that during the embryogenesis of the autonomic nervous system in the rat, the final ratio of cholinergic to adrenergic ganglia is a function of local chemical conditions existing during this brief period of growth. And Gabella (1976) notes the large interindividual variation in the size of sympathetic ganglia. It is not unreasonable to assume that psychological stress experienced by the pregnant mother during this interval might influence the local chemical environment and, therefore, the balance of cholinergic and adrenergic neurons, and, by inference, the child's temperamental tendency toward inhibition versus excitability. There is good reason to believe that the growth of the sympathetic nervous system during this early period is controlled, in part, by nerve growth factor, and that one of the sites of production of nerve growth factor is the placenta. Since the chemical composition of the placenta can be influenced by maternal infection, disease, and stress, it is not unreasonable to assume that biological or psychological stress during the first six weeks of pregnancy might affect the balance of cholinergic to adrenergic ganglia in the sympathetic system.

Because of the nontrivial variation among children in vulnerability to inhibition and apprehension, we are unlikely to make serious theoretical progress unless the variation associated with temperament is acknowledged and evaluated and made a part of every analysis that attempts to relate home experience to behavior. The data on the inhibited and uninhibited children summarized earlier, which are based on Garcia-Coll's (1981) doctoral research, reveal two different types of children who showed uncertainty. During the separation episode, some children stopped playing, became quiet, and cried. These children tended to be the same ones who were very inhibited in the other five stressful situations. But there was a second group who did not stop playing or cry, but who went to the door after maternal departure, and who approached the parent when she returned to the room. These children, who appeared to be coping with their uncertainty, were less likely to be seriously inhibited in the other uncertain situations.

An inhibited style of responding to an acute stressor might be preserved for some time. Of the many variables quantified over the first three years of life in the Fels Longitudinal Study (Kagan & Moss, 1962), inhibition was the only disposition that had predictive correlates with behaviors during later childhood and adulthood. The boys who were most inhibited during the first three years of life were, as adults, more dependent on love objects ($r = .47$,

$p < .05$) and more likely to show stable heart rates during a relaxation interval prior to test procedures. (Recall the relation in children between a stable heart rate and vulnerability to inhibition.) These inhibited infant boys also avoided dangerous activity, were minimally aggressive with peers, conformed to parents, and were relatively timid in social situations during the period 6 to 10 years of age. As adults they avoided group sports and other traditional masculine activities. The 4 boys who were most inhibited over the first six years of life chose intellectual careers as adults (music, physics, biology and psychology). The 4 least inhibited boys chose more traditional masculine vocations (football coach, salesman, engineer).

Development and Vulnerability to Stressors

The emphasis on the child's interpretation of events that might be potential stressors implies that there should be, across developmental stages, differential receptivity to specific events because of the lawful changes in cognitive functioning that occur over the first dozen years of life. But in order to name potential stressors, it is necessary to be explicit about outcome, for almost any event can elicit an unpleasant affective state in the child and adult; hence any event is a potential candidate for the category stressor.

In order to limit the discussion, we shall concentrate on the affect state that follows failure to assimilate the unexpected or the unpredicted, failure to meet standards, and the inability to resolve inconsistency in beliefs or between beliefs and standards. These states are popularly named fear, anxiety, shame, and guilt.

During the first six months, the most frequent and perhaps the most potent incentive for a state of uncertainty is a discrepant event. Events that are partial transformations of established schemata alert the infant, lead to inhibition of motor and vocal responses, and, on occasion, produce crying. It is reasonable to suppose that frequent changes in feeding and sleeping routines could produce the state of uncertainty. I do not claim this uncertainty will have long-lasting effects, only that unanticipated changes in the routine of the young infant can produce this emotional state.

By 4 to 6 months of age, the infant has created schemata for his or her caretaker's face, voice, and form, and if the infant is cared for by only one adult, it might be expected that a change in caretaker would elicit uncertainty. A great deal of research on the perceptual and neurophysiological functioning of the infant suggests that there is an important stage in central nervous system organization between 8 and 12 weeks of age (Dreyfus-Brisac, 1979). It is after this reorganization that the child behaves as if he or she recognizes the primary caretakers. By contrast, exposure to several caretakers might mute the discrepant quality of a change in caretaker because the infant's experience will have led to the expectations of variety.

The next significant change occurs at 9 to 12 months of age when a major cognitive competence emerges. Toward the end of the first year, the infant frequently displays an increase in attention to a variety of discrepant events, more prolonged attention than he did when he was 4 to 6 months old, and generalized motor inhibition to unexpected events. There is also a dramatic increase in the likelihood of facial expressions of wariness and crying in response to an event whose major characteristic is that it is a discrepant transformation of a schema for an earlier or immediately past experience. I suggest that the temporal concordance of increased attentiveness to discrepancy, inhibition, wariness, and distress to discrepant events is due to the emergence of several related cognitive competences. These include the child's ability to retrieve a schema related to his present experience, despite minimal incentive cues in the immediate field, and the child's ability to retain that schema in active memory while he compares the retrieved structure with the present event in an attempt to resolve the discrepancy or inconsistency. These suggestions are supported by several experiments (Brody, 1981; Fox, Kagan, & Weiskopf, 1979; Kagan & Hamburg, 1981; Szpak, 1977).

I believe that the major differences between the cognitive functioning of a 10- and 3-month old are that the older infant can establish a schema more quickly, can retrieve a representation of the prior event with minimal incentive in the immediate field and after a longer temporal delay, and can hold the representations of the event and his schema in short-term memory for a longer period of time. As a result, the 10-month-old shows both more prolonged attention to an event and more vulnerability to uncertainty because his ability to compare the schema with the event for a longer time permits him to work at resolving the discrepancy between the two events. If the child cannot do so, she becomes vulnerable to distress. Thus, during the last part of the first year, the infant becomes vulnerable to the stressors of separation from the caretaker and exposure to unfamiliar adults because of enhanced cognitive ability.

Recent research on the relation of indices of attachment at one and two years of age (typically the Ainsworth Strange Situation) to behavioral outcomes at one to three years of age suggests the possibility of a profound interaction between the child's temperament and the parental practices presumed to produce secure and less secure attachments (Ainsworth, Blehar, Waters, & Wall, 1978; Arend, Gove, & Sroufe, 1979). It is assumed that infants who smile easily, accept affection, and are easy to handle when raised by mothers who are physically affectionate, predictable, and nonpunitive should be most likely to be securely attached at 12 and 18 months of life;

while extremely fearful or irritable babies raised by mothers who are less affectionate and/or more punitive should be less securely attached (Ainsworth, Blehar, Waters, & Wall, 1978). The combination of a temperament prone to distress and a mother who is a less effective modulator of uncertainty should produce less securely attached children. Preliminary data suggest the latter child at age three is less likely than the former to possess the qualities valued by this culture, especially a tendency toward exploration, autonomy, and sociability, as well as a reasonable compliance to parental requests (Joffe, 1981; Arend, Gove, & Sroufe, 1979).

During the last half of the second year, children develop their first appreciation of right and wrong. The child becomes vulnerable to a special uncertainty that follows violation of standards, either imposed by others or self-generated. By four years of age, this internal state will meet the criteria for the affective construct we call guilt.

The 2- and 3-year-old child also shows evidence of awareness of self as an agent who can affect others, and of an ability to empathize with the emotional states of others (Kagan, 1981; Lewis & Brooks-Gunn, 1979). Thus, if a sibling is born at this time, in contrast to the period prior to 15 months, the child is able to realize that he or she is being treated with less attentiveness, can empathize with the state of the young sibling, and can generate ideas of displacement and disappointment. Helen Koch (1965) has suggested that the stressful potential of the arrival of a new sibling tends to be maximal when the older child is between 2 and 4 years of age.

The major changes in cognitive function at 5 to 7 years of age are a derivative of the competences that accompany Piaget's concrete operational stage. The child is now able to seriate the self, in comparison with others, on qualities that are culturally valued. The child is now capable of comparing her intelligence, popularity, or attractiveness with peers, and of experiencing the anxiety that comes from recognizing that she is less in command of a favored characteristic than are others. This competence and accompanying vulnerability occur at the time of school entrance when children are being evaluated on their academic mastery and on the degree to which they possess the behaviors that define sex-role standards.

The entrance into the stage of formal operations initiates another source of uncertainty—the recognition that one's beliefs are not logically consistent. During the years following puberty, the child acquires several profound intellective capacities. First, she gains an ease in dealing with hypothetical premises that may violate reality. The young child, unlike the adolescent, does not appreciate the discontinuity between the self-contained information in a hypothetical problem and the egocentric information she carries for more practical challenges. To appreciate that problems are self-contained entities, solved by special rules, is a magnificent accomplishment not usually attained until early adolescence. Second, the adolescent can assume a relativistic view, and is not troubled by the fact that the acceptability of a lie depends on both the situation and the intentions of the actor.

Of special relevance is the fact that the adolescent is disposed to examine her beliefs in sets and to search for inconsistencies among them and between her beliefs and related actions. Thus 14-year-olds brood about the inconsistency, for example, among the following three propositions: (1) God loves people. (2) The world contains many unhappy people. (3) If God loved people He would not make so many of them unhappy. The adolescent, unlike the 10-year-old, notes the contradictions, and can either deny one of the premises, assume that the conclusion serves an ulterior purpose, or deny the original hypothesis.

The adolescent must deal with the temptations of sexuality, independence, and hostility to parents; each of these violates earlier conclusions. Old assumptions are challenged by noting inconsistencies, and the resulting incompatibility is often resolved by delegitimizing the earlier premise. The questioning of old beliefs and a search for a new set of premises make the adolescent vulnerable to events which become stressors for the first time. Occasionally, the adolescent is left temporarily without a commitment to any belief, and this can produce a state of uncertainty and a need to resolve it. The ideational rebellion that has become definitional of adolescence serves not only hostility, but also the more pressing need to persuade the self that its mosaic of wishes, values, and behaviors derives from a personally constructed ideology. If what one believed were less central to the identity of the American young adult than it is at the present time, the clash of values between child and parent might not occur with such ferocity.

There are, undoubtedly, additional lawful relations between cognitive competences and vulnerability to distress that are the result of new interpretations of events that had been background during earlier stages. The main point of this section is to alert the reader to the fact that some aspects of the profile of distress are linked to uniform, ontogenetic changes in cognitive functioning.

Both theory and data imply that the potential for an external event to generate affect is a function of the cognitive interpretation imposed by the person. This principle is as valid for the stressors of divorce, desertion, poverty, and abuse as it is for encounter with strangers at 8 months of age. The poverty experienced by contemporary inner-city families in America might not have the same consequences as the poverty that was pervasive during the economic depression of 1930 to 1938 because of different assumptions of the causes of the privation and different expectations held by the two groups of economically disadvantaged citizens. We must always expect an interaction between the event and the psychological surface it strikes.

Although changes in cognitive function during the adult years do not have the degree of discontinuity characteristic of early childhood, modern essays on life-span development present persuasive arguments for the introduction of new adult premises generated out of reflections upon experience (Brim & Kagan, 1980). The loss of ambition, the appearance of apathy for loved ones, and boredom with vocation generate a dysphoric mood, but, as with young children, the ability to implement a coping reaction is therapeutic. As temperament monitors the degree of distress displayed by infants, economic conditions, and, therefore, the ability to cope, seem to be important monitors of outcome in adults.

Epilogue: An Evaluative Bias in the Concept of Stress

The word "stress" is a new addition to the scholar's vocabulary; it does not appear in 19th-century treatises on the psychology of the child or adult. However, the word "uneasiness" does. Both John Locke and Benjamin Franklin regarded uneasiness as the basic origin of goal-related behavior. I believe that 18th- and 19th-century theorists were more concerned with reasons for the adaptive behavior of the many than with the bases for the maladaptive behavior of the few. They conceived of the former as caused by internal motivations, and made the state of uneasiness a central motive for the profile of successful behaviors.

When scholars want to explain normative or universal properties, they typically look to the inherent characteristics of the entity. Thus water flows because of its inherent structure; infants attach to caretakers because of their natural dependence on adults. But when the entity violates its inherent script (the water does not flow), the scholar usually calls upon an efficient cause. Therefore, when a person's behavior deviates from what theorists assume is normative, they too call upon an efficient cause. In the present historical moment, that cause is often named a stressor. Thus, stress is most often invoked to explain the occurrence of less frequent, maladaptive reactions. It is counterintuitive to posit an inherent motive to being poor, socially ostracized, technically incompetent, hospitalized, or imprisoned. The use of stress, in this context, presupposes that asocial reactions are not an inherent property of humans, but—abnormal events requiring an efficient cause—a profound supposition about human nature.

Scholars writing in different historical periods vary in their conception of the natural properties of children and adults. Enlightenment philosophers regarded human nature as inherently aggressive, selfish, and cruel, and, therefore, had to explain episodes of civility, generosity, and kindness. Had John Adams used the word stressor, I suspect he would have applied it to socialization regimens, like the parental practice of admonishing a child for destroying property. By contrast, contemporary theorists view the young child as inherently affectionate, gentle, and competent, and try to explain his or her hostility. As a result, they are resistant to labelling the socialization practices of parents as stressors, even though these practices produce anxiety and anger in children, because stress presupposes an inimical outcome. Thus, the construct of stress has an incompletely disguised evaluative component which may be obstructing theoretical advance. Certain classes of events produce the affective reactions we label anxiety, fear, anger, depression, sadness, and hopelessness. Depending upon other conditions, these events and their accompanying reactions lead to socially adaptive or maladaptive behavior. The latter outcome is as much a function of the other conditions as of the incentive event. We cannot base our classifications of an incentive on the nature of the outcome for that judgment cannot be made a priori, only a posteriori. Reconstructive explanations can use the word stressor when the end of the story has been revealed, but prediction, which is central to theory, does not have that advantage.

REFERENCES

Adelson, E., & Fraiberg, S. Gross motor development in infants blind from birth. *Child Development*, 1974, *45*, 114–126.

Ainsworth, M. D. S., Blehar, M. C., Waters, E., & Wall, S. *Patterns of attachment*. Hillsdale N.J.: Lawrence Erlbaum Associates, 1978.

Arend, R., Gove, F., & Sroufe, L. A. Continuity of individual adaptation from infancy. *Child Development*, 1979, *50*, 950–959.

Brim, O. G., & Kagan, J. Constancy and change: A view of the issues. In O. G. Brim, & J. Kagan (Eds.), *Constancy and change in human development*. Cambridge, Mass.: Harvard University Press, 1980.

Brody, L. R. Visual short-term cued recall memory in infancy. *Child Development*, 1981, *52*, 242–250.

Bronson, G. W. Infants' reactions to unfamiliar persons and novel objects. *Monographs of the Society for Research in Child Development*, 1972, 37,(Serial No. 148).

Décarie, T. C. *The infant's reactions to strangers*. New York: International Universities Press, 1974.

Dollard, J., & Miller, N. E. *Personality and psychotherapy*. New York: McGraw-Hill, 1950.

Dreyfus-Brisac, C. Ontogenesis of brain bio-electrical activity and sleep organization in neonates and infants. In F. Falkner, & J. M. Tanner (Eds.), *Human growth* (Vol. 3). New York: Plenum, 1979.

Fitzgerald, R. D. Involvement of vagal activity in the unconditioned heart rate response of restrained rats. *Physiology and Behavior*, 1976, *17*, 785–788.

Fox, N., Kagan, J., & Weiskopf, S. The growth of memory during infancy. *Genetic Psychology Monograph*, 1979, 99, 91–130.

Fraiberg, S. The development of human attachments in infants blind from birth. *Merrill-Palmer Quarterly*, 1975, *21*, 315–334.

Gabella, G. *Structure of the autonomic nervous system*. London: Chapman and Hall, 1976.

Garcia-Coll, C. *Behavioral inhibition and heart rate variability in two-year-olds*. Unpublished doctoral dissertation. Harvard University, 1981.

Gellerman, R. G. *Psychological development of the Vietnamese child in the second year of life*. Unpublished doctoral dissertation. Harvard University, 1981.

Golden, M. *Aspects of childhood in classical Athens*. Unpublished doctoral dissertation. University of Toronto, 1981.

Gunnar, M. R. Control, warning signals and distress in infancy. *Developmental Psychology*, 1980, *16*, 281–289.

Jacobson, J. L. Cognitive determinants of wariness toward unfamiliar peers. *Developmental Psychology*, 1980, *16*, 347–354.

Jameson, J., & Gordon, A. *Separation protest in children with the failure to thrive syndrome*. Unpublished paper, 1977.

Joffe, L. S. *The quality of mother-infant attachment and its relationship to compliance with maternal commands and prohibitions*. Paper presented at the meeting of The Society for Research in Child Development, Boston, Massachusetts, April, 1981.

Kagan, J. Emergent themes in human development. *American Scientist*, 1976, *64*, 186–196.

Kagan, J. *The second year*. Cambridge: Harvard University Press, 1981.

Kagan, J., & Hamburg, M. The enhancement of memory in the first year. *Journal of Genetic Psychology*, 1981, *138*, 3–14.

Kagan, J., Kearsley, R. B., & Zelazo, P. R. *Infancy: Its place in human development*. Cambridge: Harvard University Press, 1978.

Kagan, J., & Moss, H. A. *Birth to maturity*. New York: John Wiley, 1962.

Katona, P. G., & Jih, F. Respiratory sinus arrhythmia: Noninvasive measure of parasympathetic cardiac control. *Journal of Applied Physiology*, 1975, *39*, 801–805.

Koch, H. L. Attitudes of children toward their peers as related to certain characteristics of their siblings. *Psychological Monographs*, 1965, *70*.

Lewis, M., & Brooks-Gunn, J. *Social cognition and the acquisition of self*. New York: Plenum, 1979.

Light, K. C. Cardiovascular responses to effortful active coping. *Psychophysiology*, 1981, *18*, 216–225.

Lusk, D. *Social cognition in the preschool years*. Unpublished doctoral dissertation. Harvard University, 1978.

Martin, B. The assessment of anxiety by physiological behavioral measures. *Psychological Bulletin*, 1961, *58*, 234–255.

Patterson, P. H., Potter, D. D., & Furshpan, E. J. The chemical differentiation of nerve cells. *Scientific American*, 1978, *239*, 50–59.

Phoenix, C. H., Goy, R. W., & Resko, J. A. Psychosexual differentiation as a function of androgenic stimulation. In M. Diamond (Ed.), *Perspectives in reproductive and sexual behavior*. Bloomington: Indiana University Press, 1968.

Plomin, R., & Rowe, D. C. Genetic and environmental etiology of social behavior in infancy. *Developmental Psychology*, 1979, *15*, 62–72.

Rheingold, H. L., & Eckerman, C. O. Fear of the stranger: A critical examination. In H. W. Reese (Ed.), *Advances in child development and behavior* (Vol. 8). New York: Academic Press, 1973.

Rorty, R. *Philosophy and the mirror of nature*. Princeton, N.J.: Princeton University Press, 1979.

Sackett, G. P., Ruppenthal, G. C., Fahrenbruch, C. E., Holm, G. A., & Greenough, W. T. Social isolation rearing effects in monkeys vary with genotype. *Developmental Psychology*, 1981, *17*, 313–318.

Spring, B., & Coons, H. Stress as a precursor of schizophrenic episodes. In R. W. J. Neufeld (Ed.), *Psychological stress and psychopathology*. New York: McGraw-Hill, 1982.

Suomi, S. J., Kraemer, G. W., Baysinger, C. M., & DeLizio, R. D. Inherited and experiential factors associated with individual differences in anxious behavior displayed by rhesus monkeys. In D. F. Klein, & J. Rabkin (Eds.), *Anxiety: New research and changing concepts*. New York: Raven Press, 1981.

Szpak, M. P. A *study of infant memory and play*. Unpublished honors thesis. Harvard University, 1977.

Tennes, K., Downey, K., & Vernadakis, A. Urinary cortisol excretion rates and anxiety in normal 1-year-old infants. *Psychosomatic Medicine*, 1977, 39, 178–187.

Thomas, A., & Chess, S. Development in middle childhood. *Seminars in Psychiatry*, 1972, 4, 331–341.

Thomas, A., & Chess, S. *Temperament and development*. New York: Brunner/Mazel, 1977.

Zaslow, M. A *study of social behavior*. Unpublished doctoral dissertation. Harvard University, 1977.

CHAPTER 8

SOCIAL-EMOTIONAL DEVELOPMENT AND RESPONSE TO STRESSORS

ELEANOR E. MACCOBY
PROFESSOR OF PSYCHOLOGY
STANFORD UNIVERSITY

INTRODUCTION

The chapters in this volume have made clear that there is great variation at any given age in the vulnerability of individuals to disruption by potential stressors. My purpose here, however, is not to enter into the discussion of factors that govern individual differences, but rather to focus attention on developmental change. I will attempt to describe a set of developmental progressions, occurring in most children in a fairly predictable sequence, which are likely to have a bearing on the nature of stress and coping.

Necessarily, the account will be speculative. With notable exceptions (e.g., Murphy, 1962; Haan, 1977) the concept of stress has not occupied a central place in the work of developmental psychologists. Indeed, to people like myself who are outsiders to the work on stress, the term has something of a bad reputation. It is known to have many surplus meanings. And as the other papers in this volume have made clear, "stress" has been used to describe several quite different elements in a chain of events. Yet there seems to be fairly good agreement about the nature of this chain: it begins with an arousing event which disrupts the organism's equilibrium; alerting responses occur, which are usually accompanied by strong affect; and the organism engages in a set of problem-solving efforts, which either return the organism to the prior organizational status or produce a new organization. In the worst case, a state of disorganization persists. While events differ in their power to arouse or alert the organism, it has been frequently noted that there is no such thing as an event which is stressful for all people at all times under all conditions. While the intensity of a stimulus appears to be an important factor in its arousal potential, it is probably not the most important one. Its familiarity and predictability appear to be of especially great importance (Berlyne, 1960).

The question of the amount and affective quality of arousal is an important one, for which we do not have good answers. It is tempting to think of a continuum of arousal, with moderate levels of arousal (occurring in response to moderately intense stimulation, or stimulation that is only moderately discrepant from expectations) producing a sense of challenge and pleasantly excited affect, while higher levels produce disorganization and distress. We know that people enjoy and seek moderate levels of arousal, and it seems not unreasonable that there might be some point on the arousal scale where stimulation suddenly becomes excessive, and the affective response switches from pleasant to unpleasant. Such a concept fits our intuition that children who are laughing excitedly can easily switch to tears with only a small change in the eliciting circumstances. Yet in our own work (Stanford Longitudinal Project, unpublished report), in which we have produced mild stress in infants ages 9, 12, or 18 months by presenting a series of animated toys with increasing potential to frighten, we have not found a switch from high positive to high negative affect. Children who are pleased and interested in the toys at the lower end of the series go through a period of neutral affect in the middle of the series before they turn to mild and then stronger negative affect. For the following discussion, I shall assume the primacy of the distinction between positive and negative affect, implying (1) that these two emotional states are on opposite ends of a scale; (2) that some forms of stimulation are likely to be associated with positive, others with negative, affect; and (3) that negative affective states are far more likely than positive ones to cause or accompany disorganized states. Indeed, it might be wise to adopt a distinction similar to the one made by Antonovsky (1979) in distinguishing between *tension* and *stress*. In his usage, tension is the organism's response to potentially stressful conditions, and it accompanies coping processes; stress describes the organism's state when coping efforts are proving unsuccessful. Tension may be an affectively positive state. Stress never is.

Development and Overall Vulnerability to Stress

If the unfamiliarity of situations is an important element in their capacity to act as stressors, then the younger the person, the greater should be the probability of stress induction. The young child is a universal stranger to the world's events and lacks experience with a large variety of situations. Furthermore, if adults are protected from becoming disorganized under intense or novel stimulation by a considerable repertoire of coping skills, the young child lacking such skills should be especially vulnerable. However, there are counterbalancing factors that favor the young. We cannot be upset by events whose power to harm we do not understand; we cannot be humiliated by failure to handle problems whose solutions are someone else's responsibility; we cannot be distressed by anticipating others' contemptuous or critical reactions to our weaknesses if we are not aware of others' probable reactions and if our egos are not yet invested in appearing strong and competent. So young children are buffered against many phenomena that would produce distress in older people. We should not overlook the possibility that some of this buffering is built into the organism, in the sense that the onset of being able to perceive certain kinds of threat may be part of a very specific developmental timetable. The early observations of Hebb (1946), and the more recent ones of Sackett (1966), and Suomi (1977) with monkeys and apes, have indicated that there are stimuli (e.g., snakes; or threatening gestures from other animals) that do not initially produce emotional reactions in young animals, but which come to be fear- or anger-producing at a fairly predictable age even for animals that have had no prior exposure to them. There is no reason to believe that humans are immune to being governed, to some degree, by such developmental timetables, although the age of onset and the overlay from learning may differ considerably by species. The onset of wariness over strange people may be an example of a preprogrammed temporal sequence in human children. Considering the factors that might make young organisms more vulnerable to stress, and those that might make them less so, we must start with this hypothesis:

1. *It is unlikely that there is any linear increase or decrease with age in vulnerability to stress.*

Having said this, we must hasten to add that the nature of the events which are capable of producing stress reactions, and the nature of the coping responses that can be mobilized, do change drastically with age.

It is also likely, as many writers have said, that individuals go through cycles, moving from periods of stabilization to periods of destabilization. An episode of destabilization may last for some time, and then be followed by a new level of stabilization. Such cycles are sometimes linked to powerful maturational changes such as the onset of walking (which brings the infant into contact with a wide range of new experiences) or, more powerful still, the onset of puberty. In other cases, the destabilization occurs in response to external events, such as the loss of a loved person.

We may assume that children's success in achieving new levels of stabilization following disruption depends, at least in part, on the skill with which their parents respond. A distressed, disorganized child imposes additional stresses upon caretakers. If the parents themselves can control their own frustration reactions and engage in their own forms of problem-solving, seeking ways to help the child reorganize, progressive rather than regressive solutions are no doubt fostered.

Internal and External "Structure"

Human attentional capacity is limited at any age, and we cannot respond stimultaneously to multiple inputs that require focal attention. However, as people grow older, more and more of their responses can be put on "automatic pilot." That is, behavioral sequences can be executed with only marginal attention. Thus, adults can walk, eat, or drive a car while participating in a conversation. Certain amounts of change and unpredictability in an unattended-to activity can be handled without requiring focal attention: e.g., an individual need not be distracted from a conversation by a change in the position of utensils at the dinner table; nor be distracted by most movements of other cars while driving. The driver can speed up or slow down as required, reacting automatically to moment-to-moment changes in perceptual inputs, and still have attentional capacity available for other enterprises. We could compile an impressive list of the activities that experienced adults are capable of carrying out with minimal attention. For young children, almost no activities have yet become automatic in this sense. The child of 12 to 14 months is greatly preoccupied by the mere act of walking. It requires attention for young children to respond to moment-to-moment perceptual changes which later will be responded to, but will not be noticed and will not interfere with other activities. It follows that young children should be able to cope with an unexpected, potentially distressing event more competently if there is little concurrent change in other aspects of the environment. Therefore, a second developmental hypothesis is:

2. *The younger the child, the greater the importance of environmental structure in reducing the child's vulnerability to behavioral disruption under potentially stressful conditions.*

Structure, of course, is a fuzzy concept, but here it means the presence of familiar routines and a predictable, understandable physical and social environment. Hypothesis 2 implies that not too many elements of the child's environment—even what seem like trivial elements—can change at once without the changes becoming stressful.

The Growth of Inhibitory Controls

Too much intense or novel stimulation overwhelms an infant, and the result is an emotional storm—an episode of crying or a tantrum—which disrupts all the infant's behavior patterns and halts problem-solving activity. Older persons can continue to carry on many organized activities even when under considerable stress and while experiencing strong negative affect. Only in rare states of outright panic do we see the degree of disorganization that is fairly common in infants and very young children. Thus the hypothesis:

3. *With an arousing event leading to strong negative affect, the younger the child the greater the likelihood of extensive behavioral disorganization.*

There is reason to believe that the maturation of the nervous system during early childhood contributes to children's increasing ability to inhibit crying and frustration reactions and to maintain behavioral organization. "Encephalization" of neural functioning continues progressively through childhood. An example from very early in the life cycle is the disappearance of spinal reflexes through inhibition by higher centers as these become functional. We can document the progressive improvement in certain behavioral processes that call for inhibition. Luria (1961) showed, some time ago, that an instruction not to act, when given to a young child who is awaiting either a "stop" or "go" signal, will act as a releaser rather than an inhibitor of the action. And though the role of inner speech (which Luria claimed was responsible for the growth of inhibitory capacities) is in doubt (Flavell, 1977; Miller, Shelton, & Flavell, 1970), there is little doubt about the phenomenon: children improve rapidly, during the preschool years, in their ability to inhibit movements. For example, Ward (1973), asked children to slow down their normal pace of walking or drawing a line; he found an increase between the ages of 3½ and 5 years in the ability to follow this instruction. Furthermore, there is a progression in terms of the source of inhibitory signals; children can inhibit a movement on the basis of an external signal before they can do so "voluntarily"—that is, with self-given instructions. While the evidence on neural growth of central inhibitory structures is incomplete in humans, we know enough about the development of these structures in animals to surmise that they must play a role in the progressive control of impulsive behavior in human children. Altman, Brunner, and Bayer (1973), in a review paper on the role of the hippocampus in animals, write: "The hippocampus has a role in behavioral maturation by contributing to the transformation of unrestrained and rash juveniles into placid and cautious adults" (p. 581). Others have noted the role of this segment of the brain in regulating emotional states. Species vary in how rapidly the hippocampus matures, but in humans it does not achieve fully mature form until approximately the age of six years (Rose, 1976). The ability to control disorganizing emotional storms, then, may be seen as at least partially linked to physiological maturation.

Regression

We may speculate that an additional reason why young children more often experience highly disorganized states is that they lack "fallback" positions when a dominant behavior pattern is disrupted. Older persons probably derive an advantage from the progressive increases in the complexity of their biobehavioral organization, in that they have less complex, but still adequate, levels of organization to turn to at times of stress. By contrast, young children have fewer temporary, regressive solutions which could provide a breathing space for mobilizing coping efforts. If busy adults encounter additional pressures which threaten to be "the straw that breaks the camel's back," there are things they can do to simplify their lives: e.g., cancel some items on their agendas, arrange to postpone deadlines, or reduce their performance standards. The diminished parenting that occurs under the impact of stressors that are external to the parent-child relationship, wherein parents behave as though short-term child-rearing goals had become more salient and long-term ones less so (cf., Maccoby & Martin, in press, for summary), may be seen as a case of a simplifying, regressive action.

Can children also make use of regressive strategies? Since the early experimental work of Barker, Dembo, and Lewin (1941), the phenomenon of regression in childhood has received little systematic study. Wallerstein (this volume) has pointed to what she calls the "suspended agendas" of children whose parents are divorcing—agendas which are resumed when the child's network of interpersonal relationships is restabilized. Heinicke and Westheimer (1966) noted the halting of progress in language acquisition on the part of two-year-olds who had undergone painful separation from their parents; it was only after the high-anxiety portion of the reunion period was over that the children showed renewed spurts of language development. A similar phenomenon may be seen in attenuated form during studies of attachment. Often, when a young child's mother leaves the child alone in an unfamiliar room, there are periods of immobility; the duration of bouts of play declines, and sometimes there is also a switch to more primitive forms of toy usage (Maccoby & Feldman, 1972). A favorite example of regression in young children is the return to earlier modes of behavior upon the birth of a sibling. Clearly, young children can and do regress. The suggestion here is simply that young children have fewer regressive options that will serve to maintain an organized behavioral state. Their current levels of organization are built upon a weaker, simpler structure of earlier organizations.

The Role of Attachment in Coping

Others in this volume provide plentiful evidence for the importance of prepared reactions insulating individuals against behavioral disorganization under potentially stressful conditions. Young children clearly have a smaller repertoire of prepared reactions that are tailored to specific possible dangers. However, they do have an all-purpose prepared response: *in case of threat, go to attachment figures*. Our next developmental principle is:

> 4. *With increasing age, there is an increasing repertoire of situationally relevant coping behaviors, permitting a lessening of exclusive reliance on the availability of the primary attachment figure under stressful conditions.*

Brown and Harris (1978) have presented evidence that the loss of a parent (more specifically, the mother) at any time under the age of 11 may produce disruptions whose sequelae are detectable at later points in the life cycle. Developmental psychologists have been accustomed to focusing on the attachment-to-parent bond in the first few years of life. Several writers (Bowlby, 1969; Marvin, 1977) have described the transition from the early form of attachment, which requires the parent's physical presence, to the more mature form (beginning around the age of three), whereby children can derive support from more distant forms of linkage with their attachment figures. However, little attention has been paid to the forms and functions of attachment to parents in the middle childhood years. We can only assume that within the eleven-year period that Brown and Harris identify as one of heightened vulnerability to disruption of the primary attachment relationship, there are important distinctions to be made in the nature of the stress involved in loss, and in the means children have of coping with it.

Also, if proposition 4 above is true, we must assume that the older children become, the better able they are to cope with *other* stressors when the attachment figure is absent. Thus, one of the main reasons why the loss of the attachment figure is traumatic—the interference with the all-purpose prepared response that young children use to deal with a large variety of stressful situations—is attenuated with development. However, the advantage that older children have in being better able to manage on their own must be counterbalanced by a number of factors that serve to make the loss more acute. Older children understand the finality of death, and also probably are less able to transfer their affections to a new attachment figure within a brief period (see review by Schowalter, 1975).

Changing Relationships to Authority Figures

Children, of course, derive considerable protection from the watchful guidance of adults, and this includes adults outside the family as well as parents. On the whole, children are aware of benefits they derive from their relationships to adults, and, at least until adolescence, most children take an obedient stance toward adult authority. Within the age range of 4 to 10, however, there is considerable change in the way children conceive of authority—what legitimizes it, and what is the basis of their own obligation toward authority figures. Damon (1977) has charted these transitions. He shows that children of preschool age tend to deny that there is any conflict between what they want and what their parents require of them—and this is true, despite numerous instances in which children of this age overtly resist parental demands. A little later, children believe that authority is legitimized by power: might makes right, and they think that parents, teachers, and police have the right to tell children what to do because they are larger and stronger and can punish infractions. Still later, the idea emerges that persons in authority occupy their positions, and derive their rights, from the fact that they have more knowledge and are more competent. And at least in our society, as children approach adolescence, they begin to say that there are limitations on the rights of persons in authority to exercise control over others—limits having to do with the range of their knowledge and competency. The idea even emerges that there are situations in which children may know more than adults, and in which the adults should therefore follow the children's lead. Clearly these changes constitute preparation for the more active rejection of at least some aspects of adult authority often seen in adolescence. The age changes outlined above lead to this hypothesis:

5. *The obedient stance toward adult authority taken by most children during the preadolescent years constitutes a buffer against stress.*

When children are following the instructions of others whom they trust, they experience little anxiety about the outcome, and are at least partially protected from guilt or a sense of failure over negative outcomes. However, throughout the preadolescent years, there is a gradual shift from reliance on external guidance to reliance on self-regulation.

The Interface of Peer Relations and Self Concepts

A corollary of the declining importance of attachment to parents as a coping response is the increasing reliance on peers. Once the age is reached when close friendships can be formed, children, of course, are subject to being distressed by the loss or disruption of a friendship. And the lack of friendship—unpopularity—is one of the most common, and most potent, sources of distress from about school-entry age on. With age, the nature and meaning of friendships change (Youniss, 1975; Selman, 1976; Damon, 1977). In the preschool and early school-age years, a friend is simply someone with whom one plays and shares activities. Also present at this age is the notion that in friendship, one shares toys or treats. After this age, the themes of sharing thoughts, or exchanging confidences and trust, of helping one another to face troubles and to sustain a happy mood are more frequently represented. Thus:

> 6. *The nature of the distress imposed by absence or disruption of peer friendships changes with age, from loss of valued activities to loss of emotional support.*

The changing meaning of friendship implies the development of new strengths, including the ability to enter into a relationship of mutual trust and obligation, a development which lays the groundwork for satisfying relationships in adulthood. It also implies an increased consciousness of what is fair and legitimate in demands between friends, and an increasing sensitivity to being treated unfairly by friends.

The nature of quarrels with peers changes. Preschool children, when they fight, tend to do so over desired objects or the invasion of one another's space. The objective of participants in a fight, generally, is to get possession of the object or maintain dominance of the space. After about the age of 6 quarrels more and more take the form of an exchange of insults, and the objective is to hurt the victims' feelings or to make them lose status (Hartup, 1974). These changes in the quality of peer aggression signal some important developments in the nature of self concepts. The growing use of insults means that children know that other children are becoming capable of being insulted. This implies that childrens' sense of personal worth or status more and more rests on being able to display certain selected attributes to others, and leads to the hypothesis that:

> 7. *The self is progressively defined in terms of a set of aspirations, ideals, competencies, and ego investments. The child is much more vulnerable in the invested than the noninvested regions.*

A very young child will become angry if persistently called by the wrong name or given the wrong sex label, but beyond this there are few aspects of self-definition that are sufficiently well established to call for defense. With increasing age, children stake out their own territory. They make choices, though often not deliberate ones, concerning the activities they want to excel in. Childhood, and especially adolescence, are periods of trial and error, of experimentation with objectives, personal agendas, and the choice of areas for investment of effort. Ego investment entails vulnerability to stress. Failure in an uninvested area is not especially distressing; failure in an activity which has become part of one's self-definition is. Children can insulate themselves against this kind of stress by reducing the number of areas in which they aspire to competence: e.g., a poorly coordinated child can decide not to be interested in sports. A reduction in the level of performance aspired to is one of the most common forms of adjustment to academic failures (Dweck & Gilliard, 1975). To disinvest one's ego from certain areas may be a constructive move; it permits energy and coping responses to be concentrated on enterprises which offer a chance of success. But the relinquishment of too many territories can become pathological, and the growing child must find a balance between striving for too many things and striving for too few.

Failure itself changes its definition. As Ruble (1983) has shown, children in the early school years seldom define their successes or failures in comparative terms. They are relatively unconcerned, at least with respect to the activities that have been assessed, with whether their performance is better or worse than other children's, and they tend to be satisfied if they can complete a task or get the right answer to a problem. This changes, however:

> 8. *With increasing age, children make increasing use of social comparison in evaluating their own performance.*

This change, of course, entails a new vulnerability. Now it is not enough merely to finish a task. It must be done better or faster than other children can do it. Thus a fifth-grade child who has strong academic aspirations can be distressed by being only the second-best student in the class, while as a first- or second-grader this child would probably have been unconcerned about rank order, and satisfied with his or her own performance.

Young children are relatively unaware of how they are seen by others, but:

9. *With age, there is increasing sensitivity to, and understanding of, the reactions of others to the self.*

Selman (1976) has charted a series of developmental changes in children's ability to take the perspective of others toward the self. As these changes occur, children begin to tailor their activities so as to make certain impressions on others. They have an image which they wish to project. They therefore become vulnerable to being humiliated or shamed if they behave in public in a way that is not seen as consistent with their desired image. They begin to take great pains about their appearance, and they become skilled at devising a cover story which will rationalize any discrepancies between how they want to be seen and the way they fear others may interpret their actions. An implication of principles 7 and 8 above is that the nature of stressors becomes more individualized. In older children, the definition of danger can be quite personal, and can depend on the nature of the identity or territory the individual has chosen to defend. Of course, there continue to be more universal threats as well.

The Growth of Self-Appraisal and Other Cognitive Strategies

The increasing awareness of one's image as perceived by others is part of a larger growth process, which has come to be called "metacognition" (Flavell, 1979):

10. *At about the age of school entry, children begin to develop skills at monitoring their own thought processes and performances.*

This means that they begin to ask themselves how much they know about something, and how much they need to learn; how ready they are to take a test; or how well they have understood the instructions they have been given. Metacognitive skills imply both a new order of coping skills, and a new vulnerability. Self-testing enables individuals to prepare themselves more efficiently for forthcoming situations, and hence reduces the likelihood of failure. It also implies increasing awareness of one's own weaknesses as well as strengths. Metacognition is also involved in impulse control. Mischel and Mischel (1976) have shown that the ability to delay gratification is related to the strategies children use during a waiting period. Whereas young children are unaware of what their own strategies are, or which ones are likely to work best, older children know that they ought to remove temptations from view and distract themselves during the waiting period. Thus, they begin to monitor their own frustration state in a way that contributes to their ability to cope with it.

Cognitive science, and specifically the science of cognitive development, has burgeoned so rapidly in the past decade that it would be beyond the scope of this paper (and the competence of the writer) to list all the aspects of cognitive development that are relevant to stress and coping. Some major themes can be mentioned, however. Piaget (1958) claimed that children, in the stage of formal operations, are capable of forms of problem-solving (e.g., systematic trial and error in testing a hypothesis) which younger children do not employ. Since Piaget formulated this view, there has been a great deal of work on problem-solving and how it changes with age. Although there is now considerable skepticism concerning Piaget's stage-like progressions (Flavell, 1982), and considerable evidence that many children develop some of the skills presumably linked to formal operations at a much earlier age than Piaget claimed, there is little challenge to the idea that problem-solving skills do undergo development. The increasing use of metacognitive processes has already been mentioned. In addition:

> 11. *With age, there is increasing avoidance of premature closure.*

This means that children are increasingly aware that there may be a range of solutions to a problem extending from barely adequate to excellent, and that they are increasingly willing to persist in a search for the better solutions (Messer, 1976; Wollman, Eylon, & Lawson, 1979). Also:

> 12. *Problem-solving strategies become more planful, in the sense that (1) they are organized sequentially so that earlier steps provide information needed for later steps; (2) there is less redundancy; and (3) probable events farther in the future are taken into account.*

Older children, when they take in information, are more likely to take active steps to prepare for subsequent recall. For example, they use more rehearsal at the time of information input. In playing the game of twenty questions (work summarized by Flavell, 1977), instead of beginning by guessing a specific object, as a younger child would, they move to a sequential strategy which is hierarchically organized, asking a series of preparatory questions which do not reveal the required answer but serve to reduce subsequent errors drastically. They are increasingly able to plan several moves ahead in games such as chess, which do not allow for actual trial and error but where consideration of alternative moves must be done mentally. Their increasing future orientation is clearly shown in a recent study by Lewis (1981), in which adolescents participated in a simulated peer-counselling session and offered advice to peers concerning the solution of real-life sorts of problems. In the age range 12 to 18, there was increasing mention of possible risks and potential future consequences of various solutions. As Flavell has noted (1977), these improved decision strategies are something which children themselves bring to the problem-solving situation, not something inherent in the problems being presented. Indeed, as Sternberg and Powell (in press) point out, "executive processes" assume increasing importance as intellectual development proceeds.

We may presume that the increased planfulness and strategic organization which older children bring to contrived experimental situations are also employed in ways whereby they manage the sequential structure of their own lives. They become capable of "nesting" plans of action in complex ways, so that a short sequence of actions (e.g., studying for a weekly exam) is undertaken to serve an intermediate-range goal (doing well in a course), which is in turn a subgoal of a still more global plan (doing well in high school and becoming eligible for college).

What are the implications for stress and coping of these changes in cognitive strategies? Along with the more mature problem-solving strategies, the development of a future orientation fosters increasingly enduring, rather than temporary, problem solutions. However, it also means that children become more and more aware of possible risks, with the result that many older children experience increasing anxieties about events which they can now foresee but feel unable to protect themselves against. We do not know how the increased awareness of risks and the increased sense of efficacy in problem-solution balance out in most children. The most we can say is that there are great variations among individual children in the extent to which these two consequences of cognitive development proceed in synchrony.

Social Cognition

We should not underestimate the contribution of the sheer accumulation of knowledge to the development of coping skills. Recent studies of "expertise" (cf., Chi, 1978; Brown & DeLoache, 1978) have shown how experienced persons not only make finer perceptual distinctions but encode incoming information in a more organized way, thus fostering its subsequent retrieval. Experience also shapes the interpretation of social encounters. One has only to think about how a football game looks to a visitor from a foreign land, or a cricket game to an American visiting England, to realize the importance of the prior knowledge one brings to a situation in determining what is understood about the interactions of persons. As Schmidt (1976) has pointed out, cognitions about other people's actions always involve inferences concerning their intentions. The experienced viewer knows that when the quarterback moves backward surrounded by a group of other players, he is falling back to pass, and that the players surrounding him intend to protect him from probable efforts by opposing players to sack him behind the line. The action can only be understood by reference to the sequential plans we know players have. Any of us who have traveled in countries whose cultures are quite unlike our own are aware of how much effort is involved in trying to decipher the meaning of social actions when we do not have the experience to know the intentions of others. Like other "foreigners":

13. *The young child tends to process social information in small chunks and neither to cognize other persons' motives nor to understand the continuing consequences of interpersonal acts (see Collins, in press).*

Thus, for children, there is a great deal that is confusing in the actions of others, causing events to seem capricious which to older persons are lawful. As in the case of the development of problem-solving strategies, children's increasing social awareness carries both costs and benefits. Children are protected from the stresses that come from sensitivity to the meaning of others' actions—for example, they may not perceive slights unless they are quite blatant, nor do they feel humiliated over a failure to perceive another person's strategy in a negotiation in which both are involved. On the other hand, their defenses are poor against being manipulated by others, and they may not be able to take advantage of early signs of impending interpersonal crises in such a way as to forestall them.

The growing skill in understanding others' intentions is especially important as children pursue goals that cannot be accomplished alone. When children are young, the adults of a society are willing to adapt themselves to children's limited skills for cooperating with others in a social network, but this tolerance fades as adulthood is approached. Thus, it becomes necessary for the adolescent to know how to cooperate, how to persuade others to adopt his or her own plan of action, and how to enter into a system of mutual obligation that sustains joint enterprises. Considering the great value of improved social cognition for these enterprises, it seems likely that the benefits of developmental change in this system greatly outweigh the costs.

Overview

I have listed a series of developmental principles, some of which rest on a secure empirical foundation, and others which have more the status of hypotheses. In concluding, let us return briefly to the primacy of affect and some of its implications. We know that an individual's current behavior is greatly influenced by mood. Experiments in which a positive mood is artificially induced, sometimes by so simple an operation as asking the individual to recall a pleasant instead of an unpleasant event, show that people are better able to postpone gratification (Gregory, Yates, Lippett, & Yates, 1981), more willing to comply with others' requests, and more likely to be altruistic (cf., Isen, Horn, & Rosenhan, 1973; Masters, Felleman, & Barden, 1981). It has also been shown that experiences can have affective tags when stored in memory. Thus, current moods bias later recall. People who are sad or depressed tend to recall previous saddening or depressing events, whereas when in a positive mood, they are more likely to recall previous successes or good fortune (Bower, 1981). It follows that good moods induce optimism about one's self and one's future, and probably make more likely the undertaking of positive coping activities rather than the retreat into defensive postures. However, some recent studies suggest that healthy personality organization involves a somewhat unrealistic optimism and an exaggerated view of the self's own capacities, whereas depressed people seem to have a more accurate view of their own strengths and especially weaknesses (as judged by others) than do well-functioning persons (Alloy & Abramson, 1979; Lewinsohn, Mischel, Chaplin, & Barton, 1980). There is little systematic knowledge about the relationship of moods to developmental levels, other than that moods vary widely at any level. It is not unreasonable to believe that since episodes of agitated distress diminish with age, there are progressively fewer occasions on which the distresses of early childhood will be recalled and woven into appraisals of current situations. However, it is clear that older children are capable of sustaining moods, both good and bad, over longer periods than younger children are. We have no reason to believe that the experiences of middle childhood are systematically biased in one direction or the other.

In adolescence, the child moves from the relatively restricted milieu of home and classroom into a broader social environment. Even if personal experience is somewhat restricted, children become progressively more aware through public information sources of societal conditions that may possibly affect their own fate. What do these broadening perspectives do to the chances of an adolescent sustaining a positive mood? Here we must sound a somber note. Messages frequently received by young people are dolorous: the world is becoming more and more overpopulated; human beings are using up their resources too fast; crime is increasing; political institutions are incapable of solving national and international conflicts without violence; and the type of violence that can be unleashed is destructive beyond imagination. In addition, there is a continual disillusionment with, or disparagement of, heroes. Presumably, adequate coping requires hope. It must be difficult indeed for youth to sustain coping efforts directed toward social institutions and public issues in the face of these strongly negative messages about the future. It remains to be seen what coping and defensive maneuvers contemporary youth will increasingly employ as they face the transition to adulthood.

REFERENCES

Alloy, L. B., & Abramson, L. Y. Judgment of contingency in depressed and non-depressed students; sadder but wiser? *Journal of Experimental Psychology: General*, 1979, *108*, 441–485.

Altman, J., Brunner, R. L., & Bayer, S. A. The hippocampus and behavioral maturation. *Behavioral Biology*, 1973, *8*, 557–596.

Antonovsky, A. *Health, stress and coping*. San Francisco: Jossey-Bass, 1979.

Barker, R., Dembo, T., & Lewin, K. Frustration and regression; an experiment with young children. *University of Iowa Studies in Child Welfare*, 1941, *18*. Adapted for a briefer report in R. G. Barker, J. S. Kounin, & H. F. Wright (Eds.), *Child behavior and development*. New York: McGraw-Hill Book Company, 1943.

Berlyne, D. E. *Conflict, arousal and curiosity*. New York: McGraw-Hill Book Company, 1960.

Bower, G. Mood and memory. *American Psychologist*, 1981, *36*, 129–148.

Bowlby, J. *Attachment*. New York: Basic Books, 1969.

Brown, A. L., & DeLoache, J. S. Skills, plans and self-regulation. In R. Siegler (Ed.), *Children's thinking: What develops?* Hillsdale, N.J.: Lawrence Erlbaum Associates, 1978.

Brown, G. W., & Harris, T. *Social origins of depression: A study of psychiatric disorder in women*. New York: The Free Press, 1978.

Chi, M. T. H. Knowledge structures and memory development. In R. Siegler (Ed.), *Children's thinking: What develops?* Hillsdale, N.J.: Lawrence Erlbaum Associates, 1978.

Collins, W. A. Social effects of children's processing of televised social narratives. In E. T. Higgins, & D. N. Ruble (Eds.), *Developmental social cognition: A socio-cultural perspective*. New York: Cambridge University Press, in press.

Damon, W. *The social world of the child*. San Francisco: Jossey-Bass, 1977.

Dweck, C. S., & Gilliard, D. Expectancy statements as determinants of reactions to failure: Sex differences in persistence and expectancy change. *Journal of Personality and Social Psychology*, 1975, *32*, 1077–1084.

Flavell, J. H. *Cognitive development*. Englewood Cliffs, N.J.: Prentice-Hall, 1977.

Flavell, J. H. Structures, stages and sequences in cognitive development. In A. Collins (Ed.), *Minnesota symposium on child psychology* (Vol. 15). Hillsdale, N.J.: Lawrence Erlbaum Associates, 1982.

Flavell, J. H. Metacognition and cognitive monitoring. *American Psychologist*, 1979, *34*, 906–911.

Gregory, C. R., Yate, R., Lippett, M. R., & Yates, S. M. The effects of age, positive affect induction, and instructions on children's delay of gratification. *Journal of Experimental Child Psychology*, 1981, *32*, 169–180.

Haan, N. *Coping and defending: Processes of self-environment organization*. New York: Academic Press, 1977.

Hartup, W. W. Aggression in childhood: Developmental perspectives. *American Psychologist*, 1974, 29, 336–341.

Hebb, D. O. Emotion in man and animal: An analysis of the intuitive processes of recognition. *Psychological Review*, 1946, 53, 86–106.

Heinicke, C., & Westheimer, I. *Brief separations*. New York: International Universities Press, 1966.

Isen, A. M., Horn, N., & Rosenhan, D. L. Effects of success and failure on children's generosity. *Journal of Personality and Social Psychology*, 1973, 2, 239–247.

Lewis, C. How adolescents approach decisions: Changes over grades seven to twelve and policy implications. *Child Development*, 1981, 52, 538–544.

Lewisohn, P. M., Mischel, W., Chaplin, W., & Barton, R. Social competence and depression: The role of illusory self-perceptions. *Journal of Abnormal Psychology*, 1980, 89, 203–212.

Luria, A. R. *The role of speech in the regulation of normal and abnormal behavior*. New York: Pergamon Press, 1961.

Maccoby, E. E., & Feldman, S. S. Mother-attachment and stranger-reactions in the third year of life. *Monographs of the Society for Research in Child Development*, 1972, 37, No. 146.

Maccoby, E. E., & Martin, J. A. Parent-child interaction. In E. M. Hetherington (Ed.), *Manual of child psychology: Vol. 4. Social development*. New York: John Wiley and Sons, in press.

Marvin, R. S. An ethological-cognitive model for the attenuation of mother-child attachment behavior. In T. Alloway, P. Pliner, & L. Krames (Eds.), *Attachment behavior*. New York: Plenum Publishing Company, 1977.

Masters, J. C., Felleman, E., & Barden, R. Experimental studies of affective states in children. In *Advances in clinical child psychology* (Vol. 4). New York: Plenum Press, 1981.

Messer, S. Reflection-impulsivity: A review. *Psychological Bulletin*, 1976, 83, 1026–1052.

Miller, S. H., Shelton, J., & Flavell, J. H. A test of Luria's hypothesis concerning the development of verbal self-regulation. *Child Development*, 1970, 41, 651–665.

Mischel, W., & Mischel, H. A cognitive social-learning approach to morality and self regulation. In T. Lickona (Ed.), *Moral development and behavior*. New York: Holt, Rinehart and Winston, 1976.

Murphy, L. B. *The widening world of childhood: Paths toward mastery*. New York: Basic Books, 1962.

Piaget, J. *The growth of logical thinking from childhood to adolescence* (translated by A. Parsons, & S. Seagrin). New York: Basic Books, 1958.

Rose, D. H. *Dentate gyrus granule cells and cognitive development: Explorations in the substrates of behavioral change*. Unpublished doctoral dissertation. Harvard University, 1976.

Ruble, D. N. The development of social comparison processes and their role in achievement-related self-socialization. In E. T. Higins, & D. N. Ruble (Eds.), *Developmental social cognition: A socio-cultural perspective*. New York: Cambridge University Press, 1983.

Sackett, G. P. Monkeys reared in visual isolation with pictures as visual input: Evidence for an innate releasing mechanism. *Science*, 1966, *154*, 1468–1472.

Schmidt, C. F. Understanding human action: Recognizing the plans and motives of other persons. In J. S. Caroll, & J. W. Payne (Eds.), *Cognition and social behavior*. Hillsdale, N.J.: Lawrence Erlbaum and Associates, 1976.

Schowalter, J. E. Parent death and child bereavement. In B. Schoenberg, I. Gerber, A. Wiener, A. H. Kutscher, D. Peretz, & A. C. Carr (Eds.), *Bereavement: Its psychosocial aspects*. New York: Columbia University Press, 1975.

Selman, R. Social-cognitive understanding: A guide to educational and clinical practice. In T. Lickona (Ed.), *Moral development and behavior*. New York: Holt, Rinehart and Winston, 1976.

Sternberg, R. J., & Powell, J. S. The development of intelligence. In J. H. Flavell, & E. M. Markman (Eds.), *Handbook of child psychology: Cognitive development* (Vol. 3). New York: John Wiley and Sons, in press.

Suomi, S. J. Development of attachment and other social behaviors in rhesus monkeys. In T.

Alloway, P. Pliner, & L. Krames (Eds.), *Attachment behavior*. New York: Plenum Publishing Company, 1977.

Ward, W. *Development of self-regulatory behaviors*. Report of the Educational Test Service. Princeton, N.J., 1973.

Wollman, W., Eylon, B., & Lawson, E. Acceptance of lack of closure: Is it an index of advanced reasoning? *Child Development*, 1979, *50*, 656–665.

Youniss, J. Another perspective on social cognition. In A. Pick (Ed.), *Minnesota symposium on child psychology* (Vol. 9). Minneapolis: University of Minnesota Press, 1975.

CHAPTER 9

STRESS: A Change Agent for Family Process

GERALD R. PATTERSON
RESEARCH SCIENTIST
OREGON SOCIAL LEARNING CENTER
EUGENE, OREGON

STRESS: A CHANGE AGENT FOR FAMILY PROCESS

The main assumption is that the daily accumulation of hassles and crises can have a significant impact on certain microsocial processes making up social interactions. The impact is ordinarily short-lived, but, under certain conditions, what begins as a short-term deflection in an ongoing process can unfold into permanent shifts in a relationship. For example, all dyads in families of social aggressors are significantly more coercive than are comparable pairs within normal families (Patterson, 1982). While these dyads presumably arrive at such high levels of performance by slow increments, this slow process of change into increasing pathology is facilitated by the impact of daily hassles and crises impinging upon the dyad. In effect, familial crises are disrupters of normal family process. It is assumed that the significant covariation between familial crises and antisocial child behavior is brought about by the disruptive effect of the crises.

The idea that stressors—such as prolonged illness or economic crises—often have a detrimental effect on a relationship is, of course, a commonplace one: however, it has never been clear just how one might go about demonstrating this effect. For this reason, one focus of the present report is on searching for a reliable measure of the microsocial process sensitive to day-by-day changes in the stressors impinging upon the dyad. The question is, which aspects of social interaction are affected by stressors, and which are not? How are these changes to be measured?

Understanding how crises may have an impact on family process and child deviancy requires a reformulation of what is meant by the concepts of *trait* and *social interaction*. Some forms of child pathology, such as social aggression and, perhaps, depression and withdrawal, are thought to be, in part, the outcome of a process, and in part, traits (i.e., they represent dispositions generalizable across time and settings). Certainly, the recent reviews of the research literature (Olweus, 1980; Patterson, 1982) show this to be the case for antisocial behavior in children. However, there are several facets of such a trait that are usually ignored. It is hypothesized that a single variable determines the stability of the disposition; this same variable is thought to determine the level or rate at which it is performed. The hidden variable(s) concerns the irritable reactions of other people to the behavior of the child. The definitions of some traits, such as aggression, require that the behavior of both members of the dyad be included. It requires descriptions of both the disposition of the child to initiate aggressive reactions from family members, and the disposition of family members to initiate and provide reactions maintaining an ongoing deviant interaction. There is, then, a mutuality of effects. One family member's high level of social aggression defines a system providing reactions maintaining these behaviors. By the same token, the aggressive child is a master at eliciting the very reactions that will extend and maintain his aggressive initiations (Patterson, 1981, 1982).

The variables defining these mutual effects also define what is meant by a bilateral trait. They will be discussed in detail in a later section. However, as will be shown, one of the key reactions determining the child's antisocial behavior is the disposition of the mother, and secondarily the father, to react to the child in an irritable fashion. The greater the likelihood the parent will react irritably, the greater the likelihood the child will display high rates of social aggression (Patterson, 1981, 1982). It is thought that the parental disposition to react irritably produces the problem. Furthermore, the disposition of parents to react irritably disrupts the family's efforts to solve conflicts among its members, and this same disposition correlates not only with poor quality of resolution for family problems, but also with the number of crises impinging upon the family. The disposition of the parent to react to the child in an irritable fashion covaries with levels of child deviancy, poor familial problem-solving, and the rates with which crises impinge from outside the family.

The hypothesis to be examined is that a measure of the disposition of the mother to react irritably to the child will provide a reliable and sensitive indication of the impact of external familial crises. The mother-irritability measure stands, then, at the interface between what happens at a microsocial level and what occurs at a macrosocial level, outside the dyad. The data relating to these assumptions will be detailed in later sections.

Implications

The analysis of the interface between microsocial and macrosocial variables has some interesting implications for the construction of theories on coping and stress. These hypotheses have not been directly tested by the writer, or by anyone else. The formulation has to do with two general problems. The first is to define a stressor, and the second is to define the impact of a stressor on the individual.

In this formulation, stress is given a neutral valence, as stress does not necessarily disrupt psychological functioning: it can have a variety of effects, positive or negative, or no effect at all. Whether or not stress alters psychological adjustment depends on two general factors. First, is the individual an isolate, or is he a member of a group? If isolated and subjected to prolonged or severe stress, such a person is at risk for certain, largely negative, outcomes. Given that he or she is a member of one or more groups, I think the risk for negative outcomes may be generally reduced. In fact, the outcomes may even be positive (i.e., growth experiences). The determining factor here is whether the stressor alters the microsocial processes for key relationships. If, as in the case of the problem child and mother, the process shifts and becomes more pathological, then stress can be said to have a negative outcome for that dyad. However, it is conceivable that for some, extreme stress may increase the cohesiveness of the support group. For these individuals, the positive microsocial processes are facilitated, not disrupted. The bomber crew, the pioneer family, and the family living in cities bombed regularly during World War II did not invariably reflect a negative outcome.

I think the missing moderating variable in stress research has been that of *interactional processes*. This is not to deny the importance of individual differences in physiological tolerance for stress, or in coping and the perception processes, but the role of microsocial processes has been largely overlooked in the studies done to date. Methods are needed for measuring these variables, determining stress-related alterations, and then in turn, their correlations with positive, negative, and neutral outcomes. The present report is intended as a very modest redress of this oversight. Because of the data set on hand, the analyses focus on families of antisocial children. It will become clear in the following discussions that the concept of stress plays an important role in altering the interactions of members of these families.

EFFECTS OF STRESS ON MICROSOCIAL PROCESS

My primary interest is in understanding the conditions under which stress produces disruptions in family processes that are, in turn, related to pathological outcomes. Therefore, my perspective has a rather narrow focus. In general, it represents what Cairns (1979) calls a social interactional position. As used here, it is analogous to the view that the social milieu functions as a buffer (see Levine, this volume). It differs from that position primarily in its emphasis on a more microsocial level for the analyses of interaction. This includes a heavy reliance on a sequential analysis format.

Since its dramatic introduction into the psychiatric literature by Selye in the mid-1950s, the concept of stress has received very little attention from investigators studying social interaction at a microsocial level (Bell & Harper, 1977; Cairns, 1979; Gottman, 1980; Lamb, Suomi, & Stephensen, 1979; Raush, 1965; Sackett, 1977). I think that it is now time to move away from the last decade's effort to erect a general theory of stress and to focus instead on identifying critical parameters that characterize specific stress situations.

I doubt we are going to develop a useful general theory of stress. First, it is not clear just what is meant by the general term *stress*. At a general level it means that some unpleasant stimulus impinges upon the individual. It also implies that the stressor *may* produce a reaction that has negative implications for the long-term adjustment of that individual. The case for the functional relation between stressor and pathological reaction may rest upon the findings from tightly organized laboratory studies summarized by Levine and Ciarenello (this volume); but it also refers to the loosely correlated relations between stress and psychiatric symptoms based on retrospective data (Brown & Harris, 1978; Dohrenwend & Dohrenwend, 1974; Holmes & Masuda, 1974). The definitions of stressor also vary: noxious physical stimuli (Selye, 1976); separation of mothers from infants (Levine, this volume); death of the mother (Brown & Harris, 1978); divorce (Hetherington, Cox, & Cox, 1980; Wallerstein, this volume); concentration camps (Segal, this volume); infantry combat (Robins, 1981). A stressor has also been defined in terms of life change (Holmes & Masuda, 1978); perturbations in development during infancy (Lipsitt, this volume); presenting a stranger to an infant (review by Kagan, this volume); or the impact of a premature infant on the mother (Leiderman, this volume). Most writers express disbelief in the utility of constructing a taxonomy of stressors (Eisdorfer, 1981; Kagan, this volume; Rutter, this volume). The consensus of the steering committee for Research

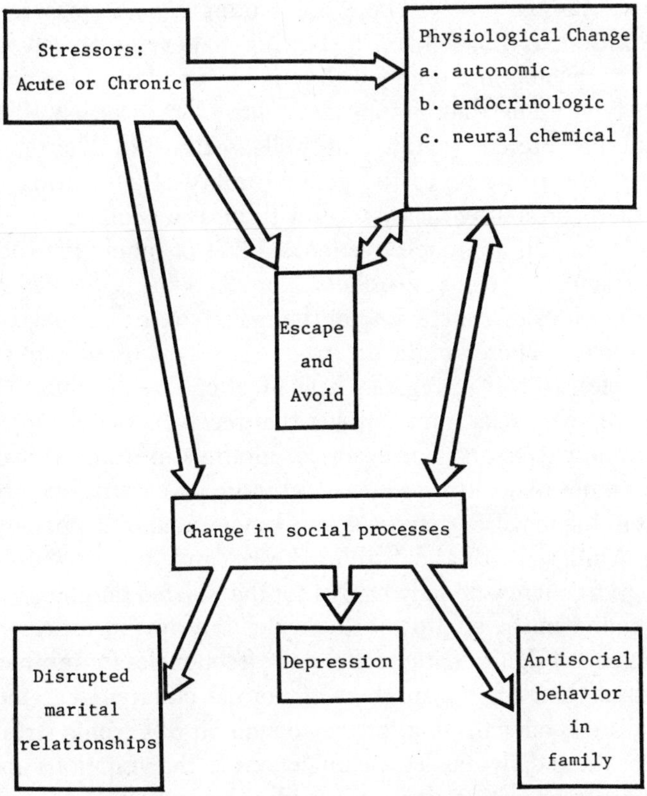

Figure 9-1. Stress as a process variable.

on Stress in Health and Disease was that "after thirty years no one has formulated a definition of stress that satisfied even a majority of stress researchers" (Eisdorfer, 1981, p. 1).

What, then, is a stressor? There seems to be no general answer to that question. However, I believe that if one limits one's vision to some subset of the various phenomena related to stress and stress reactions, one may make some progress in these matters (i.e., construct a theory about some manageable subset of this larger question). In the present report, the focus for this more modest enterprise will be the study of the impact of stress on family interaction processes. While these terms will be discussed in detail in following sections, suffice it to say here that the term *process* refers to structures that change over time. *Structure* describes the functional (statistical) relation between one behavioral event and some other event that precedes or follows it.

It seems reasonable to begin by emulating the productive procedures employed in the retrospective studies of Brown and Harris (1978) and

Holmes and Masuda (1974). There are a number of studies reviewed by Sarason, Johnson, and Siegal (1978) showing that events perceived as negative tend to correlate more highly with long-term pathologic outcomes than do Holmes-type items that simply assess life change per se. The studies reviewed in the present volume, as well as those in Dohrenwend and Dohrenwend (1974), attest to the general utility of measuring *major* life crises and then correlating these scores with measures of adjustment. However, I think such an approach overlooks a fact of family life that may be potentially useful to stress researchers: caretakers are subjected to a daily round of *minor* hassles. These are not the major stressors one would discuss with one's analyst. These are the day-to-day crises discussed with a friend (if one is available). In the aggregate, their effect can be profound.

There are, of course, some families that receive a richer supply of both major and minor stressors. For example, mothers in lower socioeconomic classes have more major stress events and more psychiatric symptoms than do mothers in higher SES groups (Myers, Lindenthal, & Pepper, 1974). The findings of Wahler (1980) and Wahler, Leske, and Roberts (1977) demonstrated a high frequency of daily hassles for the isolated families of antisocial children who live in the ghettos of Knoxville. Our own measures of familial daily hassles reveal significantly higher daily frequencies for mothers of antisocial children than for the mothers of normal children. For the former, such daily distress adds up to a low-key condition of chronic stress.

Some of these daily hassles are analogous to the visitations upon Job—they can neither be anticipated nor avoided; but others can be potentially brought under our control. A modicum of anticipatory planning or shared problem-solving can, I think, reduce their number considerably. In our view, the mothers of antisocial children are generally unskilled persons. Their daily fare of crises constitutes an uncontrollable segment of their environment. In keeping with the findings reviewed by Cohen (1980) and Levine (this volume), the mother's lack of skill produces an increase in the number of crises they experience; the lack of control further enhances the impact of such critical incidents.

Events or Processes?

At first glance, there is no compelling reason to introduce the concept of stress-initiated *process*. One can proceed in a correlational manner to identify a stressor, and then look for a correlation in the incidence of a psychiatric syndrome. The study by Brown and Harris (1978) is a case in point. They interviewed several hundred women to identify, retrospectively, those who recalled a severe life crisis. The severe event was defined as something that disrupted the individual's life for a week or more. For the normal sample, about 25% of the women had experienced at least one such event during the prior nine months. This compared with 61% of the depressed women, who recalled that such an event had occurred prior to the onset of their depression. They found that the combination of early loss of the mother by death and a later severe event or difficulty significantly differentiated depressed from normal women. The problem is that these second-order conditionals described 5% of the depressed group, and the proportion of false negatives for this index was 95%. That is not to say the finding is trivial. It is, in fact, a useful piece of information to know that early loss of the mother followed later by a second severe event places one at risk for depression. However, the same data set showed that if the conditional was loss of *father* followed by a later severe event, the difference between the clinical and the normal groups was not significant. Why should the death of the mother be a more pathogenic stressor than the death of the father? Post hoc explanations may be challenging, but they do not resolve the issue.

The stress literature is replete with puzzling findings of this sort. For example, most studies agree in showing that *most stressed persons do not evidence any discernible psychiatric or medical complications*. Why is this so? This seems to hold even for prolonged and extreme stress, such as infantry combat (Robins, 1981). Certainly the loss of sleep, extreme physical discomfort, intermittent artillery barrage, and the random death and mutilation of one's friends seem to fulfill all the requirements for chronic stress. Why, then, did the long-term sequelae fail to differentiate combat from noncombat veterans when controls were introduced to match for background factors prior to induction into the armed forces?

Obviously, some additional variables are needed to help us understand the failure to differentiate between stressed and nonstressed persons. For example, one could assume that not all participants view the stressor in the same way. These differential perceptions or appraisals, to use Lazarus' term, could very well determine whether or not there would be long-term sequelae to a stressful experience (Lazarus et al., 1980). Another reasonable alternative is to assume individual differences in coping ability (Garmezy, this volume). A third set of variables often mentioned as a potential mediator is the presence or absence of a support system (Cassel, 1974). Cassel's review and Levine's chapter (this volume) document the fact that animals stressed in isolation show more long-term pathological signs than do those stressed in the company of litter mates, mothers, siblings, etc.

Levine's programmatic work demonstrates that having the stressed mother squirrel monkey in the same cage with her infant is associated with significantly lower plasma cortisol levels. Mothers stressed in isolation show higher endocrine reactions to the stress. By way of illustration, let us assume that this stress was repeated every other day for a month: Would some mother-infant dyads demonstrate changes in the structure of their interactions? Are such changes a step in the development of adjustment problems for the infant? The point is that the traditional laboratory work on the buffering concept may lend itself to an analysis of microsocial process as it mediates stress outcomes.

A follow-up study by Meyer and Haggerty (1962) provides a good illustration. One hundred children provided a throat culture for streptococci every two weeks. The parents also kept a diary of upsetting events and illnesses. They found that documented inflammations, as well as clinical symptoms of illness, were significantly correlated with the incidence of upsetting events. However, only about one-fourth of the infections had been preceded during the prior two weeks by such events. This study lends itself nicely to questions about interactional process. For example, why is it that some stressors were associated with infection, but others were not? Why were some families affected, but not others? I would hypothesize that some of these stressors may have produced changes in family interaction processes that magnified the effect of the stressor upon the immune system. In other families, I would expect a microsocial analysis to show no stress-related changes.

As I noted earlier, the emphasis is on examining a continuum of familial stressors ranging from severe events (Brown & Harris, 1978) to daily household hassles. The latter is in keeping with the position of Lazarus et al. (1980). We are also in agreement in our joint emphasis on the possibility that the long-term outcome of stressors may be *either* positive or negative. The effect of a stressor may be to alter the dynamics of the family, or the small group, in such a way that the long-term consequences may be quite positive (i.e., a growth experience). (The summertime experiences of several thousand participants in Outward Bound programs are consistent with this notion.) It is for this reason that I view stress as a potential *change* agent. For example, the five-man infantry squad provides a process that partially determines whether the individual's reaction to combat stress will be positive or negative. If the squad is partially destroyed, then one can anticipate an increase in psychiatric and/or medical sequelae correlated with stress. Similarly, as long as the family was intact, the process initiated by the repeated bombing and shelling of such cities and London or Dresden was capable of producing long-term *positive* changes.

If the system or the dyad is already disrupted, then I suspect the effect of outside stress may be to further disrupt the interaction. The key lies in our understanding of interactional processes in such small groups as the family, infantry squads, or friendship groups; but developing such understanding involves a series of steps. First, how does one measure slight shifts in interactional processes brought about by minor or major stressors? Second, what are the parameters that determine if a minor perturbation in process will generate long-term changes in interactional patterns? Third, what is the relation between these interaction patterns and long-term changes in coping skills? Fourth, which patterns relate to risk for negative outcomes? For example, are there differences between familial group interactions following the death of the mother as compared to the father? Brown and Harris's (1978) fascinating data suggest that there will be. What determines the manner in which processes unfold?

There are two sets of problems to be considered. The first concerns the question of how one can conceptualize social interaction at a microsocial level. Specifically, what are these variables, and how does one measure them? The second concerns the matter of how one studies the interface between microsocial and macrosocial events. Each of these questions will be considered in turn.

A MICROSOCIAL ANALYSIS OF CHILD AGGRESSIVENESS

It is traditional to view a trait score as a summary of past commerce between the child and his or her social environment. In keeping with that tradition, the present formulation holds that a molecular analysis of what a child is reacting *to* (i.e., the social environment) would provide a kind of mirror image of what is meant by any given social trait. In the case of a trait such as child aggression, a molecular analysis of sequences of family interaction would identify each member in the role of both *reactor and initiator*. Each person, then, is embedded in a context defined by the reactions of other family members. Measures of each member's disposition to react aggressively and to initiate aggression constitute a description of the social environment with which the child must cope.

If one proceeds to define aggressive reactions and initiations by *both* members of a dyad, then, in an important sense, the behavior of one person constitutes a list of determinants for the behavior of the other. At one level, this means the aggression scores for a dyad must intercorrelate. This, in fact, is the case for samples of both normal and antisocial families (Patterson, 1982). At another level, such a bilateral definition for a trait implies that the level at which a trait is performed could be altered by changes in the disposition of the *other* member of the dyad to either initiate aggression or to react aggressively to the first member's aggression. This altered definition of a trait provides a means for studying the impact of variables from outside the dyad.

One of the hypotheses tested in the present report is that familial crises alter the social interaction patterns of mother and child. It is assumed that for most families the disruption produces increases in antisocial child behavior.

Structure

I am assuming that major forms of child deviancy, such as depression, withdrawal, and antisocial behavior, are in part the outcome of a process. This process is defined by interaction sequences that are, in turn, made up of structured components that change over time. *Structure* is the correlation of one behavioral event with another adjacent event in the sequence. In the context of child aggressiveness, the structure has two general components that are of interest: intrasubject and intersubject. The two components together define what is meant by a microsocial analysis of family interaction.

Intrasubject simply means that what the child is doing at a given time ($time_1$) may correlate with an immediately preceding time ($time_{-1}$) or ensuing ($time_{+1}$) aggressive act. To study this, we began by constructing a 29-category code system recording the sequential interactions of one family member with another (Reid, 1978). The data, collected in the home over a series of six to ten sessions, are recorded every six seconds by highly trained observers, who then enter the data for computer analyses. The methodological studies concerning observer agreement, observer bias, reactivity, test-retest reliability, and validity are summarized in Reid (1978).

The first step in the analysis of intrasubject components is to define the base rate of a target event, such as Physical Negative (PN). Physical Negative would include such responses as push, shove, grapple, kick, or strike with an object. Given a total of about 600 interaction events per session, what is the likelihood of a target event such as Physical Negative? In a sample of 37 children referred for treatment as social aggressors, this event occurred at .3% during their interactions with mother and 1.3% during their interactions with male siblings.

If the problem child engaged in a Physical Negative (PN) event once, what is the likelihood she or he will be doing it again in the next 6-second time interval? Summing across interactions involving all family members, the conditional probability of a second PN, given the first, was .286. A PN at $time_1$ was functionally related to the problem child's PN at $time_{-1}$.

What does this tiny bit of structure analysis mean? To place it in context, the data from a matched sample of normal boys were analyzed in the same fashion. For them, the conditional probability for a second PN, given a first, was zero. That is not to say that normal boys did not engage in Physical Negative behavior with male siblings. The base rate was .001, but after one event, *they stopped*. This is a fundamental difference in intrasubject structure between normal and distressed families. In fact, it was one of the first significant differences noted between antisocial and normal boys (Patterson,

1976). As a general case, problem children tend to persist in their aggressiveness for longer periods of time. All other family members also share this disposition. They are significantly more likely than their counterparts in normal families to engage in extended coercive interactions. The measure of this disposition is described as $P(A_2/A_1)$; that is, the probability (P) of a second aversive event (A_2) given that the first (A_1) has occurred. In fact, the problem child's disposition to extend his own coercive behavior correlates .76 ($df = 15, p < .001$) with his overall level of coercive performance (Patterson, 1977). As we shall see, the mother's disposition to continue the aggressive sequence accounts for more variance in the child's performance than does any other family variable. A family comprised of people characterized by a disposition to continue being irritable once started constitutes an operational definition of anarchy. The parent and the child are roughly equal in coercive power.

As pointed out by Thomas and Martin (1976) and Martin, Maccoby, Baron, and Jacklin (1981), there are both intrasubject and intersubject components to interaction structure. In the present context, this second, or intersubject, component refers to the functional relation between the behavior of one family member to another. Again, the structure is defined by immediately adjacent events in an ongoing sequence.[1] For example, in the social aggressor sample, the likelihood of the problem child's reacting with a PN to a male sibling was .010. However, given that the sibling's prior behavior had been a PN, the likelihood of the target child reacting with PN was .269.

The next step is to examine adjacent structures in a coercion sequence. The variables identified by these analyses are used to study the interface between microsocial process and such macrovariables as stress.

The Irritability Cycle

A decade's work of analyzing various intersubject structures found in families of antisocial and normal children emphasizes the simple fact that aversive behavior elicits aversive reactions. Members of antisocial families

---

[1] In pursuing intersubject structure, it is clear that there are some functional relations that reappear again and again across families. There are, in fact, patterns of coercive responses controlled by shared networks of antecedents (Patterson, 1977). The same study that identified the classes of responses controlled by shared networks of antecedents, also found that the responses elicited common sets of consequences from family members. The fact that the same intersubject structures were found across families raises some interesting questions about how such cultural programming comes about.

I think that, as a general case, parents who invariably react in an irritable fashion tend to also be less skilled in family management. The variables describing such skills include: setting house rules, monitoring deviant child behavior, punishing deviant behavior, and using problem-solving skills (Patterson, 1982). We think these four measures of parenting practices are the major determinants of the three irritability values for the mother. The hypothesis is that the irritability probability values are very large in families of antisocial children because the parents have set aside the practice of certain family-management skills.

are significantly more likely to initiate and/or react aversively than are members of normal families; once started, they are likely to continue. At each juncture in the aversive exchange, members of antisocial families demonstrate an increased likelihood that the next reaction will be aversive.

There are three measures of these irritable reactions that are pertinent to the present discussion. The first variable, *crossover*, describes the likelihood that things will "start up." If one person, such as the problem child, is being neutral or prosocial, how likely is another family member, perhaps the mother, to initiate an aversive exchange? The second variable is *counterattack*. If the other member initiates an attack, how likely is the subject to react aversively? The third variable is *continuance*. If the subject initiates an aversive exchange, how likely is he or she to continue being aversive? One can, of course, continue to search for such structure through as many junctures as the data will allow, but each step introduces an increasing number of zero entries in the sample, particularly for normal children and their families. For this reason, most of our analyses involve only three measures of the irritability cycle for each member of the dyad. Problem children and their mothers were significantly more likely than their normal counterparts to respond in all three ways (Patterson, 1982).

It is thought that these dispositions define a "fight cycle." One variable defines the likelihood for start-up. The next defines the likelihood that the other will continue it by reacting aversively. The last one defines the disposition to continue a fight, no matter how the other person reacted. Families of antisocial children are characterized by more cycles, and by cycles of longer duration (Patterson, 1976; 1982).

Each of these three measures of irritability may serve very different functions. Which contributes most heavily as a determinant of antisocial child behavior? Do each of them contribute equally in determining whether the child performs at very high or very low rates of coerciveness? In a series of analyses, the three measures of irritability were correlated with the Total Aversive Behavior (TAB) score for the target child. This score summarizes the overall level of the child's aggressivity as he or she interacts with family members. This has been shown to correlate significantly with the child's disposition to fight at home and at school.

The analysis was done separately for fathers, mothers, and siblings as reactors (Patterson, 1982). It was the probability of the continuance measure for both parents that correlated significantly with the TAB score for the child. The continuance measures also correlated with a score measuring the daily occurrence of antisocial symptoms. The parents reported these data by daily telephone interviews.

As a result of these studies, the mother's probability of continuance was selected as the most promising microsocial variable for the present study.

The next step is to determine whether it sensitively reflects the impact of daily crises on caretaker behavior.

Before leaving this issue, it is important to note that the level of the children's aggressiveness can be changed in two general ways. One way is to alter the child's disposition to continue. This is the reason that an important feature of our treatment is training parents to use effective punishments (Patterson, Reid, Jones, & Conger, 1975). Punishment effectively reduces the likelihood of a given behavior. Second, one can also train parents to reduce their own, and sibling, dispositions to start, and to continue, fights; that is, give the problem child less reason to react aggressively.

In the discussions that follow, the implicit assumption is that changes in the mother's irritable reactions will produce changes in the child's coerciveness. A number of single-subject experiments demonstrated such an effect (Patterson, 1982). In a group design, Johnson and Lobitz (1974) also demonstrated this effect. Twelve parents of normal families were instructed to make their preschool children "look bad" for three observation sessions, and "look good" in three alternate sessions. On "bad" days the parents increased their rate of commands: the rates of deviant child behavior increased in a commensurate fashion. The effect has been replicated in a second study (Lobitz & Johnson, 1975).

Covariation of Stressors and Microsocial Measures

I emphasized the point earlier that stress and microsocial variables covary. The implication was that stressors cause a disruption in microsocial process. At the very least, this form of the hypothesis requires a demonstration that the stressors and the microsocial variables covary over sessions. In the present context, it is assumed that the day's accumulation of hassles alters the likelihood of the mother's continuance.

The design involved a small sample of mothers observed in their homes on a daily basis for a period of several weeks. Each mother-child dyad is observed for each of, say, twenty sessions. It is a straightforward matter to calculate the child's level of aggressivity, and the probability value for mother continuance for each session. The mother is also asked to fill out a checklist of familial crises each day, describing the accumulation of hassles, large and small, occurring in the last 24 hours. High stress days should be consistently associated with some sort of change in the probability of mother's continuance. On days when stress is low, the conditional probability value should also reflect that change. If stress and the probability of continuance covary, a correlation across days for each dyad should demonstrate it.

I suspect that testing for covariation across time is a more powerful means of testing hypotheses on cause and effect relationships than is the across-subject correlation. If one finds across-trial correlations between variables x and y, it is, I think, safe to say that the relation will also be found in across-subject analyses. However, the reverse is not necessarily true. Of course, it goes without saying that hypotheses about causality eventually require experimental manipulations, but I see the across-session correlational analysis as being an efficient first step in screening for those variables worth pursuing further.

Before examining the findings, there is a question that needs to be addressed: how can the mother's probability of continuance be viewed as both a stable trait and as a measure fluctuating from day to day? The data in Figure 9-2 illustrate the assumptions and the problem. "Spring" was a preschool child. She and her mother were observed in the home for a series of 17 days; each session lasted roughly an hour. The analysis of the mother's disposition to continue reacting aversively provided a mean probability value of .37. That is, if the mother reacted aversively to Spring, then 37% of the time she continued being aversive in the next time interval. However, as shown in Figure 9-2, any one day's observation session may give a score markedly different from this mean value. My assumption is that these fluctuations in the measure are not errors of measurement; rather, they are multiply determined. It is hypothesized that, in part, these fluctuations covary with crises and other macrovariables from outside the family. One way to support the hypothesis would be to demonstrate that these fluctuations are indeed systematic, that is, that they covary in a significant fashion with some other variable(s).

With no long-term major shifts in reinforcement or punishment provided by Spring for the mother's behavior measured by probability of continuance, the slope for the probability values should remain at zero. Theoretically, if Spring could somehow react so that mother's probability of continuance no longer worked, the slope would then reflect a general decrease in average probability values. If, on the other hand, Spring increased the reinforcement for this reaction, there should be a gradual increase in these probability values.[2] As shown in Figure 9-2, the values fluctuate about their mean value of .37. There is no systematic trend toward increases or decreases: the slope is zero.

How is one to decide whether these fluctuations are random errors of measurement or systematic shifts? One step would be to demonstrate that the measure is internally consistent. In that negative findings would not lead to a rejection of the hypothesis, this is a weak test. A positive outcome would,

[2] Actually, this is a very complex issue. The impact on the probability of the mother's continuance would more likely be relative to the reinforcement provided for other behaviors in the mother's repertoire. The effect is relative to what is available for other competing responses. The work of Herrnstein (1970) and others on the matching law relates to this issue.

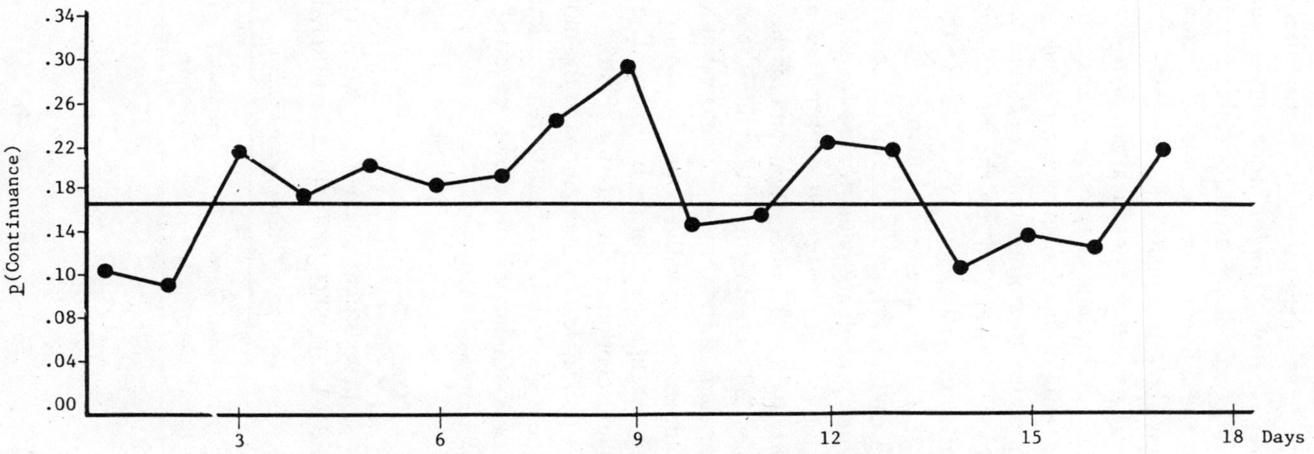

Figure 9-2. Day to day fluctuations in irritability for one mother.

however, be reassuring. A sampling of odd-numbered days for Spring showed a mean probability value of .39, as compared to .35 for even-numbered days. Comparable calculations for the five mother-child dyads produced a reliability coefficient of .70 for the probability of continuance. Seven or more sessions seem to provide a reasonably stable estimate for the mean probability value. In the following section, we will examine the extent to which the fluctuations about the mean value are systematic.

There remains one more methodological problem. To what extent does the mother's disposition to continue sample a generalized trait for irritability? In part, our understanding of this variable requires that it relate in a meaningful way to other measures of mother traits. An earlier across-subject analysis showed a median of .40 ($p < .001$) for the intercorrelations among the four measures of irritability (Patterson, 1982), but do these variables also covary across sessions? It seems wise to reassure ourselves that across-session measures of mother irritability do, indeed, sample a generalized disposition. If a mother showed high probability values for crossover but not for continuance, it would suggest that crossover and continuance are controlled by different sets of determinants. The interaction data for the five mother-child dyads were reanalyzed. The conditional probability values were calculated for each day, and for each of the three irritability variables. Each variable was then correlated across sessions with each of the other two measures. The analyses were carried out separately for each subject. The findings showed that, with the possible exception of the data for "Pluto," all three measures covaried (see Table 9-1). Day-to-day fluctuations in the mother's probability of continuance define a general disposition to react irritably. Notice, too, that the probability of continuance more closely covaried with the disposition to counterattack than with crossover.

TABLE 9-1
CORRELATIONS ACROSS SESSIONS AMONG MEASURES OF THE MOTHER'S DISPOSITION TO REACT IRRITABLY

		Correlation of likelihood for		
Family Code Name	*Number of Days*	*Continuance & Counterattack*	*Continuance & Crossover*	*Counterattack & Crossover*
Spring	17	.62†	.70†	.57*
Eclipse	13	.71†	.32	.53
Pluto	16	.38	−.01	.22
Tofu	14	.68†	.53	.27
Pumpkin	12	.56	.34	.12

* $p < .10$
† $p < .01$

The next question concerns the feasibility of accounting for day-to-day fluctuations around this mean value. It is assumed that each day's value is comprised of three components. Given that observation sessions were on consecutive days, and that the setting remained the same, the probability value for any given day would actually reflect the history of yesterday's exchange. This component is combined with information about the general basal level for that dyad (i.e., the level characterizing them for the past few days). In effect, a probability value reflects variance attributable to basal level (grand mean) and, in addition, the unique contribution of yesterday's history. The third component reflects the contribution of conditions outside the dyad, macrovariables, that may have a temporary effect on the probability values for one or both members. The list of candidates for status as a macrovariable is brief indeed. At present it consists of two conditions for which primitive assessment devices could either be constructed or are available. These included a daily measure of household stress/crises, and a daily measure of contacts with adults in the community. We also added a measure of day-to-day changes in mother's mood. Whether to classify mother's mood as a macro- or a microvariable is uncertain. It was included because of a general interest in the relation of caretaker role, depression, and aversive experiences.

The next question concerns the means for measuring macrovariables. The following sections explore the relation of these measures to the measure of the mother's probability of continuance and to the child's deviancy.

MACROVARIABLES

The hypothesis is that the daily accumulation of minor crises may alter the irritability of the mother's reactions to the child. The mother's efforts to cope with these mundane stressors may include problem-solving discussions with a friend, her husband, or the family. The importance of these efforts to cope with crises lies in their potential impact on the duration and the recurrence of the crises. Effective problem-solving should mean that the same crises are less likely to last for extended periods, and are less likely to recur tomorrow or next week. However, even if dealt with effectively, the crisis may still function as a stressor on the day it occurs, e.g., the mother may effectively cope with the child who is very ill, but, nevertheless, find it a stressful experience. In the present formulation, I am emphasizing the contribution of problem-solving to the reduction of the immediate impact of crises and their long-term resolutions.

The network of hypotheses is as follows. My a priori expectations were that days characterized by a large accumulation of crises would be days that should have a high value for probability of continuance, though it may be that some persons become more distant and withdrawn from social interaction when stressed, while others became more irritable, as suggested by a colleague, M. S. Forgatch. With the present limited state of our knowledge, the best statement would be that we are searching for covariations between stress and the probability of continuance, rather than testing one hypothesis or another. First, whether or not effective coping occurs, the daily fare of stressors will covary with the mother's probability of continuance. Second, parents who have effective problem-solving skills will have fewer crises. Third, parents who lack these skills, and a support system, will tend to have many more recurring crises.

Measures of Stress

Interviews by Tonge, James, and Hillman (1975) documented the overwhelming frequency and intensity of the crises encountered by multiproblem families seeking assistance from community agencies. The method used to assess these familial crises, in the present study, was based, in part, on the procedures developed by Holmes and Rahe (1967). The Family Event List was composed of items thought to occur in normal, as well as in distressed, families. In the study reported here, the mothers filled out the checklist daily, describing events from such general categories as Household, Transportation, Economic, Health, Employment, and School. It included such specific items as bills to pay, arguments with spouse, someone ill, car broke down, or a ruined dinner.[3] The checklist was filled out daily by five mothers, each of whom participated in the extended baseline studies. The range was from a mean of 1.6 to 5.6 hassles per day for the sample (Patterson, 1982).

Insularity

As stated earlier, I believe that effective coping reduces the likelihood of crises recurring in the future. We have, however, no information on the impact of other reactions to stressors (e.g., talking about the problem to a spouse or to a good friend). How important is the support network? How often is it used as a means of coping with stressors, and is it effective? Wahler, at the University of Tennessee, has constructed an ingenious and

---

[3] The earlier checklist has been revised and extended. This revised checklist was used in the study of problem-solving by Forgatch and Patterson (in preparation). It now includes 101 items. Each item is rated for intensity on a scale ranging from −3 to +3. Mothers and fathers independently described their impressions about crises occurring in the past 24 hours on each of the three days. Data are now available for over 100 normal families who have filled out the checklist.

simple means of obtaining data related to these issues. He measured the insularity of families of antisocial children by studying daily records kept by the mothers, describing contacts with the community. Wahler's first sample of eight families at high risk for treatment failure showed an average of 2.6 community contacts per day; of these only 30% involved friends (Wahler, 1980; Wahler et al., 1977). This was in contrast to an average of 9.5 contacts per day for low-risk families. For the latter sample, 58% of the contacts were with friends.

Our insularity data for the extended baseline studies did show three to five daily contacts with persons outside the family. These contacts could be either a telephone call or personal contact; roughly half were positive in valence. There was also a surprising range in the amount of time involved in these contacts: an average of 42 to 430 minutes per day.

Measure of Mood

Prior to each observation session, the mother completed one of the three alternative forms of the Lubin Mood Scales[4] (Lubin, 1963). The scales measured the mother's mood from euphoric to dysphoric. It was expected that there would be sizable shifts in the mood scores from one day to the next. It was also assumed that, for some mothers, these scores would covary with the frequency of crises. In the first set of analyses for three of the five mothers, there were, in fact, correlations in the .33 to .55 range across sessions between mood and crises (Patterson, 1982). Frequent crises covaried with the mother checking a larger number of negative adjectives when describing her current mood. The mood scores also correlated across days with the number of the mother's positive contacts. The greater the number of positive contacts, the more positive the mood. However, these correlations were of a very modest magnitude and held for only three of the five mothers.

COVARIATIONS OF MICRO- AND MACROVARIABLES

The hypothesis, central to our discussion, concerned the covariation between daily measures of crises and the probability of the mother's continuance. The across-session correlations in Table 9-2 showed consistent support

[4] The scoring consisted of a tabulation of the number of dysphoric adjectives checked each day as being self-descriptive. Other investigators using this instrument have used somewhat different scoring procedures (e.g., the proportion of dysphoric items checked).

TABLE 9-2
CORRELATION ACROSS DAYS FOR CRISES AND LIKELIHOOD OF THE MOTHER'S CONTINUANCE

Family Code Name	*Correlation of Probability of Continuance and Frequency of Crises*	*Multiple R**
Spring	.45	.73
Eclipse	.61†	.76
Pluto	.58†	.67
Tofu	−.45	.69
Pumpkin	−.70‡	.72

* The Multiple R's combine data for crises, mood, and three measures of insularity to predict the probability of continuance.
† $p < .10$
‡ $p < .01$

for the idea that the two variables covaried. Even with the small number of trials involved, the covariation was significant for three of the five families.[5]

From the viewpoint of the child, it was evident that, for some, family crises made things worse (e.g., for Spring, Eclipse, and Pluto). On days fraught with hassles, the mother was more likely to react irritably. These increases were presumably accompanied by counterreactions from the child, and a concomitant increase in risk for high-amplitude aggression.

Note that, for Tofu and Pumpkin, crises and the probability of continuance covaried, but in a negative direction. One post hoc construction is that, for these two mothers, crises and stress related to a general withdrawal from social interaction, including a reduced irritability. In principle, this is a testable proposition, but, as yet, we have not followed it up. In any case, it is obvious that the conclusion that stress causes increased irritability simply does not apply to all mothers. As they stand, the findings provide moderate support for the idea that the day-to-day fluctuations in the probability values for mother continuance are systematically, rather than randomly, determined.

The next question asked what would happen if the other macrovariables were added: Could they account for additional variance in the fluctuations of the probability of mother continuance? The daily scores for crises, mood, frequency of community contact, valence of contact, and number of min-

[5] The data were not usually collected on consecutive days. However, it seemed wise to investigate the possibility of serial dependency for both the dependent and independent variables. Autocorrelations (Lag 1) were calculated separately for each variable for each subject. None of the values exceeded .30. It was concluded, therefore, that the problems of serial dependency would not seriously hamper efforts to estimate either the magnitude or the level of significance for the correlations in Table 9-2 (Hoffman, 1967).

utes of contact all served as independent variables in a multiple regression format. Mother *p*(Continuance) served as the criterion variable. In that the number of sessions was only four or five times larger than the number of variables, these results must be interpreted with a good deal of caution. The findings are illustrative of what might be done with more adequately designed studies sampling 40- or 50-day base lines. As shown in Table 9-2, the independent variables accounted for about one-half the variance in the criterion measure. The standard partial-regression coefficients showed, in each case, that the frequency of crises scores made either the largest, or second largest, unique contribution to the criterion. If one were to accept these results at face value, they strongly suggest that the daily fluctuation of microsocial variables may be systematically determined.

In a survey study of a London borough, Brown and Harris (1978) found that stressful events were more likely to occur in the lives of working-class women than middle-class women. However, the long-range impact of these crises was ameliorated if the women had a close friend, husband, or relative available with whom crises could be shared. In support of this position, Kohn (1973) and others have noted that it is not solely the amount of stress or the number of crises, it is also the individual's resources for coping with crises that determines the long-term impact. Kohn makes the interesting observation, in his review, that, at any given level of stress or crisis, people from the lower social classes are more likely to manifest breakdown symptoms than are middle- or upper-class members in similar straits. However, he points out that, with the same amount of stress, the lower-class person has available fewer community, financial, and inner coping resources. As noted earlier, Wahler has also confirmed the isolated status of families of many antisocial children (Wahler, 1979; Wahler et al., 1977).

The interview study by Tonge et al. (1975) graphically portrays the feelings of alienation and mistrust that characterize members of multiple-problem families in their perception of neighbors; relatives; agencies of school, government, and police; and the welfare system. They tended to have few contacts with friends, neighbors, or family. Contacts, when they did occur, were largely aversive in nature. This is certainly in accord with our clinical experience in treating families of thieves, social aggressors, and multiple-offending delinquent adolescents. For these families, there is a relative lack of support networks, and a concomitant difficulty in coping with crises. These factors seem to be related at a clinical level. Problems accumulate and eventually become the concern for a committee of case workers from a half-dozen agencies. These families seem to be more mobile than other families. Their increased shifts from one location to another is perhaps a convulsive effort to escape from the mounting crises and largely abrasive communications received from members of the community.

The primary hypothesis investigated in this section concerns the relation between familial problem-solving skills and frequency of crises. Conflicts among members are routine within any given family. In like fashion, minor crises and hassles from outside are also standard fare. It is the responsibility of the parents to cope with both kinds of intrusions. In the present context, the term *coping* refers to a set of problem-solving skills identified by investigators in widely disparate areas. From a social learning viewpoint these coping skills usually include several steps. As an example, Jacobson & Margolin (1979) list the steps taught couples who are in severe conflict:

1. Clearly stating the problem in neutral terms
2. The partner paraphrasing to show he or she has heard what the problem was
3. Brainstorming a discussion of alternative ways of proceeding
4. Negotiating some sort of compromise that is then written down as a means of reducing future conflicts over what was agreed upon
5. Agreeing upon a set of positive consequences for both members if the agreement is kept, and punishments if it is not.

I assume that parents of antisocial children do not typically seek out a friend or relative with whom the problem can be discussed in detail. If such support is sought, it is unlikely that the discussion proceeds to an in-depth consideration of alternative courses of action. The problem is not solved. If it is discussed at all, it is "talked around." The crises reappear and accumulate. In a 1981 study, the amount of familial crises reported by the mother was shown to be greater in families of "fighters" than in non-fighting families (Patterson, 1981). The revised checklist of familial crises was filled out by mothers of 25 fourth-, 27 seventh-, and 21 tenth-grade boys. These scores were then correlated with a composite score measuring physical aggression. The latter consisted of standardized scores summing across ratings by parents, teachers, and peers about the incidence of physical fighting. The correlation for the fourth-grade sample was .32 ($p < .10$); .23 (n.s.) for the seventh-grade sample; and .63 ($p < .01$) for the tenth-grade sample. The higher the incidence of familial crises, the greater the likelihood of physical aggression.

However, these correlations do not prove that the parents of antisocial children are inept problem solvers. It is hypothesized that parents of antisocial children are significantly less effective in their use of problem-solving skills than are parents of normal children. In a general sense, much of their coping behavior could be described as maximizing immediate payoffs. If there is a sibling conflict, shout at them, hit them, or threaten. There is a chance that such an irritable expression will produce a temporary alleviation of the problem. Incidentally, if the parent's irritable reaction produces a termination of the sibling conflict, it increases the likelihood the parent will employ it again. The alternative is to take the time to set up house rules that will reduce the likelihood of future sibling conflicts, and also to take the time to press home a punishment for misbehavior. This trait of irritability is the major contribution to parents' lack of skilled performance in coping with crises internal to family interaction and to those from outside the family, and is one of the outstanding characteristics of parents of antisocial children (Patterson, 1981, 1982). It occurs in conjunction with a tendency to avoid confrontation.

The effect of the short-term escape strategy is that conflicts mount within the family, and unsolved crises accumulate. The studies of distressed couples showed significantly more conflicts per week and significantly more areas in which change was sought (Vincent, Weiss, & Birchler, 1975). Prinz, Foster, Kent, and O'Leary (1979) found that families of distressed adolescents desired more areas of change. The mothers wished for about 20 areas of change, and about 24 areas of change were desired by the adolescents. What also differentiated samples of distressed from nondistressed adolescents was the intensity of the feelings of both the parent and the adolescents about these issues. These findings for intensity of feelings were replicated by Robin and Weiss (1980). They also found a significantly greater frequency for the areas of change desired by the mothers of the distressed adolescents, in comparison with mothers of nondistressed offspring.

The strong feelings about problems that require negotiation and the general disposition by all family members to react irritably create an unlikely atmosphere for effective problem-solving. The earlier studies of distressed couples showed them to be significantly more likely to introduce aversive events during problem-solving interchanges (Patterson, Weiss, & Hops, 1976), and these findings have been replicated by other investigators, such as Gottman (1980). These studies were based on videotapes of couples attempting to solve some of the problems that were disrupting their marriages. Robin and Weiss (1980) extended the same problem-solving format to distressed adolescents interacting with their mothers. They also adapted the Marital Interaction Coding System used in the earlier work with distressed couples (Hops, Wills, Patterson, & Weiss, 1976) to provide a better fit to the interchanges of distressed adolescents with their mothers. Their analysis of the frequency data for the code categories showed ten times more Put Downs and four times more Commands for the distressed, than for the nondistressed, dyads. There was also significantly less Specification of Problem, Humor, Assent, Agree, and Accept Responsibility.

Did the increased use of Put Down and Command sidetrack the use of effective problem-solving behaviors for the distressed dyads? To test this and related hypotheses, 90 normal families participated in the videotape problem-solving procedure developed by Forgatch and Wieder (1981). The problem-solving interchange took place in the laboratory. A complex code was then used to assess several dimensions of the interaction. One-third of the sample were single-parent families (father absent). There are three parts to this procedure. First, one of the parents brings up something she or he would like to have changed in the family. Second, the child brings up something he would like to have changed. Finally, the family is asked to plan an activity for the weekend. Each section of the procedure lasts about 10 minutes. The videotaped interactions are then coded for a number of composite scores. The most relevant one for the present hypothesis was labeled *Irritable*. It was the sum of the proportion of interactions for the mother taken up by each of the following categories: Blame, Command, Complain, Criticize, Disagree, Disqualify, Guilt Trip, Leading Question, Mind Read, Threat, and Why. The Negative Verbal score was obtained by observers scoring the videotaped interaction. At the end of the session, each observer was asked to complete an Observer Impression Checklist (Forgatch & Wieder, 1981). Included among the checklist items were global judgments rated on an 8-point scale about the overall quality of the solutions reached by the family. Figure 9-3 summarizes the assumed relationships among the variables. As shown there, crises are thought to covary directly with antisocial child behaviors. This effect was demonstrated in the study of Forgatch and Patterson (in preparation) reviewed earlier. In that study the hypothesis, also tested, was that crises would covary with Mother Irritability during problem-solving. The correlations were supportive of this hypothesis, but of only borderline significance. They were .21 (n.s.) for the fourth-grade sample, .32 ($p < .10$) for the seventh-grade sample, and .29 (n.s.) for the tenth-grade sample.

Presumably, in these families, the irritable reaction of one member elicits a synchronous reaction from the other, and the goal—to solve a conflict—becomes lost in the ensuing melee. The findings were in keeping with this hypothesis. The Mother-Irritability scores were correlated with the coder's ratings for the quality of problem solution. For the fourth-grade sample the correlation was .38 ($p < .01$), for the seventh-grade sample .35 ($p < .01$), and for the tenth-grade .09 (n.s.). Similarly, the correlations between the coders' ratings for the chaotic quality of the interaction and Mother Irritability were .23 (n.s.) for the fourth-grade sample, .33 ($p < .01$) for the seventh-grade sample, and .09 (n.s.) for the tenth-grade sample.

As shown in Figure 9-3, Mother Irritability and quality of problem-solving are both assumed to covary with criterion measures of antisocial child behavior. In the Forgatch and Patterson (in preparation) study, general support was found for both hypotheses. Irritability during problem-solving and poor quality of solution showed low-level correlations with observed

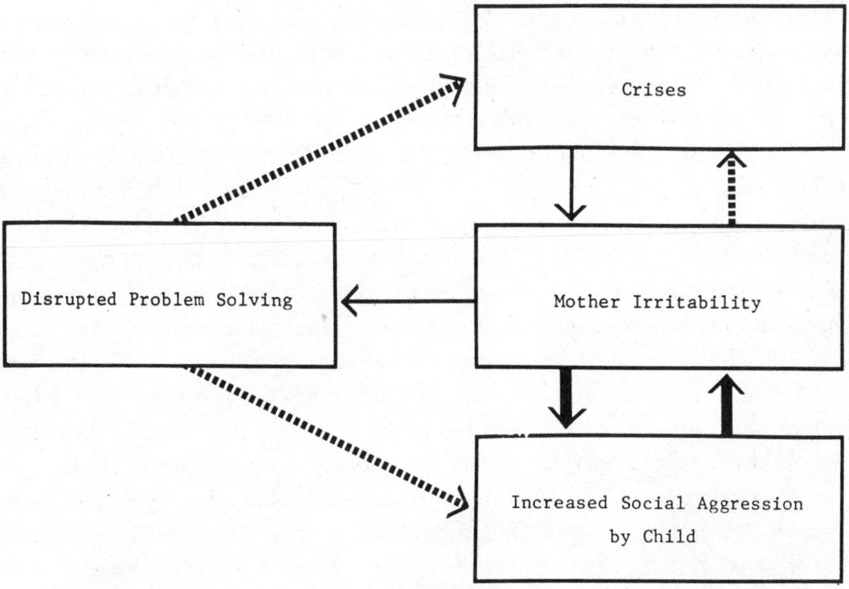

Figure 9-3. A triad of variables for the coercion process.*

* Dotted lines refer to correlations of about .25 to .35; thin lines to correlations of about .36 to .50; and thick lines to correlations of over .51.

child coerciveness in the home, on the one hand, and with measures of child lying and delinquent lifestyle, on the other. The correlations support the network of hypotheses presented in Figure 9-3. As already noted, the one exception is the hypothesis that disrupted problem-solving produces more crises. As things now stand, these findings have direct relevance to the treatment of these families. One of the first steps in training family members in the use of negotiation skills is to control their use of negative reactions during problem-solving (Patterson & Forgatch, 1975).

SOME SPECULATIONS ABOUT STRESS AND FAMILIES

This general formulation was intended to be illustrative of how one might proceed to study the interface between microsocial and macrosocial variables. As they stand, these preliminary findings suggest that it is feasible to think the daily fare of stressors impinging on the caretaker may function as a change agent. In one study, these prosaic familial stressors, plus community contacts and mood swings, accounted for most of the variance in the mother's observed behavior. The pattern of variables that made the largest contribution invariably included the crises measure. Now we must go on and design studies that provide a tighter fit to these ideas. But before we speak to these issues, it is reasonable to question the implications of this approach for the concepts of stress and child pathology.

The primary implication is that it is not children who are directly at risk because of stress: it is the family system. We can only learn which systems are at risk, and which are not, by studying them at the microsocial level. It is not the child who is vulnerable or invulnerable; it is, rather, the system in which he or she resides that determines eventual adjustment. Parents living in a ghetto may produce a nondelinquent child, if their child-management practices function effectively (i.e., are not frequently disrupted by crises with which the parents cannot cope). The family with a schizophrenic parent may produce an adequately adjusted child, if the adults can maintain effective child-management skills in the face of recurring psychotic bouts.

At another level, we have need for a theory about family development vis-à-vis stress, coping, and adjustment. To construct a proper theory would require answers to a series of questions. For example, is it the case that the young parent of a toddler encounters different types and intensities of stress, than the parent of a child entering school for the first time? What are the stressors encountered by adults and children as the family moves through its various phases? Even more to the point, what do members of normal families do about these stressors that erupt from within the family as well? What does in vivo problem-solving look like? Can five minutes on the telephone with a friend or relative partially neutralize the impact of a new crisis? What techniques reduce the likelihood of a crisis recurring? Does the child learn his or her primary coping procedures from parents or peers? Why is it that some stressors—such as a serious illness or a death in the family—facilitate positive microsocial processes?

The literature on personality traits, values, and interest patterns demonstrate a surprising consistency from ages 16 through middle age. People do not change a great deal. Why does change not occur more often? I think that each of us selects settings, friends, and employment that support our existing response repertoire. In this cocoon, the microsocial processes support the status quo. Change is brought about because circumstances are such as to force us to react to some new challenge (i.e., a stressor). It is odd to think of change as being largely a function of reaction to stress, or to the biology of maturation. That is an oversimplification of the true state of affairs, but it does put the concept of stress/aversives at center stage as a critical area to be studied. It does not account for all change in family development (e.g., the aging of parent and child must also relate to change); however, most rapid changes in behavior are stress/aversive related. Sending the child to school is a stressor to which all children respond, and I suspect it is associated with rapid changes in child behavior. Divorce is another stressor that is associated with massive changes in both the parent and the child (Wallerstein, this volume; Hetherington, Cox, & Cox, 1980).

Much of my own clinical and theoretical work has been focused on families of antisocial children. It is certainly clear that the problem of aggression is not localized initially in the child; it is in the family. It is also apparent that a good part of the problem lies outside the family itself. The would-be therapist must help the parents overcome one crisis after another while teaching them relatively simple child-management skills. For example, as noted earlier, the mean crises scores correlated with the measures of the child's antisocial behavior. Families are vulnerable, and some are more vulnerable than others. The fact that these families can be changed, and that the effects can persist through at least 12 months of systematic follow-up (Patterson & Fleischman, 1979), provide indirect support for this formulation. The parents, when taught family-management skills including crisis and child management, are able to bring about profound changes in the preadolescent, antisocial child. The next step is to demonstrate that these changes in the child and siblings correlate with reductions in crises and parent irritability.

As noted in Figure 9-3, the triad of variables and its product, child deviant behavior, includes several interlocking positive feedback loops. All of them feed the process. The best understood components are the relations between deviant child behavior and mother irritability. An increase in one is followed by an increase in the other. The mother's irritability was also shown in several studies to covary with the daily round of crises. As presented in Figure 9-3, her increased irritability is thought to mediate the impact of crises. Increases in crises increase the mother's irritability, in turn increasing the child's social aggressive problems. This is further exacerbated by her irritable reactions during problem-solving efforts. When stressed, she reacts more irritably during problem-solving, and presumably the unresolved crises are likely to reappear. Does a support system reduce the immediate impact of stressors?

The coercion triad has the outlines of a kind of psychological perpetual motion machine. How does it stop? Did it all begin because of the mother's disposition to be irritable? I do not think so. It is more likely an interaction effect produced by a very unskilled parent having a difficult child and being unable to cope with a multitude of crises. An extended series of defeats in managing the child may provide the base for increasing irritability in the mother's confrontations with the child. Many of these parents have poorly developed survival skills. They manage neither children nor crises very well. Their life seems to be out of their control. Therapy must help the parents cope with their out-of-control children and with their own out-of-control crises at the same time, for crises and antisocial families seem intimately related.

REFERENCES

Bell, R. Q., & Harper, R. V. *Child effects on adults*. Hillsdale, New Jersey: Lawrence Erlbaum Associates, 1977.

Brown, G. W., & Harris, T. O. *Social origins of depression: A study of psychiatric disorder in women*. New York: The Free Press, 1978.

Cairns, R. B. *The analysis of social interactions: Methods, issues, and illustrations*. Hillsdale, New Jersey: Lawrence Erlbaum Associates, 1979.

Cassel, J. Psychosocial processes and "stress": Theoretical formulation. *International Journal of Health Service*, 1974, *4*, 471–482.

Cohen, S. After-effects on stress of human performance on social behavior: A review of research and theory. *Psychological Bulletin*, 1980, *88*, 82–108.

Dohrenwend, B. S., & Dohrenwend, B. P. (Eds.), *Stressful life events: Their nature and effects*. New York: John Wiley & Son, 1974.

Eisdorfer, C. *Conceptual issues in stress*. A research perspective paper presented at the Conference on Stress, Coping, and Development, Center for the Advanced Study in the Behavioral Sciences. Stanford, California, March 1981.

Forgatch, M. S., & Patterson, G. R. *Maternal problem solving and antisocial child behavior*. In preparation.

Forgatch, M. S., & Wieder, G. *The Parent Adolescent Naturalistic Interaction Code (PANIC)*. Unpublished manuscript, 1981. (Available from the Oregon Social Learning Center, 207 East 5th, Suite 202, Eugene, Oregon 97401.)

Gottman, J. M. *Marital interaction: Experimental investigations*. New York: Academic Press, 1980.

Herrnstein, R. J. On the law of effect. *Journal of the Experimental Analysis of Behavior*, 1970, *13*, 243–266.

Hetherington, E. M. Children and divorce. In H. Henderson (Ed.), *Parent-child interaction: Theory, research, and prospect*. New York: Academic Press, in press.

Hetherington, E. M., Cox, M., & Cox, R. *Stress and coping in divorce: A focus on women*. Unpublished manuscript, 1980.

Hoffman, W. H. Statistical models for the study of change in the single case. In C. Harris (Ed.), *Problems in measuring change*. Madison, Wisconsin: University of Wisconsin Press, 1967.

Holmes, T., & Rahe, R. The social adjustment rating scale. *Journal of Psychosomatic Research*, 1967, *11*, 213.

Holmes, T., & Masuda, M. Life changes and illness susceptibility. In B. S. Dohrenwend, & B. P. Dohrenwend (Eds.), *Stressful life events*. New York: John Wiley & Sons, 1974.

Hops, H., Wills, T., Patterson, G. R., & Weiss, R. Marital Interaction Code System (MICS). In G. R. Patterson (Ed.), *Some procedures for assessing changes in marital interaction patterns*. *Oregon Research Institute Bulletin*, *16*(7). Eugene, Oregon: Oregon Research Institute, 1976.

Jacobson, N., & Margolin, G. *Marital therapy: Strategies based upon social learning and behavior exchange principles*. New York: Brunner/Mazel, 1979.

Johnson, S. M., & Lobitz, G. K. Parental manipulations of child behavior in home observations. *Journal of Applied Behavior Analysis*, 1974, *7*, 23–31.

Kohn, M. L. Social class and schizophrenia: A critical review and reformulation. *Schizophrenia Bulletin*, 1973, *7*, 60–79.

Lamb, M., Suomi, S., & Stephenson, G. *Social interaction analyses*. Madison: University of Wisconsin Press, 1979.

Lazarus, R. S., Cohen, J. B., Folkman, S., Kanner, A., & Schaefer, C. Psychological stress and adaptation: Some unresolved issues. In H. Selye (Ed.), *Guide to stress research* (Vol. I). New York: Van Nostrand Reinhold Company, 1980.

Lobitz, G. K., & Johnson, S. N. Parental manipulation of the behavior of normal and deviant children. *Child Development*, 1975, *46*, 719–726.

Lubin, B. Adjective checklist for measurement of depression. *Archives of General Psychiatry*, 1963, *12*, 57–62.

Martin, J., Maccoby, E., Baron, K., & Jacklin, C. *The sequential analysis of mother-child interaction at 18 months: A comparison of several analytic methods*. Manuscript submitted for publication, 1981.

Meyer, R. J., & Haggerty, R. J. Streptococcal infections in families. *Journal of Pediatrics*, 1962, *29*, 529–549.

Myers, J., Lindenthal, J., & Pepper, M. Social class, life events, and psychiatric symptoms. In B. S. Dohrenwend, & B. P. Dohrenwend (Eds.), *Stressful life events*. New York: John Wiley & Sons, 1974.

Olweus, D. The consistency issue in personality: Psychology revisited with special reference to aggression. *British Journal of Social and Clinical Psychology*, 1980, *19*, 377–390.

Patterson, G. R. The aggressive child: Victim and architect of a coercive system. In E. Mash, L. Hamerlynck, & L. Handy (Eds.), *Behavior modification and families*. New York: Brunner/Mazel, 1976.

Patterson, G. R. A three-stage functional analysis for children's coercive behaviors: A tactic for developing a performance theory. In D. Baer, B. C. Etzel, & J. M. LeBlanc (Eds.), *New developments in behavioral research: Theories, methods, and applications. In honor of Sidney W. Bijou*. Hillsdale, New Jersey: Lawrence Erlbaum Associates, 1977.

Patterson, G. R. *A bilateral definition for the social aggression trait*. Manuscript presented at the Conference of Relations between Developmental and Social Psychology, Vanderbilt University, June 1981.

Patterson, G. R. *A social learning approach, Vol. 3: Coercive family process*. Eugene, Oregon: Castalia Publishing Company, 1982.

Patterson, G. R., & Fleischman, M. J. Maintenance of treatment effects: Some considerations concerning family systems and follow-up data. *Behavior Therapy*,1979, *10*, 168–185.

Patterson, G. R., & Forgatch, M. S. *Family living series*. (Five cassette tapes to be used with *Living with Children* and *Families*.) Champaign, Illinois: Research Press, 1975.

Patterson, G. R., Reid, J. B., Jones, R. R., & Conger, R. *A social learning approach to family intervention, Vol. 1: Families with aggressive children*. Eugene, Oregon: Castalia Publishing Company, 1975.

Patterson, G. R., Weiss, R. L., & Hops, H. Training of marital skills: Some problems and concepts. In H. Leitenberg (Ed.), *Handbook of behavior modification*. Englewood Cliffs, New Jersey: Prentice Hall, 1976.

Prinz, R. J., Foster, S., Kent, R. N., & O'Leary, K. D. Multivariate assessment of conflict in distressed and nondistressed mother-adolescent dyads. *Journal of Applied Behavior Analysis*, 1979, *12*, 691–700.

Raush, H. L. Interaction sequences. *Journal of Personality and Social Psychology*, 1965, *2*, 487–499.

Reid, J. B. (Ed.) *A social learning approach to family intervention. Vol. 2: Observation in home settings*. Eugene, Oregon: Castalia Publishing Company, 1978.

Robin, A. L., & Weiss, J. G. Criterion related validity of behavioral and self-report measures of problem-solving communication skills in distressed and nondistressed parent-adolescent dyads. *Behavioral Assessment*, 1980, *2*, 339–352.

Robins, L. N. *What effect did Viet Nam have on veterans' mental health?* Unpublished manuscript, 1981.

Sackett, G. P. The lag sequential analysis of contingency and cyclicity in behavioral interaction research. In J. Osofsky (Ed.), *Handbook of infant development*. New York: John Wiley & Sons, 1977.

Sarason, I., Johnson, J., & Siegal, J. Assessing the impact of life changes: Development of life experiences survey. *Journal of Consulting and Clinical Psychology*, 1978, *46*, 932–946.

Selye, H. *The stress of life* (Rev. ed.). New York: McGraw Hill, 1976.

Thomas, E., & Martin, J., Analysis of parent-infant interaction. *Psychological Review*, 1976, *83*, 141–156.

Tonge, W. L., James, D. S., & Hillman, S. Families without hope. *British Journal of Psychiatry*, 1975, Special Publication 11.

Vincent, J. P., Weiss, R., & Birchler, G. R. A behavioral analysis of problem solving in distressed and nondistressed married and stranger dyads. *Behavior Therapy*, 1975, *6*, 475–487.

Wahler, R. G. The insular mother: Her problems in parent-child treatment. *Journal of Applied Behavior Analysis*, 1980, *13*, 207–219.

Wahler, R. G., Leske, G., & Roberts, E. *The insular family: A deviance support system for oppositional children*. Paper presented at the Banff International Conference on Behavior Modification, March 1977.

CHAPTER 10

CHILDREN OF DIVORCE: Stress and Developmental Tasks

JUDITH S. WALLERSTEIN
EXECUTIVE DIRECTOR
CENTER FOR THE FAMILY IN TRANSITION
CORTE MADERA, CALIFORNIA

INTRODUCTION

The intent of this chapter is threefold: first, to delineate the attributes of divorce as a stressor for the child and adolescent in the divorcing family; second, to present a conceptual structure of the psychological tasks that the child and adolescent must perform in meeting the complex challenges and threats which marital rupture poses to developmental progress and psychic integrity; and, finally, to suggest some linkages between developmental factors and the child's subsequent characteristic responses and efforts at mastery that emerge under the initial impact of the acute divorce stress and its aftermath.

I will rely primarily on the observations made during an extensive clinical investigation of 131 children and their parents from 60 predominently white, middle-class families in Northern California who were followed for a five-year period after the decisive marital separation[1] (Wallerstein & Kelly, 1980a). All data drawn from the year prior to the legal divorce, and the observations about school-age children and adolescents throughout the divorcing experience are drawn entirely from our research, and have not yet

[1] A 10-year follow-up study of the same population is currently underway.

been replicated elsewhere. However, many of these observations have been corroborated by Hetherington and her co-workers (Hetherington, Cox, & Cox, 1976, 1978, 1979a, 1979b). Theirs is the only other longitudinal study of divorced families that has been reported. Based in Virginia, the investigation focused on 36 preschool children and their divorcing parents and 36 control families who were studied for a two-year period following the legal divorce.

The systematic acquisition of knowledge regarding the impact of family rupture on children is only now getting underway. Although, annually, the incidence of children in newly divorcing families throughout the United States has remained at one million or more since 1973, the topic has been largely neglected by social and behavioral scientists. The interest that is germinating now is severely hampered by the lack of conceptual clarity regarding the links between childhood experiences and subsequent psychological development, as well as by many perplexing issues related to individual variation in response to what appears to be a similar stressful experience (See Rutter, 1971). Studies are hampered by the dearth of systematic longitudinal observations that might shed light on the short-term or long-term impact of divorce or other types of stressful experiences during childhood.

These issues have become critical as community concern at the high incidence of divorce has mounted, and the pressure to develop intervention programs has increased. Children from divorced families have appeared on the intake lists of clinics and consulting offices throughout the land in numbers that far exceed their proportion in the general population. It has been estimated that these children of divorce make up 50 to 75% of the child patient population (Kalter, 1977). Schools, too, have reported a higher rate of disrupted learning, erratic attendance, and school dropout, as well as increased tardiness and deteriorated social behavior among these youngsters (Brown, 1980).

One potential danger is that the wish to provide help for these children may push communities into undertaking hasty ill-conceived interventions. Lacking an appropriate knowledge base, such programs may be shaped to fit the current professional mode or draw on experience gained from other groups of children, such as those who have suffered parental loss through death or abandonment. Unfortunately, we have found that intervention methods developed to assist children to cope with one form of stress may be poorly fitted to another.

Moreover, interventions that are suitable for adults who have undergone a particular stress experience may be ill-suited to children and to adolescents in similar circumstances. Time and again, events reported as traumatic by other family members have proved not to be equally stressful for the child. Obversely, the child may react with terror to an aspect of an experience that has eluded the adult entirely. Thus, a child's perceptions and experience are often significantly different from those of the adult. Additionally, the responses of the child and the immediate, as well as the lasting, consequences of the stressful experience appear to be profoundly influenced by developmental factors in ways which are still insufficiently identified or understood.

Because the concept of stress has presented recurrent problems of definition and meaning, it may be important to clarify the use of the term as it is used here. I have used stress in two ways: as a stimulus event, a "stressor," and as a disequilibrating event, "stress," that requires change or adaptation on the part of the exposed individual (Rutter, this volume). The context of the discussion will clarify the intended usage.

The first part of this paper examines the many components of the divorce experience from the perspective of the child, and thus employs the concept of divorce as "stressor." Viewing divorce as a stressor provides a convenient rubric that enables the researcher to bring together the many complex components of the divorce experience that separately and together evoke acute distress in the child. It permits us to distinguish the divorce experience from other stressors, and to compare it with other disturbing events along a range of dimensions which may include their respective time trajectories, the expectable sequence of stages, and the availability or absence of supports.

By contrast, the discussion of the child's responses to an experience which must be met treats "stress" as a disequilibrating event, or series of events, that demands change and adaptation. This usage has enabled me to array various disequilibrating events which the child must master in the course of development. These are the coping tasks that accompany the divorce experience. This same use of stress as a disequilibrating event has been helpful in distinguishing among individual differences in children's initial responses to marital rupture, and their relationship to developmental factors.

Thus, although employed in these different ways, the concept of stress can fill a needed role both in the ordering of observations about the divorce experience, and in the construction of hypotheses regarding the effect of that experience on children's adaptation.

DIVORCE AS STRESSOR

Although designed as a social remedy for an unhappy marriage, divorce has only gradually and reluctantly been acknowledged to be severely stressful for children and adolescents, as well as for many adults. Holmes and Rahe (1967) and others who have developed or utilized the life events rating method have considered marital rupture to be second only to death of a spouse in terms of both its intensity as a stressor and the length of time required to accomodate to it. Their perspective is fully in accord with the findings of a large national survey indicating that the American public considers the marital relationship central to their assessment of the quality of life, and second only to physical health in being accorded the highest priority (Campbell, Converse, & Rodgers, 1976). In a comprehensive review of the psychological, psychiatric, and medical literature relevant to the adult divorced population, Bloom and his coworkers (1979), using a range of indices including admission to mental hospitals, concluded that the severe consequences of divorce-induced stress can be expressed in a surprisingly wide variety of physical and emotional disorders.

Observations of children and adolescents at the time of parental separation also reflect the acuteness of their distress. A comprehensive review of research on children at the point of the marital rupture (Wallerstein & Kelly, 1979) reveals considerable agreement among researchers from different parts of the United States regarding the severe impact that such an experience generates in children and adolescents.

Still, it is rather ironic that divorce should even be considered from such a clinical perspective. Presumably, the *intended* effect of divorce is to relieve marital stress and to reduce psychopathological outcomes in family members. The *unintended* effects are those that are generated not only by separation, but by new stressors. Thus, from the outset, divorce belongs in a special category, representing as it does both solution and problem. The tension and balance between these two seemingly antagonistic consequences provide the singular context for its examination.

Unlike other distressing experiences of childhood, such as child abuse, the goal is not to eliminate the stressor nor to reduce its incidence unless such a reduction can be reliably linked to enhanced marital contentment. Unfortunately, we know very little about how to achieve such linkage. Several researchers have found that discordant marriages are more disturbing to children than divorce and have, as a consequence, viewed the latter as the preferable alternative (Despert, 1962; Rutter, 1971). They have assumed, not unreasonably, that the marital conflict would end with the termination of the marriage. Our own work, however, reveals that conflict between the parents often survives the legal divorce by many years; in fact, a startlingly high proportion (approximately one-third) of the children in our study continued to experience open parental discord even five years after dissolution of the parents' marriage.

To elaborate further this elusive quality of the divorce experience, there is evidence that the father's absence leads to intense yearning and years of unhappiness for many children. Yet, in other instances, father's absence may enhance a child's development. In our study, some children in families in which the father had been abusive, overtly seductive, or significantly corrosive of the child's self-esteem, showed a marked developmental spurt at the end of the first year following the marital separation, and continued to look well several years later. Yet the child's distress at the departure of a beloved and loving father is often *not* distinguishable from the distress of the child whose father has been abusive or neglectful. Nor is the longer term outcome for the child readily predictable at that early point.

The goal of the examination of divorce as stressor is, therefore, not to seek its abolition as with other stressors of childhood, or even notably to diminish its incidence, at least at this time, but rather to understand its nature and ramifying effects in order to discover ways that will diminish the *unintended* effects which divorce brings in its wake.

It is important at this early stage of research to narrow the inquiry and to select a particular pattern of divorce within the wide spectrum of that experience. There are many such patterns in marital breakdown, and the experiences of the adults and the children within each can vary widely. I will consider here the most frequent one, namely the experience of divorce for the child reared within an intact, two-parent family prior to the rupture, and who remains subsequently in the custody of the mother. I will not include in this paper the experiences of children reared entirely within a one-parent family, or who were infants or toddlers at the time of the divorce, or whose parents select and maintain joint physical custody following the divorce. I believe that the attributes of divorce as stressor would be distinguishably different in these different groups. In these cases, the adaptive tasks required of the child would also vary significantly.

Divorce and Bereavement Compared

Divorce belongs within a particular category of stress which is initially acute, usually unexpected even if it is anticipated, and with an intensity of impact that is dreaded, since it fundamentally and irrevocably changes the child's world. Stress of this special kind engenders profound distress and is potentially disorganizing in its impact because it demands complex, rapid recognition of a major life change and a rapid adaptation to the changed circumstances.

There are several stressors that fall into this same broad category. These include the untimely death of a close family member or beloved friend, and the loss of community, imposed by exile or natural disaster. Together with divorce, these share in requiring major absorptions of loss and a psychic accommodation which can only take place over the passage of time. Such stressors differ from an acute stress in which the status quo ante may be restored, as in an acute illness. They differ from more chronic stressors such as poverty in which there is no initial and readily identifiable point to indicate the onset of the stressful experience. They differ from the intermittent or recurrent stressful experiences, such as are imposed by living with a severely ill parent who suffers periodic or continuous physical or psychological decline.

It is important not only to understand the long trajectory of bereavement and divorce as stressors but also to examine the patterning of the responses which these evoke over time. Such responses will often show a period of acute distress followed by an extended aftermath which may last for several years beyond the initial impact. The responses of the acute phase are distinguishable from those of the long period that follows, in their form, intensity, and duration. Moreover, responses during the long aftermath sometimes emerge slowly and less visibly than do responses that accompany the acute phase; yet these later emerging ones may ultimately be of greater significance.

In bereavement, the initial response, which is usually one of acute grief, overshadows all other sources of difficulty. In divorce, too, the initial response, which is usually anxiety, is intense and dominates other components of the experience. Only gradually do the multiple changes in the various domains of family life, which have been precipitated by the death or the divorce, come into view.

Writing about bereavement, Parkes (1972) noted:

> Even bereavement by death is not as simple a stress as it might, at first sight, appear to be. In any bereavement it is seldom clear exactly what is lost. The loss of a husband, for instance, may or may not mean the loss of a sexual partner, companion, accountant, gardener, baby minder, audience, bed warmer and so on, depending upon the particular roles normally performed by the husband. Moreover, one loss often brings other secondary losses in its train. The loss of a husband is usually accompanied by a considerable drop in income, and this often means that the widow must sell her house, give up her job (if she has one) and move to a strange environment. (p. 7)

Divorce, too, is not as simple a stress as it might at first sight appear to be, and it is seldom clear, during the early stages, exactly what is lost or what is gained. From the child's perspective the dissolution of the intact family brings a train of losses, and, perhaps, gains in its wake. Thus, divorce, like death, is always accompanied and followed by many other long-lasting changes. Unlike death, the long-lasting changes that follow divorce carry the promise of positive changes and relief as family stability is reestablished. For a significant number of children, losses may continue to outweigh any gains; the eventual balance is probably impossible to assess at the outset.

It may well be, in accord with Rutter's observations (see Chap. 1) regarding the potentiating effects of successive stressful experiences, that the chronic difficulties, whether socioeconomic, social, or psychological, which beset many divorced families in the several years following the marital rupture (Wallerstein & Kelly, 1980a), have a further impact on children whose vulnerability has already been increased markedly by the marital rupture. Perhaps the child's experiences during the acute phase and during the long-term aftermath should be analyzed independently, with outcome several years later regarded as a consequence of the multiple effects or potentiating interactive effects of several successive stressful experiences. There is, in fact, significant evidence in our work (Wallerstein & Kelly, 1980a) that some children maintain their good adjustment during the acute phase of the divorce, and then deteriorate markedly when exposed to the deprivations and heightened tensions in their postdivorce families.

Parental Divorce versus Parental Death

Some of the differences between bereavement and divorce as stressors are important for understanding their impact on the child, and particularly for highlighting the nature of each of these related experiences from the child's perspective. Loss due to death is final, and the lost person is irretrievable. Only the very young child or the person with a severe psychotic illness is able to deny, for any length of time, death when it has occurred. Moreover, no matter how drawn out or unanticipated, death always has an identifiable calendar date. As a consequence, the reality of death is easier to acknowledge.

In divorce, the rules are different. Finality is not present in the same way as in death, and it appears reasonable to the child that the loss can be modified at any time. As a result, the child of divorce at every age, and sometimes well into adulthood, is more likely to experience the persistent, gnawing sense that the loss lacks finality and can be undone. Our clinical experience includes a middle-aged woman patient who sought help from a male and female therapist simultaneously, and finally confessed to each her central preoccupation that she wished to bring both therapists together within the same room so that they could resemble the intact family she had lost as a young child. It proved difficult to dissuade this functioning, non-psychotic woman that the actualization of her fantasy, with the participation of both therapists, would not cure her recurrent, severe depressions.

Further contributing to the child's continuing preoccupation with the fantasy that the loss can be undone is the fact that divorce is often preceded by several separations, all of which may seem decisive but are not final separations. Furthermore, divorce typically is only a partial loss. Children may continue for many years to see the departed parent several times weekly.

There are other differences. Divorce, unlike death, is always a voluntary decision for at least one of the partners, and the participants are both keenly aware of this fact. The child knows all too well that divorce is not a natural disaster, and that its immediate cause is the decision of one or both parents to separate. Its true cause lies in the parental failure to maintain the marriage. The stress that is generated for the child, therefore, always carries the message that the divorce may have been avoided, and that someone is culpable for the unhappiness which is being experienced.

This knowledge burdens the child. Although parent and child may huddle together for mutual support in the face of the divorce storm, the child's terrible dilemma arises from his recognition that the stress has been caused by the very persons charged with his or her protection and care. The stress of divorce for the child is greatly increased by the child's *accurate* perception that the parents are the agents of his distress, and that they have become such agents voluntarily. This awareness may come sooner or later, dimly or clearly. Inevitably, however, the child's stress is greater because it poses the dilemma of knowing something that cannot be expressed without increasing the child's own anger, anguish, or sense of vulnerability. For the child also recognizes that this understanding cannot be expressed without hurting or angering the parent or parents, and thus, further imperiling his or her own position. Thus, ironically, the stress is compounded by the child's understanding of the root cause. Since its successful mastery is linked to accurate perception and understanding of the stress, the child in the divorcing family carries an extra burden in trying to cope—one not experienced by children who face the stress of bereavement following a parent's death.

Anger at both parents for their disruption of the family, or at the parent who sought divorce, is a frequent response among children, whatever their ages. And while anger is often present in bereavement—the anger of the survivor at being abandoned, or self-accusation for failure to prevent a parent's death—there is a fundamental distinction between the anger of the bereaved child with its roots in fantasy and the realistic perception of the child of divorce that one or both parents failed in time of need. The likelihood of blame or anger is always present in divorce, much more strongly than following death and may, as we have observed, last for many years with undiminished intensity (Wallerstein & Kelly, 1980a). Working through this anger becomes one of the major tasks which the child must face during the postdivorce period.

Guilt is also present in both experiences, but in different ways. The bereaved child suffers with the guilt of having failed to rescue the parent who died. The fantasy of having been able to save the dead person, if only to offer somehow to stand in the parent's place, is a persistent one, as is the notion that the anger of the moment, or the vengeful wish, was responsible for the death. During the period of mourning, the grieving child must break free of the oppressive guilt of the survivor and accompanying self-accusations by recognizing the reality of death and its true causes. Similarly, children of divorce often feel that their minor sins of omission or commission may have caused the divorce: "I played too noisy;" "I did not give Mom the message from Dad;" "My dog was naughty." All such expressions can survive for a long time, especially in the minds of young children, to explain a divorce that they cannot comprehend except in such egocentric terms. The fantasy guilt leads many youngsters to wish to undo the misdeed and restore the marriage. This wish is stronger in divorce because it is reinforced by the living presence of both parents. Therefore, guilt-drive restitution or restoration fantasies are likely to be as prevalent in divorce as in bereavement; they may even be more powerful and longer lasting.

Perhaps the greatest difference is that death, unlike other losses, is a universal experience, and each survivor, in confronting the death of another, knows this. Each person finds both terror and comfort in the recognition that the same fate awaits us all. That recognition both increases the anxiety and mutes the guilt of the survivor. Divorce, however, invites the core question: "Will fate write a similar script for me?" This question remains a perennial concern for the child of divorce, and reoccurs as the child progresses through each developmental stage, often appearing with its greatest force when the child reaches adolescence and looks anxiously at what may be ahead when the threshold into adulthood is crossed.

Finally, the social milieu and the available community support are different for the children in each of these groups. Divorce, certainly at the outset, is a lonelier road for children and adolescents in the divorcing family. Unlike the social network that rallies for the ceremonies of death and the support of the bereaved in the immediate aftermath of parental loss, when a divorce occurs such supports are often absent. More often, friends and neighbors stay away, and grandparents may take sides in the conflict or frown on the decision of the divorcing couple. Thus, divorce, as we see so many times, represents for both children and adults intense distress at a time of diminished support, despite the increased need for help at a time of great loneliness.

Children of divorce and bereavement share in their awareness that a shadow has been cast over their lives. Both experiences set off a chain of ruminative anxieties about the future. Attempts at mastery require renewed effort at each developmental stage because the questions stimulated by either the divorce or the death reoccur or continue as the absent parent or the intact family of childhood is sought anew to satisfy different needs at each successive stage of development.

THE TIME TRAJECTORY OF DIVORCE

Divorce is accurately understood as a multistage *process* of radically changing family relationships which begins with the marital rupture and its immediate aftermath, continues over several years of disequilibrium during the transition period, and finally comes to rest with the restabilization of the new postdivorce family unit.

Social scientists influenced, in part, by the legal process, have regarded divorce as a single stressful event—or as a brief period of disruption, followed by a settling in of the one-parent family. Our own observations affirm that family instabilities set into motion by the marital rupture are likely to occupy a significant portion of the child's growing-up years. The average time which the women in our study required to regain a sense of order and stability in their lives was 3 to 3½ years postseparation. These time estimates can be extended markedly in many families were we to add the instability and disequilibrium of the failing marriage just prior to the decision to divorce. The time-frame for these processes will vary, but a realistic perspective would see them occupying a period some 3 to 5 years from the separation, 2 to 4 years from the divorce. Such a span covers perhaps one-half of the life time of the 7-year-old and one-quarter of the childhood of the 12-year-old.

Stages of the Divorce Process

Although additional observations of larger samples and different demographic groups are needed, our present information enables us to conceptualize several successive stages to the divorcing process—which, despite overlap, are significantly distinguishable one from the other.

The *acute phase* is precipitated by the decisive separation of the married couple, and is usually accompanied by the legal step of filing for dissolution of the marriage, and, most often in our society, by the father's departure from the household. The duration of this phase ranges from several months to over a year from this beginning step of the legal process which, in most jurisdictions, occurs at least one year prior to the final divorce decree. The stressful, often chaotic, ambience of the acute phase is linked to the fact that the decision to divorce in families with children rarely represents a truly mutual decision, but is usually sought by only one member of the marriage and opposed or accepted reluctantly by the partner.

The *transitional phase* which follows spans a period of several years, during which adults and children embark on unfamiliar roles and relationships within the new family structure. Often the newly diminished family unit will change its residence. Mother and children may experience a reduced standard of living and a different life style, as the mother shoulders a greater share of economic responsibility. Parent-child relationships are likely to alter radically, especially within the visiting relationship (Wallerstein & Kelly, 1980b). These radical changes require complex and painful adaptations.

Finally, there follows a *stabilizing phase* in which the postdivorce family is eventually reestablished as a stable, functioning unit. The economic and social roles and the relationship patterns at this time represent those that evolved or were retained after the years of transition. Remarriage is a frequent occurrence during and following the transitional phase, and introduces additional changes in all domains of family life.

Not all families progress through this sequence of change. Some families may remain fixated at the acute phase. Such families expend their energy, and often their financial resources, in bitter, continued fighting over children or property—whether in or out of the courts. For such families, the acute stress remains high and soon becomes chronic, but it does not resolve or substantially subside.

Other families remain in a transition phase. The family may move from place to place without settling down for many years. Or the instability may remain evident in a pattern of continuing household disorder, marked by a profusion of people present in the home, and frequent job and residence changes, accompanied by a continued sense of being in midair, despite the reduction of the original high level of tension. Referred to aptly as the "chronically reconstituting family" (Hunter & Schuman, 1980) in these instances, the continued psychological, social, economic, or geographic instability reflects an incapacity to reach closure.

The Nature of Divorce-Induced Changes

The changes which occur during these years are likely to be at a very different tempo than anticipated at the time of the decision to divorce. They are likely to be abrupt—episodic yet continual—even as they gradually diminish. The changes are likely, moreover, to occur in all domains of family life: economic, social, psychological, and sexual, as well as in parent-child relationships and household spheres of functioning. Many of the changes which are reflected in school, in the neighborhood, in the home, in child-care patterns, in the availability of each parent, and in the general standard of living occur within a compressed time span during the early postseparation period. As a result, the experience of many children is that almost all aspects of their lives are in flux over a period of years, and that the world as they knew it has lost its sense of stability and order.

Of course, many such changes often occur within an intact family as well. Nevertheless, the intact family can be expected to bend rather than to break with the changes, and to provide the family members with a basic sense of coherence and stability, even in the midst of grave disorder. In fact, one cardinal function of the family system is to provide a sense of continuity and a place of comfort amidst the predictable unpredictability of life. The changes induced by the divorce are especially stressful because the protective structure of the family has been toppled. Therefore, each individual within the divorced family not only experiences more change, but also feels more exposed to danger and is more threatened by its anticipated actual impact.

The Acute Phase

During the acute phase, the changes may include new behaviors in the parents that differ greatly from their customary demeanor. Children are confronted by a marked discrepancy in images; although these bizarre behaviors are short lived when they are at their most intense, the child lacks the assurance that the more customary behaviors will reappear. These disruptive new behaviors are of many kinds, including verbal accusations, threats, and rage accompanied by violence, and depression which may include a preoccupation with suicide.

It is interesting, and not at all self-evident, to conjecture as to why so many adults experience the divorce as striking centrally at their psychic integrity, with its evocations of hurt, and even fantasies of annihilation. One explanation may be that the severity of the response of so many adults is related to the fact that the decision to terminate the marriage is rarely mutual. There is, therefore, a sense of a loss of internal control with respect to one of the major decisions that is made in one's lifetime. Although there may have been considerable accord on the sad state of the marriage, there is frequently sharp disagreement in the desire to end it. It is not unusual for a marital relationship which has been relatively lifeless or humdrum for years on end to come to life with the threat of its termination. Nor is it uncommon for people who have lived side by side for years in loneliness and without sexual contact to be stung by humiliation and rejection and galvanized into activity. Apparently nothing brings life to a marriage as quickly as the threat of its dissolution.

Often even a weak or a failing marriage may provide a structure which serves as a bedrock of safety and a source of externalized ego control. As the marriage structure fails, aggressive feelings and sexual impulses which have been held in check are suddenly released with new force and with reduced efforts to control them. The unrestrained expression of these feelings dominates many households which prior to the decision to divorce had been marked by a more circumspect and reserved way of life.

Diminished Capacity to Parent

The acute phase is one of physical dislocation, psychological change, and the diminished availability of parents. Newly employed parents are likely to leave children with new sitters, or in strange settings, or alone after school. Sometimes the burden of work is such that very young children need to prepare their own lunch, get themselves off to school, and put themselves to bed. Thus, these practical life changes take their toll in reducing the parents' time and attention available for children. Additionally, the search by parents for new relationships takes on heightened importance, and further reduces the time available for the children. The flurry of social or sexual activity that often occurs immediately following the breakup can absorb weekends that customarily have been spent with children.

The visiting or noncustodial parent's housing is often inadequate for extended visits, and early visits tend to be uneasy, tense, and may have a makeshift quality. Moreover, few visiting parents are prepared for the challenge of the visiting relationship, nor can they acknowledge how difficult this will be to initiate and to maintain over the years to follow.

Hetherington et al. (1978) has called attention to the household disorder that prevails in the aftermath of divorce with its coercive pattern of control, of rising tempers in both mother and child, of reduced competence and a greater sense of helplessness in the mother that stimulates a continuing cycle of mutually interacting and frequently destructive behaviors. Our own observations are similar. We, too, find greater disorder, poorly enforced discipline, and diminished regularity in enforcing household routines. The root causes underlying the deteriorating household order we have found to be, in addition to fatigue and overloading, the mother's fear of rejection by her children. Her wish to avoid reproach for the divorce and a fear of the children's anger lead her to yield to the children's clamor, and to retreat from the requirement that standards be maintained in the home. In a significant number of families where the father had been tyrannical, even abusive to the mother, the conflict between the parents was silently reinstated in the relationship between mother and child. Conflicts transplanted from the failing marriage immobilize the mother anew and recall her similar immobilization during the marriage.

For all these reasons, our studies indicate that during the immediate aftermath to the separation and for the first year, the custodial parent tends to be less competent as a parent, less able to maintain the structure of the household, and less available to the children. The youngsters are irritable, edgy, and often accusatory and rebellious. The result is mounting disorder, less discipline, and less caretaking, which in turn heightens the anxiety of all the participants. As one woman described it, "I feel like I'm treading water in a tidal wave."

The Child's Experience during the Acute Phase

From the perspective of the child two initial events prove to be immediately most stressful. These are first, learning about the divorce decision, usually from their parents (see Wallerstein & Kelly, 1980a, for a detailed account of the children's responses); and second, the departure of one parent from the home. Youngsters remember *both* of these events for many years and, in fact, well into adulthood with a detail that reveals their long-lasting significance. Etched in memory are the mundane events of "the day my father left." The poignant, vivid sense of recall is reminiscent of that of bereaved people, or of people who have lived through a natural disaster. These two events become the core memories for many children.

To increase our understanding of stress in childhood it is important to realize that, despite the awareness some children have of the marital conflict, it does not mute their response to the divorce when the separation finally occurs, nor does it distinguish their behavior from the significant number of children who apparently have no conscious awareness of their parents' marital unhappiness. Our observations indicate that there is little evidence that either foreknowledge or ignorance of the conflict are critical factors in predicting the child's response to marital rupture in the family. We have speculated that some events are too overwhelmingly stressful to master, even in fantasy, and that for the younger (preadolescent) child, family breakup may fall into this category. Perhaps this is also similar to bereavement, in that anticipatory mourning may be possible for the adult and even the adolescent, but, on the basis of our own data, there is no evidence that the child's ego is capable of similar anticipatory cognitions regarding divorce. There is, in fact, some evidence that anticipatory attempts to master this trauma may actually aggravate the problem by raising the child's anxiety, thus providing a reversal to the coping effort. In lieu of mastery, the child may worry for years about the divorce that he or she expects to happen. When the divorce occurs, the child may experience horror at the actualization of the feared nightmare.

The acute distress, the rage and the moderate to severe depression of one or both parents have a direct impact on the children. The parental preoccupation with their own problems substantially decreases the care or attention which the children receive. Many children are frightened and worried by the parental mood and behavior, by the intensity of the conflict, and by the physical violence that may occur in their presence. Children are rarely protected from witnessing the angry scenes and, in fact, in some families the fighting only occurs when the children are present.

Additionally, the behavior and distress of the parent increases the children's awareness that the parents are not available for help during the family crisis amid their sense of having to make use of their own resources. This realization is of major importance to the children's mode of response and evokes widely different reactions, many of which are age-related.

Observations Regarding Developmental Factors in the Child's Initial Response

Developmental factors are critical in the responses of children and adolescents at the time of the marital disruption. Despite significant individual differences, the child's age and developmental stage appear to be the most important factors governing the initial responses. Stage of development profoundly influences the child's need for, and expectation of, the parents, and the perception of the stress, as well as the child's available armamentarium of coping and defensive strategies.

We have elsewhere (Wallerstein & Kelly, 1980a) noted that a major goal of our own research was to formulate tentative models of expectable responses or norms of behavior for divorce-related reactions of children and adolescents, and the length of their duration following the marital rupture. The unavailability of such a model of developmental stages and norms has severely handicapped parents, and those who undertake to help parents, in their efforts to fashion appropriate measures which will provide comfort and relief to the children. Additionally, in the absence of knowledge regarding normative responses and the expectable duration of these responses, it has been difficult to identify those children whose behavior reflects the need for special intervention.

One of the major findings of our research has been that it is possible to delineate patterns of response that are associated with different age groups. We had expected some correspondence between the children's initial behavioral responses to the divorce and the child's age and developmental stage. Nevertheless, we were surprised to find the extent to which the children's perceptions, worries, and fantasies about the divorce, its causes and its likely consequences for them, and their major affective as well as symptomatic responses were governed by their age and place on the developmental ladder at the time of the marital rupture. The four groups which we reported, preschool children (age 2½ to 5), early school-age children (age approximately 5½ to 8), later school-age children (age approximately 9 to 12) and adolescents, did not reflect a priori groupings. We did not begin with these specific groups in mind; rather, our observations dictated them because of the commonalities which we found in the responses of children within each of these age groups.

Thus we have described that the *preschool child* following the marital rupture is likely to regress behaviorally; is likely to worry about being abandoned by *both* parents; is more likely than the older child to feel responsible for causing the divorce; is likely to become intensely aware of all separations and to be very frightened at the routine separations during daytime and especially at bedtime; is likely to develop moderate sleep disturbances; is likely to be tearful, irritable, and more aggressive; and is likely to suffer an inhibition of play (Wallerstein & Kelly, 1975; Wallerstein, 1977a, 1977b).

Findings among children within the other age groups can be similarly extrapolated from our study to suggest a range of expectable behaviors. Thus, to provide further examples, children in the *early school-age group* are likely to show moderate depression; to be preoccupied with the father's departure from the home; to grieve openly and to long intensely for his return; to fear replacement ("Will my daddy get another mommy, another dog, another little boy?"); and to experience the father's departure as rejection ("If he loved *me*, he would not have left"). Approximately half of the children in this age group experienced a disruption in their learning at school as well as deteriorated relationships with their peers during the year following the decisive marital separation (Kelly & Wallerstein, 1976).

Children in the *older school-age group*, by contrast, are, at the time of the marital breakdown, more likely to perceive one parent as responsible for the divorce and the other parent as victimized; they are likely to be intensely angry at one or both parents, often expressing this anger directly in ways that can be profoundly distressing to one parent. They are also likely to be acutely aware of the dating and sexual behavior of the parents, and to find this behavior both stimulating and distracting. They also appear more likely to develop mild somatic symptoms at this time (Wallerstein & Kelly, 1976). *Adolescent youngsters* shared in the intense anger of the preadolescent or older school-age group, but they too presented a range of specific behavioral responses which seem to reflect the impact of the divorce on adolescent developmental processes and conflicts (Wallerstein & Kelly, 1974).

It may be, of course, that the usefulness of these group descriptions will extend only to similar samples of predominantly white, middle-class children in communities where the nuclear family is the predominant family structure. Or it may be that more extensive research studies will demonstrate that major stressful experiences, such as loss, death, and divorce, are rooted in developmental factors which span broad social, economic, racial, and ethnic variations.

Our further findings regarding responses during this acute phase, which are corroborated by Hetherington et al. (1979b), reveal that sex differences in response to the stress of divorce could be distinguished. Thus, the responses of boys and girls ran a separate course; from the very beginning, the girls (in mother-custody homes) did significantly better than the boys in their overall adjustment at home and at school. The differences between the boys and the girls were especially evident during the first year and a half following the decisive separation. By 5 years, however, these early differences faded along with differences related to age and developmental achievement. However, significant subgroups did emerge at the 5-year follow-up; for example, there was a significant group of girls who, upon entering into adolescence, became acutely depressed for what appeared to be the first time. In general, however, neither age nor sex proved to be significant in separating troubled children from the children who were well adjusted at the 5-year postseparation mark. Differences among the children 5 years later appeared less tied to the impact of the divorce experience on their development and more to individual differences among the children, to the parent-child relationships which developed within the postdivorce family, and to the quality of life within the postdivorce family.

I have written primarily one account in an effort to capture the stressfulness of the acute phase of divorce, and to call attention to the various components of that experience and their complex interactions. There is, of course, not one, but multiple accounts of that same stressor. Nevertheless, I have tried to describe and include the modal experiences of the children, avoiding extremes on either side, such as those in which the stress is greatly exacerbated because parents undertake prolonged or repeated litigation over the children and, by contrast, other situations in which the divorce is relatively benign in its impact because both parents maintain their personal intactness throughout, including their full capacity to parent. Although it is difficult to estimate the incidence of families in each group, Foster and Freed (1980) have reported that approximately 10% of divorcing couples with children carry their battle over the children to the courts. In our study, approximately 15% of the total number of families seeking divorce did not experience grave emotional upheavals immediately following the separation.

THE TASKS OF ADAPTATION

Having delineated various aspects of marital rupture as severely stressful from the perspective of the child who has been reared within the two-parent family, I turn now to an attempt to conceptualize the child's responses over time. The use of *task* as an organizing construct may help to take us forward toward a next step in bridging the theoretical and experiential ground between the concepts of stress and coping. By interposing the concept of tasks, we are able to formulate more clearly questions related to the child's coping efforts by spelling out the patterns of coping. What what aspects of the stressful experience do children cope? Over how long a time span? In what temporal sequence? With what type of outcome? In encompassing both the manifest behavior of the children as well as their inner psychic experience, the concept of tasks and their mastery provides access to the psychological significance of children's responses, as well as their social context and social consequences. Additionally, it permits us to envision responses to stress not only over the period of childhood and adolescence, but in the broader context of the life-span perspective.

Its chief limitation as a concept is implicit in the dichotomy of failure *or* success in coping with the divorce experience. Therefore, it is important to bear in mind that the resolution of life's tasks is always relative and, probably, always partial. Within this framework, successful resolution can be defined as that which permits the individual to maintain a reasonable developmental progression. Alternatively, relative failure can be thought of as that which significantly hampers or distorts subsequent development.

The concept of task has its roots in Freud's early formulations about "grief work," that is, a consequence of the loss imposed on the bereaved individual. The concept identifies the psychological processes that the bereaved individual must engage in in order to integrate the stressful experience and to continue life without psychic impairment (Freud, 1917). The concept of "grief work" and related tasks was elaborated further by Lindemann (1944) and Caplan (1955) and was central to their construction of crisis theory and in the development of crisis intervention as a psychotherapeutic modality. Tasks are central, as well, to Erikson's architectural view of the course of human development (Erikson, 1950). Erikson's notion that each maturational stage in psychological development presents the growing individual with a sequence of tasks, which must be confronted and successfully achieved or failed in varying degrees, is congenial to this same view.

Both the time constraints and the temporal sequence imposed by each of the divorce-related tasks are important. Several tasks need to be addressed almost immediately, optimally within the first few months of the marital rupture, but at least within the first year. These include the first two of six tasks which are to be mastered: I identify Task I as *Acknowledging the Marital Disruption*; and Task II as *Regaining a Sense of Direction and Freedom to Pursue Customary Activities*. The child's successful mastery of these relatively immediate tasks is tied to the maintenance of his or her developmental pace and to the resumption of progress in school after an initial, expectable dip in learning effectiveness and academic performance.

Other tasks pose their challenge more benevolently, in the sense that their accomplishment has a longer delay period which may extend over the child's growing up years. These are likely to become salient only at mid-adolescence. I have included in this group Task III, *Dealing with Loss and Feelings of Rejection*; Task IV, *Forgiving the Parents*; and Task V, *Accepting the Permanence of the Divorce*.

The last task, which is most central to adolescence, depends on the efficacy of the child's resolution of the earlier tasks for its full accomplishment. This final Task VI, which I have called *Resolving Issues of Relationship*, is, in the long run, perhaps the most important task both for the child and the family, and for society. There is some recent evidence (Kulka & Weingarten, 1979) that the first decade of young adulthood between the ages of twenty and thirty may find the child of divorce still burdened by unresolved issues. The last task may indeed come fully to resolution only after that time.

THE SEQUENCE OF TASKS FOR CHILDREN OF DIVORCE

TASK I: Acknowledging the Marital Disruption

The first and simplest task for the child is to acknowledge the marital rupture and to grasp its immediate consequences independent of the frightening fantasies which have been evoked in the child's mind. A primary obstacle to the child's acknowledgment of the marital separation are the many fantasies by which he endows these changes with terrifying causes and consequences. An additional obstacle to the child's acknowledgment is the torrent of intense feelings that pose an overwhelming sense of threat. Of course, the child's strong wish to deny the rift and restore the intact family also plays a role. Success or failure will be governed by several factors: the individual's capacity and his or her developmental level in addressing both inner and outer reality, and the assistance provided to the child from the family and the social surround. Cognitive mastery, in this regard, can be considered as a function of accuracy of perception, the emotional and intellectual capacity of the child to understand the march of events, combined with a mastering of terrifying and disturbing fantasies.

For many children, the task of understanding the divorce and sorting out reality from fantasy, and, in some instances, reality from dreams, is gravely hampered by the troubled behavior of the parents that, as already described, can sometimes approach bizarre limits under the driving force of frenzied anger or depression. Added to this is the relative absence of assurance, explanation, and support from parents and other adults. In addition, the many unknowns that mark the divorcing process, and the many rapid changes that have been described, contribute to the child's heightened anxiety. The lacunae in the child's understanding and expectations attract and foster greater dependence on fantasy, blocking the capacity to make sense out of the events. Finally, the fact that the departed parent is, at the outset, vaguely located somewhere beyond the home, and whose reappearance is indeterminate, lends further power to the child's fantasy constructions. The ego regressions which are a characteristic anxiety response to the stressful marital rupture, especially among the younger children, further burdens the child's capacity to understand and assimilate the family changes and to separate reality from fantasy.

Developmental factors are relevant both to the perception and mastery of this task. Adolescents and older youngsters do not struggle as much with this problem as do their younger siblings. Nevertheless, a surprisingly large number of older children also had trouble acknowledging the reality of the divorce, and their behavior reflected their difficulty. For example, one 12-year-old boy on being told of the impending divorce by his parents ran through the house screaming, "You're trying to kill us all." A 10-year-old child began to vomit. The earliest reactions of many of these children reflected their perception of the divorce as bearing catastrophic consequences.

The task was most difficult for those children whose capacity to understand the world around them was limited by two interacting factors: their own developmental immaturity and the failure of the parents to provide an explanation of the disturbing event. For example, one 3-year-old child whose mother had impulsively departed the household refused to leave his position in the middle of the living room where he had last seen her. His father's repeated efforts to remove the child from the living room elicited wild screaming. Evidently the child had endowed that particular spot with the fantasy power to evoke the mother's return. Like a sentry, the child stood hour after hour, waiting with courage and steadfastness, dominated by the fantasy of the mother's imminent return, and entirely unable to sort out the events swirling around him.

How Did the Children Accomplish the Task of Acknowledgment?

Most children mastered their anxiety by gradually recognizing that their fears and worries for themselves and their parents, which underlay their initial panic, were unlikely to occur. One-half of the children in our study had feared at the outset that the father would abandon them; one-third expected the mother would do so; a few feared they would be placed outside their homes. As time passed and these fears proved groundless, the children were able to sort out reality from their own fantasies, to recover from their anxiety-driven regressive behavior, and to return to their customary activities.

Similarly, the children's anxiety subsided as the parent assured them of continued love and care. Sometimes the anxiety subsided dramatically when the remaining parent was able to realize the child's core concern, and then deal with it directly. When this occurred, the relationship between the parent and child was strengthened, and the child was then able to draw upon the new strength to increase his or her own capacity to deal with fantasy and fear. For example, one 4-year-old boy whose mother had left several weeks after there had been a small fire within the household, confessed to his father that he was unable to sleep at night because he was afraid that the mother had burned in the fire. He was able to make the confession only after the father had talked with the child at length, and after he had taken the child to visit the mother where they had shared an afternoon together. On the way home from the visit, the child was able to summon his courage. Relying on his closeness with his father and reassured by the visit with his mother, he began to sort out his fantasy by revealing it to the father and asking him to clarify the reality. "Daddy," said the child, "let's have another talk."

Sometimes as anxiety decreased, the child was able to approach the parent for help in clarifying the distinction between the fantasy and reality. We saw this time and again with children whose first response to the father's departure was one of panic. Several weeks later, these youngsters were able to ask the questions which clearly had troubled them from the very start. When the question was verbalized by the child, the adult's attention was directed toward answering it and providing reassurance to the frightened child that their relationship would continue.

Acknowledging the marital rupture is a task distinct from the more problematic one of acknowledging its permanence. This was a second, more difficult step for many children which will be addressed later. All of the children in our study succeeded during the first year in achieving the initial task of acknowledging the marital breakup. For most, this was done with considerable effort, and then only by modifying their perceptions and diminishing the anxiety that had been evoked by visions of a cataclysmic disaster.

TASK II: Regaining a Sense of Direction and Freedom to Pursue Customary Activities

A major task for children is the resumption of their normal pursuits, with the appropriate pleasure and commitment of energy and sustained interest, despite worry and preoccupation about the crisis at home. In order to accomplish this task, the child needs to achieve a modicum of mastery over the powerful anxieties triggered by the collapsing family structure. At the outset, children of all ages kept their attention riveted on the events of the household. Many were unable to leave home for an extended period of time, or if they did so, were likely to continue their preoccupation with family events. Therefore, the child's return to school, play, and the peer group depends on the capacity to remove the divorce from its central, commanding position in thought and feelings, and to regain sufficient composure and perspective to permit return to age-appropriate activities.

Following the marital rupture, many children develop symptoms and mood changes which seriously interfere with their capacity to carry on their customary activities. Many of the new behaviors are developmentally linked. As we have noted in our research study, the youngest children grew frightened by separation and became anxious when attending a nursery school; they were newly agitated and tearful at the many routine separations of day and evening. A significant number suffered with nightmares and awoke many times during the night, with the result that they were exhausted during the long days that followed.

For the school-age children, worry over a depressed or angry parent kept many of them from venturing away from home. Some were overcome with sorrow and withdrew mournfully to sit all day in darkened rooms. Others in this age group were preoccupied with fantasies about the sexual activity of their parents. For example, Gwen, age 10, complained that she had lost interest in school, in her friends, and in her piano lessons, "in everything since Dad left." She reported that she thought all day that he was "making out with his girlfriend." She also thought constantly about her mother together with her boyfriend and "shuddered" at the thought that her mother "might fall in love." "How," asked the child, "can I concentrate at school, thinking about Mom and Dad kissing and making love with other people?"

Approximately half of the children who attended elementary school experienced a serious disruption in concentration and their ability to learn. Many reported that they failed to make sense of the teachers' instructions because they were absorbed in thinking about the divorce. Additionally, their capacity to play was gravely impaired during this period. Youngsters reported a major inhibition in their ability to enjoy after-school activities ranging widely from athletics to ballet. Friendships were also difficult to maintain as they became tense, irritable, bossy, demanding, and manipulative with friends whom they soon antagonized or drove away.

Some adolescents took flight from both home and their usual round of activities. Such youngsters were truant from school and sought new companions, many of whom were often engaged in minor or more serious delinquencies, sexual activities and drinking, which brought them to the attention of the school authorities. Other adolescents remained at home. Included in this latter group were a few youngsters who reported that they paced the floor restlessly until the early hours of the morning whenever the custodial parent spent the evening out.

Only very few youngsters, at every age, seemed able to maintain their customary activities at the height of the crisis. The acuteness of the children's initial distress and the gravity of the learning disruption did not, however, predict which child would later resume studies successfully and which child would fail to do so. Many of the children who exhibited acutely disorganized responses at the outset were able at a later time to pick up their school work and to play with undiminished zest.

How Did the Children Accomplish This Task?

Most of the youngsters within the year following the marital breakup were able to reengage in their customary routines. Those with a history of successful achievement in many domains, children who had previously "learned well, loved well, played well, and expected well" (Grinker, 1968) found this task easier to accomplish as they resumed their earlier pattern of competent behavior. Those who had the support of patient, loyal friends and concerned teachers also found their way back more quickly and were gradually able to make use of gratifications at school and on the playground to offset deprivations at home. Others were able to return to pleasurable activities and academic pursuits only as the parents grew more calm, as their physical care was resumed, and as the routines of the household were stabilized.

Children Who Failed

A significant number of children were unable to resume their customary activities in school and playground after the divorce. They remained lonely, worried, and unhappy as they continued to experience difficulty in school and at play. These youngsters appeared unable to make sufficient use of the support available from teachers, even loving, sensitive teachers, who made strenuous efforts to engage the children and to help them in a variety of ways. These youngsters also had difficulty in maintaining friendships with peers and tended instead to retreat to their own homes after school where they could be with the custodial parent, to await her return, to watch TV, to overeat, or to play with younger children. Some of these adolescents and preadolescents remained heavily involved in activities which were not conducive to their academic or social progress. Several such youngsters remained highly stimulated by the sexual behavior of their parents. Unable to concentrate at school, they began to seek older companions. Other children continued to be actively embroiled in the parental battles, while still others spent increasing amounts of time at home in the company of the parent who remained troubled and depressed.

We have elsewhere (Wallerstein & Kelly, 1980a) distinguished various subgroups among these youngsters who failed to recover their developmental stride within the first year or two following the breakup. Some were living in families in which the acute stress had failed to subside and had become chronic. Others were residing with a depressed parent. Some of these youngsters who grew depressed following the father's departure were unable to master the sense of having been abandoned. Overall, children who came to the divorce with a history of chronic difficulties and poor achievement, and for whom the postdivorce family provided little or no improvement in the overall quality of their lives, experienced the greatest difficulty following the divorce. The age of the child at the time of the breakup was not significant in separating the children who mastered this task from those who failed to do so.

TASK III: Dealing With Loss and Feelings of Rejection

Assimilating the grief over the departure of one parent from the home, and coming to terms with the partial or total loss of that parent, is the single most difficult task for many children to master. To accomplish this task, the child is required to mourn the father's absence and to bring the mourning process to relative closure by acceptance of the loss. Additionally, the task demands that the child overcome the profound sense of rejection and humiliation which the one parent's departure so often brings in its wake. To avoid seriously diminished self-esteem consequent to the loss, the child is required to break the link which so often connects the parent's departure to the child's misbehavior or fantasied sense of being unloved or unworthy. This task often requires an extended period of continued reworking which may last several years. Moreover, the child of divorce is more heavily burdened than the child who loses a parent through death because, as we have noted earlier, divorce is a voluntary decision and the very voluntariness of the one parent's departure magnifies the complexity of mastering the loss and feelings of rejection experienced by the child.

An additional burden at the time of the marital breakup, and later as well, is the children's awareness that they need to maintain the love and attention of the visiting parent in order to assure the continuation of such visits. In this way, visitations extend this task over many years. The explanation which children found so persuasive, namely: "Had he loved me, he would not have left the family;" was easily extended to: "If he loved me, he would visit more often or spend more time with me;" a belief made especially acute by the absence of a reliable visiting pattern. As a result, the child's vulnerability to feeling rejected can persist over the years that follow.

The loss of the father's presence within the family was experienced by children of all ages as an event of far-reaching significance, even when accompanied by a sense of relief from earlier scenes of violence and fighting between the parents. Open grief, accompanied by sobbing, prolonged tears, and sighing were especially observable among the younger school-age boys. Sometimes the grief was overwhelming. "I don't have a daddy! I'll need a daddy!" sobbed one 6-year-old boy who would not be comforted.

The yearning for the departed parent was particularly painful for children who had been close to their fathers during the marriage and were accustomed to spending many hours in their company. But this yearning was not confined to such children alone. Some were hardly able to accept the father's absence and relied on a wide range of defenses, particularly denial, to mute their unhappiness. Thus, several youngsters insisted that he would return stating, "It's going to be *just* like it was." Little girls of oedipal age were especially likely to weave elaborate Madame Butterfly fantasies around the father's expected return. Often they combined this fantasy preoccupation with the insistence, "He loved me the best," attempting in this way to reverse and to undo the rejection which they experienced. Others denied the father's absence through identification. They took on his pattern of speech and intonation, wore his tie, or adopted his mode of talking with the mother, which was often unpleasant and even tyrannical.

It is probably realistic to anticipate that both divorce and bereavement leave an enduring residue of sadness. Their legacy may include continued vulnerability to subsequent loss of another loving relationship. For the child of divorce, the legacy may also include a continued vulnerability to feelings of rejection and diminished self-esteem. Successful resolution, however, would envision a coexistence of these vulnerabilities with a lively capacity to enjoy life and a realistic self-confidence.

How Did Children Accomplish This Task?

The task in its two-fold challenge was accomplished most readily when the loss was only partial, and when father and child successfully and collaboratively established a reliable, mutually gratifying visiting relationship. Many fathers and children were able to do this, including those who grew closer following the divorce. Within such relationships, the child's grief was aborted. In fact, the child's self-esteem was likely to be enhanced by the knowledge that the father chose voluntarily to visit and remained constant in his efforts to do so, despite the formidable obstacles of time and space.

A few youngsters were able to deal successfully with sporadic, even erratic visiting, by turning their attention elsewhere and becoming involved in school, developing attachments to friends, teachers, an extended family member, or the custodial parent. Seemingly, after a period of an acute response to the departure of the father, they appeared able to turn their attention elsewhere without evident conflict, especially when the father's residence was a distant one. By and large, youngsters in this group were especially well supported by loving, competent adults both within and outside their families.

When they reached adolescence, a few youngsters appeared able to mount a counter-rejection of a father who had abandoned them. They acquired at adolescence new strengths which enabled them to take a vigorous, independent stand and to deal successfully with their earlier feelings of hurt and humiliation at having been abandoned. Their counter-rejection or repudiation usually took the form of a new perception of the father as an undesirable ego ideal, and they consciously turned away in anger, coupling this with the conscious choice of a mentor elsewhere. Whether this conscious disowning of a central relationship will continue into adulthood, and whether it will enable the young person to move successfully into the tasks of that stage, is at this time unknown.

Children Who Failed

Unfortunately, most children who experienced significant loss of one parent following the divorce and were disappointed by the visitation patterns over the years did not succeed in overcoming their own dejection and sense of being unlovable or unworthy. Their low self-confidence burdened their learning effectiveness and their peer relations. A goodly number were clinically depressed. Madame Butterfly fantasies which had developed as their earliest response to the marital breakup were consolidated and strengthened in those who remained preoccupied with fantasies of the father's return, while acutely aware of the unlikelihood of this occurrence. Nevertheless, they seemed unable either to believe, or to renounce, the fantasy of his expected return which preempted their daydreams. Older youngsters who failed to resolve their acute feelings of rejection were likely to show anger and aggressiveness.

Developmental factors were relevant to the child's capacity to accomplish this particular task of dealing with loss and feelings of rejection. Oedipal-age children were more likely to hold onto the fantasy of the father's return to the family, and seemed to suffer the loss more intensely. At the same time, children of all ages who had enjoyed a close, loving relationship with the father during the marriage also suffered intensely, encountered grave difficulty in assimilating their loss, and often were unable to do so. These children who failed utterly to master the loss, typically were exposed to poor parental practices by the remaining parent. The emotional valence of the absent parent did not, therefore, stand entirely on its own but was related to the range of gratifications in the child's current life, including other available relationships.

TASK IV: Forgiving the Parents

A major task for children in the process of recovery from the acute reactions precipitated by the marital breakup was working through the intense anger they felt toward one or both parents. Such anger not only alienated the child from the parent, but often led the child, especially the preadolescent and adolescent youngster, into mischievous acting-out behaviors aimed at harassing and punishing the parent they accused of causing the divorce. Contrapuntal to the anger was the child's love and dependence on the parent, and the mutual need of parent and child for reconciliation, forgiveness, and partnership in the postdivorce family. In this task, we address one of the central and more painful dilemmas of the divorcing process, namely that the child often experiences the divorce as opposed to his own best interests. Therefore, the child's anger was most often linked to accusations that the parents were indifferent to the child's needs, and that they were acting only out of a selfish concern for their own interests. A recurrent theme in the playroom at the time of the marital rupture was one of adults only caring for adults while children, in turn, cared only for children.

Accusations were sometimes very bitter. Parents were regarded as having failed in their primary responsibility as parents; as corrupt in preaching morality to the children while following different guidelines in their own conduct; as exploitative of the children's powerlessness; as cruelly rejecting of the children's love and friendship; as unfeeling and unconcerned about the children's unhappiness; as cowardly and weak, unable to deal with adversity except by taking flight; as powerful figures who needed to be overtly appeased and secretly resisted. The anger which accompanied these accusations was often intense and dominated the youngster's mood in its fierceness and pervasiveness. Tantrums, screaming for hours on end, and threats of violence directed at property and person occurred. Sometimes the anger spilled over into other domains of life as children fought with their friends on the playground or got into trouble with teachers and other adults in authority.

How Do Children Resolve This Task?

It is important to distinguish between the full resolution of angry feelings and the reduction of such anger so that they no longer exercised a major influence on the child, or dominated the parent-child relationship. Perhaps one must recognize realistically that some residue of this anger remained unresolved. Children remained aggrieved, in some measure, feeling for many years that a significant portion of their growing up had been burdened by the parental failure. A goodly number of these youngsters perceived the inability or unwillingness of their parents to remain faithful within the marriage. Such anger which was rooted in accurate perceptions of the parents' infidelity was unlikely to disappear over the years, although the intensity diminished with time.

For some youngsters, the task of forgiving one or both parents was achieved within the context of a newly close or reaffirmed relationship with one parent. The friendship between parent and child, which grew during the crisis out of a mutual need, served, thus, not only to offset the child's unhappiness and loneliness, but also to mute the intense angers which had been evoked. Within the framework of the new mutuality and interdependence, children acquired a more realistic perspective regarding the divorce and a better understanding of the distribution of responsibilities on both sides. Such relationships also fostered maturity in the child. In fact, some of the special helpfulness which youngsters provided their parents following the divorce may have had its roots in several factors: compassion for their burdened parents; a constructive effort to deal with the underlying intense anger which they experienced; and the effort to reverse or undo that anger by building a constructive alliance within the postdivorce family.

Some of the children's intense anger came under control as they were able to observe improvement in one or another parent following the separation. As children grew in their understanding of this change, they began to recognize the parents' needs as different and distinct from their own, and they were able to say with a calm perspective, "The divorce is better for my mother, although it is not especially so for me." Finally, as the household stabilized and the children experienced a diminution of their anxiety and a greater sense of comfort, their anger also diminished correspondingly.

Children Who Failed

A significant subgroup of youngsters continued for many years to be angry with one or both parents. Some of these youngsters became involved in delinquent activities and sexual promiscuity. Others appeared to adjust well to the external demands of school and social life. Nevertheless, the continuation of their intense anger appeared to keep major aspects of the divorce experience fully alive, and revealed the child's inability to relegate the divorce to the past. The divorce-related anger appeared to have extraordinary staying power, especially when it brought together parent and child in an alignment against the other parent.

Although children at all ages experienced a rise in irritability at the time of the marital breakup, the continuation of the anger was most evident in the preadolescent and adolescent youngsters. Their aggression appeared to be compatible with the psychological needs and conflicts that typify young people of this age group in their relations with their parents.

Guilt

Although guilty feelings about having precipitated the divorce was not a universal phenomenon, it was very burdensome for those children who saw themselves as responsible for the divorce and attributed to themselves both a sense of power and of evil. One such child confessed that she was a witch, giving as examples of her power her grandmother's death and her parents' divorce.

The incidence and outcome of these self-accusations were developmentally linked. Most self-accusations occurred in younger children in whom they had a different meaning and a different degree of fixity than for the older child. Thus, when the self-accusation had its origins in the cognitive immaturity of the child, it appeared to dissipate in the natural course of development as the child's capacity to understand the nature of cause and effect increased.

When the self-accusation was present in older youngsters, the likelihood of its enduring was far greater; in fact, guilt over having caused the divorce did not appear to be a task which the older child could accomplish unless aided by psychotherapy. Educational measures by parents and others seemed to provide little relief.

TASK V: *Accepting the Permanence of the Divorce and Relinquishing Longings for the Restoration of the Predivorce Family*

Closely related to the successful mastery of the feelings evoked by the father's departure was the gradual acceptance by the child of the permanence of the divorce. This acceptance emerged as critical in the child's capacity to maintain a good adjustment in the postdivorce or the newly remarried family.

A major inner struggle for the child at the onset, and one that endured for many years for many children, was the strong pull exerted by the wish and need to deny the divorce versus the evident lasting reality of the marital rupture. We have earlier attempted to describe the great attraction of denial for the child in the divorcing family, and how such denial was reinforced by the ready availability of both parents, as well as by the child's anger and guilt at the time of the marital break.

We note here that there was no discernable connection between the very early use of denial at the time of the marital rupture, and the child's eventual capacity to deal with the permanence of the divorce. In fact, even at the outset, in some cases denial went hand in hand with an acute perception of reality. I would suggest that the child's early denial is often the first step of a coping process which is like a screen that alternately is lowered and raised until the child is able to confront the full reality of the marital break without undue anxiety. Sometimes youngsters who recognized the permanence of the divorce continued to hope for a reconciliation. Such hope, if it did not deny the reality, did not interfere with developmental progress.

The strength of the child's wish to turn the clock back to the time of the intact marriage cannot be underestimated. Vigorous attempts to restore the broken marriage with bribes, demands, threats, and angry tears abounded at the time of the breakup. Younger and older children alike fully expected the divorce to give way to their efforts to reconcile the parents. Sometimes, the refusal to accept the divorce outlasted the remarriage of one or both parents, as children saw magical omens of the forthcoming reunion in the most casual smiles or handshakes between the divorced parents.

How Did the Children Resolve This Task?

In the main, the idea of permanence was absorbed over several years, as hope for the restoration of the marriage gradually yielded to reality. This recognition did not come easily. Rather, many youngsters worked assiduously at this task, assessing the state of the divorce, continually revising their expectations, accepting new evidence carefully, and reformulating their ideas with painstaking care. We have elsewhere described the hyper-alertness of the child of divorce to the status of the postdivorce or remarried family and the intense concern with issues of permanence and transience within the remarried family (Wallerstein & Kelly, 1980a).

For example, Danny, age 11, said thoughtfully, five years after the marital rupture, that he had just recently figured out that divorce is "something like if you break a glass and pick up the pieces right away they will fit back perfectly, but if you take one piece and sand the edge, it will never fit again." Danny had clung to his strong reconciliation fantasy during the two years following the marital breakup. Only several years later did he fully accept the permanence of the divorce with his own words that "the two pieces of glass will never fit again." Clearly, prolonged thinking had generated this child's later reformulation.

The acceptance of permanence within the divorce often went hand in hand with the child's current satisfactions. Thus, the divorce became acceptable as permanent when it no longer stirred acute anxieties, and as it became associated with relief from conflict, or with gratifications within the present. The child's acceptance of the divorce as permanent was also related developmentally to the child's ever-increasing capacity to separate psychologically from the parent and to perceive the parent's needs, experiences, and motivations as different from his or her own.

Children Who Failed

A significant group of children remained unable to accept the divorce as final. Five years after the marital rupture they continued to await the restoration of the intact family. Some youngsters spent many hours daily in fantasies about the restoration of the parents' marriage. A significant number of these children were clinically depressed.

Many of the children who failed at the 5-year mark to believe in the permanence and irreversibility of their parents' divorce were living in families which were emotionally depressed, as compared with the image of the intact family as they had known it. Some youngsters were confused by the behavior of parents who continued to have many contacts with each other, and gave the children mixed messages regarding their intentions to reunite.

Developmental factors were relevant to the accomplishment of this task. The younger children worked at it for many years as they matured, and often encountered great difficulty in relinquishing the fantasy which remained so attractive and persistent. Older youngsters found the permanence of the divorce easier to accept, but sometimes felt their loyalty to a parent was tied to the fantasy of the restored marriage. In addressing this task, another factor of continued importance was the extent to which one or both parents continued to long for the restoration of the marriage. Such adult fantasies reinforced the fantasies of the children, and tended to fix them in place. The balance of gratifications and deprivations within the postdivorce family, as compared with the earlier intact family, continued to be of importance to young people of all ages.

TASK VI: Resolving Issues of Relationship

A major task for the children of divorce which is shared with all other growing children, but to which these children bring greater anxiety as well as a heightened potential for cynicism, is to reach, sustain, and support the personal vision that love, mutual understanding, and constancy are expectable components of human relationships. Perhaps the major developmental task posed by divorce is this: *To achieve realistic hope regarding future relationships and the enduring ability to love and be loved*. In order to reach this sense of psychic wholeness, the children of divorce will spend years of childhood and adolescence working to understand their parents' marital failure. Over the years they will revise and reformulate their judgments many times as to what really happened and why it did, and who was to blame, and how to forgive.

These youngsters, whom we came to know so intimately, worked very hard to evolve strategies which might safeguard them from failure. They thought about morality and the rules which should govern conduct between men and women: "My parents cheated and lied, but I have decided I would never do that." They laid careful plans for avoiding impulsive marriages: "I will live with a guy for a long while. I won't rush in." They sought explanations: "They should both have been more considerate." And they passed judgment, sometimes harshly so: "My mother is selfish, and my father should never have married."

None of the youngsters in our study were entirely optimistic and, in fact, all were worried about their future entry into adulthood. Especially as they went through the additional pain and anxiety of the adolescent years, each young person was consciously aware of the parental failure, and the fear of its repetition in their own lives. The powerful spectre which they struggled consciously to exorcise was, "Will it happen to me as it did to my parents?"

Perhaps this task which enables the child of divorce to restore his bruised sense of self and to strive to achieve a sense of wholeness and integrity is, in the long run, as I have noted earlier, the most important task both for the children and their families and for society. Ultimately, over the many years of growing up, the children of divorce will serve their own best interests by rescuing a vision of love and constancy in human relationships to which they can aspire in their adult lives. Then, in turn, their task is to transmit these values to their own children.

How Was the Task Accomplished?

Although children worked for many years on various aspects of their relationship in their view of the future, the challenges inherent in this task rose to full consciousness and intensity in adolescence. It is proper to consider this task as one primarily located within the domain of the adolescent youngster.

The demands were complex and varied with the particular circumstances of the family, the behavior of the adults, and the background causes for the divorce. Where the parents had behaved with consideration for each other and for the children, the task proved easier for the youngster. Where the divorce had been rocked by bitter anger, dishonesty, and aggression by the parents, the task was infinitely more difficult.

One practical issue in assessing success or failure in this task is the absence of information about the eventual adjustment these youngsters will make during the course of their adult lives. But, those who entered later adolescence and early adulthood with greater confidence and age-appropriate achievements included the youngsters who had been able to place the parental divorce within a frame of reference which made sense of the parents' decision. Rightly or wrongly, these young people had arrived at an explanation which not only helped them to obtain closure, but enabled them in some specific way to differentiate themselves from their parents. Others were able to find within themselves a sense of compassion and a new understanding which enabled them to forgive their parents for past failures, to give up their own participation within the parental combat zone, to cool long-standing resentments and battle allegiances. Others, as we have noted, needed to repudiate a parent or both parents whose behavior they consciously chose not to follow. All of these youngsters had in some significant way made use of their cognitive abilities and their new emotional maturity to separate psychologically from the parents and to declare their independence, albeit perhaps more self-consciously than do their counterparts from intact families.

Those who succeeded in this task often were able to draw on figures outside the nuclear family as models or as mentors for support and encouragement. These young people had the capacity to reach out to the world around them, to step-parents, teachers, friends, parents of friends, and grandparents, to maintain some sort of family structure following the divorce. Such children were able, with their own sense of power or their responsiveness, to build substitute value systems, or to find people to love who loved them in return. It may well be that to accomplish this requires both a greater personal appeal and greater courage than is expected from youngsters in intact, nurturant families.

Children Who Failed

Youngsters whose adjustment was otherwise adequate foundered on this more subtle task. For example, Jay at age 14, expressed cynicism about all relationships: "Dad left because Mom bored him. I do that all the time." Others, as they approached adulthood, confessed they might never marry, and revealed how convinced they were that their own marriage would fail or how little they trusted their ability to choose more wisely than did their parents. Still others became caught in a web of promiscuity and low self-esteem and spoke cynically and despairingly of ever achieving a loving relationship or any of their other goals. Several of these youngsters dropped out of school. Some became severely depressed in adolescence as they relived the sadness of the divorce within this new age context and experienced acutely the sense that their own important relationships would likely come to grief because of their powerlessness to influence significant aspects of their own lives. One subgroup among those who failed were youngsters who were still unable to make sense of the divorce, and continued to regard their parents' decision to part as capricious or frivolous.

In addressing this task, the child of divorce resembles his or her counterpart in bereavement. In the same way that the child who loses a parent through death must learn to take a chance on loving with the full and reinforced knowledge that humans are mortal and that all relationships will indeed end, so too the child of divorce must take a chance on a loving relationship, despite the realistic concern that it may fail. In order to achieve this, children of divorce will need to have acquired some confidence in their own abilities and self-worth, as well as their ability to love and to be loved; they will have had to come to terms with the permanency of the parental divorce and to relinquish longings for the restoration of the family. Finally, they will have had to have long given up the early anger or guilt potentiated by the marital rupture and to arrive at some understanding, forgiveness, and compassion for their parents. This task, therefore, is built on the successful negotiation of those five tasks that preceded the final one.

We were increasingly impressed with the significance of adolescence for this final resolution, as well as for the full-dress reworking of the divorce experience. Youngsters were motivated and able at adolescence to take a new look at themselves and at their parents, and to question and modify earlier attitudes, identifications, and alliances. In accord with the conception of adolescence as providing "a second chance" (Blos, 1962), many children radically revised their earlier relationships with both parents and step-parents, siblings and step-siblings.

Adolescence, as might be expected, also proved to be a period of greater vulnerability. A significant subgroup of youngsters, consisting largely of girls, became acutely depressed during adolescence as they reexperienced the divorce-related feelings of earlier years. Several, who had adapted well, worried intensely about the possibility of being disappointed in their relationships with men. It appears that the second chance which adolescence provides can lead not only to progress, but to regression as well. Nevertheless, the potential healing power of the adolescent years is significant because it emerges as a natural recovery period, as well as a time for potential consolidation of earlier gains provided by the developmental process. Adolescence may, therefore, be especially important for children who have experienced severe stress during their earlier years.

Coping with the multiple impact of parental divorce during childhood encompasses all of the tasks we have described and perhaps others as well. Each task requires a complex interweaving of abilities within the child, within the child's family, and within the social surround. In some tasks, mastery or failure proves to be closely associated with the level of developmental maturity of the child, as for example in the child's ability to grasp the meaning of the divorce and to separate reality from fantasy. In other tasks, the quality of life within the child's current family is a major determinant of outcome, as for example in the child's ability to relinquish preoccupation with the restoration of the original family. Overall, the contribution of developmental factors varies, and the diversity of the configurations that emerge are striking.

SUMMARY

I have proposed a broad framework for the examination of short- and long-term effects of marital rupture on the child. For this purpose, I have selected from within the wide range of divorce experiences the child whose family was intact prior to the divorce. Obviously, even within a predominantly middle-class sample, there exist marked individual differences in children's perceptions of an event and in their accompanying adaptive capacities. Furthermore, since the divorce event, too, varies widely within each household, so each experience can occupy a unique placement along many dimensions. Within this pattern of variation, I have tried to hold to the expectable vision of the child exposed to a fairly typical parental divorce as a tentative base from which to construct a model of the effects of such a stressful experience upon children. Further, I have tried to distinguish this experience from the one faced by the child whose parent has died.

My intent in describing the complexly interwoven components of the child's experience is to call attention to the uniqueness of marital rupture as a stressor, and to its important differences from even closely related stressors such as bereavement. To this end, I have described the conflict and sexuality that marks the divorce-engendered ambience, the diminished capacity and diminished judgment of the marital partners in their parenting roles, and the crescendo of change these induce in all domains of family life.

Divorce has been portrayed as a multistage process of radically changing family relationships and family circumstances that begins with an acute phase, undergoes several years of transition, and eventuates in the establishment of a postdivorce family. Many of the changes that mark the acute phase that extends over the first year or two after the decisive separation are profoundly stressful. The total impact, however, for adult and child is greater than the sum of its parts.

Using the concept of stress as a disequilibrating event requiring adaptation and change, I have described how the children's initial responses are governed largely by age and developmental factors and, to a lesser extent, by sex differences. These responses are consistent with the child's perceptions, especially the modal one of having been placed in grave danger as a result of the marital rift and the accompanying diminution in parental care.

I have proposed, however, that the child's successful mastery of the divorce-engendered stress is only, in part, related to these initial responses, and is directly related to the child's long-term capacity to address the coping tasks posed by the divorce. Divorce by its very nature as a stressor, and as a precipitant of acute and enduring radical family change, poses particular tasks for each child to address at different stages of the divorcing process. In the course of this confrontation with change, children will vary in the degree of mastery they attain, or in their failure to do so. Fortunately, it appears that children have many opportunities during their years of childhood and adolescence to succeed; unfortunately, this period may repeat and consolidate failure, as well as success.

The coping tasks of the child have been seen as interrelated, overlapping, and temporally sequential. They represent the efforts of the youngster to hold to the developmental pathway to overcome the perceived hazards. As formulated, these tasks are six in number. They fall into a sequence with varying attached time spans for the accomplishment of each task.

The hazards which the child experiences have been portrayed as the dark side of tasks whose resolutions require sustained work, and reach closure in late adolescence. These tasks, when failed, expose the child to the dangers which they were designed to prevent, namely developmental arrest and fixation at the level that had been achieved at the time of the marital rupture. Such arrest can result in flawed reality testing, poor self-esteem, the continuation of intense sorrow, anger and feelings of rejection, and a never-ending search for the absent parent (Tessman, 1978). On the other hand, these tasks, when completed, are likely to carry the child successfully into adulthood without significant psychological inhibition or behavioral deviance arising from the trauma of the parental divorce.

One problem which should be noted is that the child of divorce, in this view, must address the tasks imposed by the divorce experience, in addition to and within the context of the expectable, ordinary tasks of development. These special tasks are likely to add to the child's burdens. Their successful resolution should lead the child to a well-earned sense of mastery, a pride of independence, and a committed sense of connectedness toward other people, especially for those children for whom life has been in some measure burdened. These are indeed, happily, the characteristics of many of the children we have seen at the 5-year mark following the parental separation.

The many research tasks aimed at understanding these multifaceted phenomena, of patiently collecting observations over time, of distinguishing among stressors, of teasing out the particular impact, as well as the tasks which each stressor may impose, of discovering the many factors associated with achievement or failure, these are the responsibility of scientist and clinician. It is likely that these tasks will require our joint attention for a long period of time.

REFERENCES

Bloom, B. L., White, S. W., & Asher, S. J. Marital disruption as a stressful life event. In G. Levinger, & O. C. Moles (Eds.), *Divorce and separation*. New York: Basic Books, Inc., 1979.

Blos, P. *On adolescence: A psychoanalytic interpretation*. New York: The Free Press of Glencoe, 1962.

Brown, B. F. A study of the school needs of children in one-parent families. *The Phi Delta Kappan*, 1980, *61*, 537–540.

Campbell, A., Converse, P., & Rodgers, W. L. *The quality of American life: Perceptions, evaluations and satisfactions*. New York: Russell Sage Foundation, 1976.

Caplan, G. (Ed.). *Emotional problems of early childhood*. New York: Basic Books, 1955.

Despert, J. L. *Children of divorce*. Garden City, New York: Doubleday, 1962.

Erikson, E. *Childhood and society*. New York: W. W. Norton and Co., 1950.

Foster, H. H., & Freed, D. J. Joint custody: Legislative reform. *Trial*, 1980, *16*, 22–27.

Freud, S. (1917) *Mourning and melancholia*. London: The Hogarth Press, Standard Edition, 1957, *14*, 237–258.

Grinker, R. R. (Quoting Whitehorn in) Psychiatry and our dangerous world. In *Psychiatric research in our changing world*. Proceedings of an International Symposium, Montreal, 1968. Excerpta Medica International Congress Series, No. 187.

Hetherington, E. M., Cox, M., & Cox, R. Divorced fathers. *Family Coordinator*, 1976, *25*, 417–428.

Hetherington, E. M., Cox, M., & Cox, R. The aftermath of divorce. In J. H. Stevens, Jr., & M. Mathews (Eds.), *Mother-child relations*. Washington, D.C.: National Association for the Education of Young Children, 1978.

Hetherington, E. M., Cox, M., & Cox, R. Play and social interaction in children following divorce. *Journal of Social Issues*, 1979a, *35*, 26–49.

Hetherington, E. M., Cox, M., & Cox, R. Family interaction and the social, emotional and cognitive development of children following divorce. In V. Vaughn, & T. Brazelton (Eds.), *The family: Setting priorities*. New York: Science and Medicine, 1979b.

Holmes, T. H., & Rahe, R. H. The social readjustment rating scale. *Journal of Psychosomatic Research*, 1967, *11*, 213–218.

Hunter, J. E., & Schuman, N. Chronic reconstitution as a family style. *Social Work*, 1980, *6*, 446–451.

Kalter, N. Children of divorce in an outpatient psychiatric population. *American Journal of Orthopsychiatry*, 1977, *47*, 40–51.

Kelly, J., & Wallerstein, J. The effects of parental divorce: Experiences of the child in early latency. *American Journal of Orthopsychiatry*, 1976, *46*, 20–32.

Kulka, R. A., & Weingarten. H. The long-term effects of parental divorce in childhood on adult adjustment. *Journal of Social Issues*, 1979, *35*, 50–78.

Lindemann, E. Symptomatology and management of acute grief. *American Journal of Psychiatry*, 1944, *101*, 141–148.

Parkes, E. M. *Bereavement: Studies of grief in adult life*. New York: International Universities Press, 1972.

Rutter, M. Parent-child separation: Psychological effects on the children. *Journal of Child Psychology and Psychiatry*, 1971, *12*, 233–260.

Tessman, L. H. *Children of parting parents*. New York: Jason Aronson, 1978.

Wallerstein, J. Some observations regarding the effects of divorce on the psychological development of the pre-school girl. In J. Oremland, & E. Oremland (Eds.), *Sexual and gender development of young children*. Cambridge, Mass.: Ballinger Press, 1977a.

Wallerstein, J. Responses of the pre-school girl to divorce: Those who cope. In M. F. MacMillan, & S. Henao (Eds.), *Child psychiatry: Treatment and research*. New York: Brunner/Mazel, 1977b.

Wallerstein, J., & Kelly, J. The effects of parental divorce: The adolescent experience. In E. J. Anthony, & C. Koupernick (Eds.), *The child in his family* (Vol. 3). New York: John Wiley and Sons, 1974.

Wallerstein, J., & Kelly, J. The effects of parental divorce: The experiences of the preschool child. *Journal American Academy of Child Psychiatry*, 1975, *14*, 600–616.

Wallerstein, J., & Kelly, J. The effects of parental divorce: Experiences of the child in later latency. *American Journal of Orthopsychiatry*, 1976, *46*, 256–259.

Wallerstein, J., & Kelly, J. Children and Divorce. A review. *Social Work*, 1979, *24*, 468–475.

Wallerstein, J., & Kelly, J. *Surviving the breakup: How children and parents cope with divorce*. New York: Basic Books, 1980a.

Wallerstein, J., & Kelly, J. Effects of divorce on the father-child relationship. *American Journal of Psychiatry*, 1980b, *137*, 1534–1539.

CHAPTER 11

UTILIZATION OF STRESS AND COPING RESEARCH: Issues of Public Education and Public Policy

JULIUS SEGAL

FORMER DIRECTOR, DIVISION OF SCIENTIFIC AND PUBLIC INFORMATION

NATIONAL INSTITUTE OF MENTAL HEALTH

INTRODUCTION

In 1975, over 300 consultants concluded an intensive analysis of the twenty-five-year history of federally-sponsored research programs in mental health, and made recommendations for future priorities in the field. Their report (Segal, 1975) includes the following observation:

> Mental health research is not an end in itself. It acquires value only when its findings are used, whether the users are scientists, science administrators, practitioners, social agency managers, or the general public. Integral to the conduct and support of research itself, then, is the support of programs to disseminate and promote the use of knowledge that arises from it. (p. 393)

Publication of findings in scientific journals, however important to cadres of professionals, does not make research information readily available to many important potential users—among them mental health practitioners, policymakers, and the general public.

Lynn (1978) has described the issue as it applies to research funded by the United States government. In 1976, the United States invested more than 1.8 billion dollars in social research and development projects—including controlled experiments, epidemiological surveys, and program demonstrations and evaluations relating to the identification and solution of social problems. Although the need for large-scale federal support of social science research has traditionally been widely accepted by the scientific community and—at least until recently—by the political community as well, questions concerning the relevance of such research, and its practical application to the development of social policy, continue largely unanswered.

The general issue of the practical applications of social and behavioral research is especially relevant to the field of child development. The federal outlay for research in child and family mental health has for many years represented a major proportion of the nation's total mental health research effort. During fiscal year 1980, for example, the National Institute of Mental Health (NIMH) provided grant support for 228 projects whose primary emphasis was in child mental health. The Institute's portfolio in this area has traditionally been boosted further by additional projects involving "studies of stress effects and the implications of varied experiences or their lacks during critical developmental periods" (Fishman, 1980). Private foundations add considerably to the support of child development studies.

Although it is generally agreed that few areas of behavioral research carry as much potential for public education and the development of social policy as does research in child development, considerable disagreement exists regarding the degree to which such utilization has been achieved. Many view the gap between what is known and what is applied as inordinately wide, among them Zigler (1973), Fraiberg (1977), and Keniston (1977). The blame for this gap is attributed largely to political and legislative inertia.

Others, however, question the degree of specific guidance and direction possible—whether to families or lawmakers—from existing bodies of behavioral science data, including findings from the field of child mental health. Davis (1965), for example, concluded that the reason for lack of progress in research utilization lies not in the medium or the audience, but in the message. It is not, he argues, that dependent variables are difficult to measure, that audiences would be resistant to accepting information provided, or that the delicacy of the content might require special communication, personnel, or techniques. "Rather, the major problem appears to be this: mental health educators have little or nothing specific or practical to tell the public" (p. 138).

Many in the field would disagree with Davis's verdict. As part of the work of the NIMH Research Task Force (Segal, 1975), for example, child development experts led by Marian Radke Yarrow identified "an impressive array of applications to society" growing out of the cumulative body of child development research, among them a number that have altered dramatically approaches taken in the rearing and education of our young. Cited, for example, is research on the development of levels of aspiration, along with studies on the effects of success and failure and of praise and reproof on performance—all of which have had the cumulative effect of changing the attitudes and methods of educators in motivating children. Cited too are studies of the gifted child that have altered a set of stereotypes which pictures the genius as weak and eccentric, introducing a new image of the gifted child; research on the effects of institutionalization leading to radical reforms in the care of children without parents; research on cognitive and language development contributing vitally to changes in the educational system, particularly the adaptation of curricular structures to the capacities of the children; and laboratory research on operant conditioning, begun with animals, leading to behavior modification techniques that now have many practical applications in schools and clinics, and in parent education. The report offers an optimistic view of the potential applications of accumulated knowledge of how children think and learn; how they are influenced by punishments, incentives, and knowledge; and how environmental conditions influence their motives, values, and achievement. "This knowledge is directly relevant and applicable to family living, education, psychiatry, institutional management, manufacture of toys, writing of children's books, city planning, and understanding of intercultural conflicts" (p. 113). It should be added that much of this knowledge is potentially relevant, as well, to continuing efforts to clarify the role of stress in early development and to minimize its deleterious consequences.

The actual extent of the utilization of child development studies is probably neither as narrow nor as abundant as described above; certainly the potential implications described by Yarrow have not, in many cases, been translated into actual policy changes. In any case, this chapter is devoted to a discussion of a few of the many issues that arise in attempts to exploit the results of child development research in public education and public policy initiatives related to child mental health—especially of research on stress and coping. (In a few places references will be made to more general efforts in the stress and coping field other than those relating specifically to children; these have been chosen to emphasize or elaborate a particular point at issue.)

History of Public Education Efforts in Child Mental Health

American efforts in public education related to child mental health are hardly new. Publications on child care were imported into the United States from Europe prior to 1800, and, as early as 1815, parents in Portland, Maine, and subsequently other communities held meetings to exchange experiences and ideas on childrearing (Croake & Glover, 1977).

Examples of early nineteenth-century American literature on childrearing may be found in *Mother's Magazine*, first published in 1832, *Mother's Assistant* in 1841, and an earlier version of *Parent's Magazine* begun in 1840 (Sunley, 1955). The Rev. John Abbott's *Mother at Home*, which appeared in 1833, was probably the first popular parenting manual, emphasizing in typically Puritan tones the child's tyrannical nature, and *Godey's Lady's Book*—a nineteenth-century woman's magazine—offered advice to mothers long before *Redbook*. With the publication of John Holt's classic, *The Care and Feeding of Children*, in 1894, and the Yale studies of child development by Arnold Gesell beginning a few decades later, parents—and particularly mothers—were transformed into consumers of "how-to" approaches to childrearing (Segal & Yahraes, 1978).

The diversity of childrearing manuals from which modern parents can now choose is overwhelming. It has been estimated that most bookstores today stock an average of 30 such manuals, ranging from James Dobson's (1970) *Dare to Discipline*, which recommends pinching and other methods of inflicting pain, to Haim Ginott's (1965) *Between Parent and Child*, which stresses that parents must learn to communicate with, rather than judge, their children.

The government's role in public education in mental health has been growing steadily. In the past few years, for example, a single agency, NIMH, has produced over 50 books and pamphlets—a high proportion of all its publications—written for parents and other caretakers. They provide both information and advice on a wide range of topics, among them emotional development, birth order, temperament, genetics, learning disabilities, schizophrenia, depression, delinquency, and many more. In addition, NIMH has been engaged in the production of a weekly radio program, and of several films for general audiences, many of these dealing with child development.

With the passage in 1964 of the Community Mental Health Centers Act, regulations were developed requiring community mental health centers to offer, among other services, public education to residents in areas served by the centers. Later, the primary goal of such mental health education efforts was defined as promoting positive mental health by helping citizens acquire knowledge, attitudes, and behavior patterns that foster and maintain their well-being.

The considerable public and private effort—only briefly described here—increases the importance of assessing the viability of initiatives designed to translate existing data in the child development field into public education initiatives.

Public Education to Improve Children's Coping Skills

This section raises a pair of related issues impinging on public education programs in the field of childhood stress and coping: Is sufficient relevant information available on which to base such programs? And what are the impediments to their success? A discussion is also presented of activities specifically designed to educate children, themselves, in techniques for coping with the stresses encountered during their growth and development.

The Information Base: Quantity versus Quality

Interested parents today can choose from a vast array of magazine articles, books, and films intended to teach adults how to improve their skills as parents and caretakers. Many of these deal specifically with the stressors children face; they are designed to aid parents in helping their young cope with crises such as bereavement, divorce, and hospitalization, or with more universal but often stressful problems of early development.

It must be acknowledged at the outset that such materials are often based not on research evidence, but rather, on the idiosyncratic views of a particular author, or on insights gained from limited clinical experience. There continue to be many disagreements on the "best" methods of parenting, arising primarily from convictions rather than from persuasive data about the relationship between parental interventions and subsequent child behavior.

Given our present state of knowledge of risk events and their consequences, is it at least theoretically possible to engineer sound, research-based mental health education programs designed to strengthen the coping capacities of children? An affirmative answer would go far in meeting the generally agreed-upon criteria for successful pursuit of the primary prevention task. While Cowen (1980) and other authors have used slightly different language to define the concept of primary prevention, all such definitions are equally relevant to mental health education programs, most especially to those programs designed to facilitate the healthy psychological development of children and to help children to cope successfully with stresses they encounter.

The design of effective public education materials to meet prevention criteria requires the availability of at least two essential bodies of information: first, an identification of the specific stressors that challenge the coping capabilities of children; and second, a specification of the characteristics and environments of children who appear resistant to such stressors. Such data would help mental health education personnel to begin defining both the key target audiences for their communications and the messages to be contained in them.

Given the expanding body of evidence regarding specific stressors correlated with later developmental difficulties, we now appear to be responding to the first challenge. Rutter (1979), for example, has identified some of the family variables strongly associated with child psychiatric disorder; these include severe marital discord, low social status, overcrowding or large family size, paternal criminality, maternal psychiatric disorder, and admission of the child into the care of the community.

Moreover, there is some evidence to suggest that we can begin to identify those children who are especially at risk. Children encountering only one of the array of risk factors identified above, for example, were found by Rutter to be no more likely to suffer psychiatric disorders than children experiencing no risk factors at all. On the other hand, when any two of the stresses occurred together, the risk increased by a factor of four; and with still more concurrent stresses, the risk climbed further still. In other words, "the stresses potentiated each other so that the combination of chronic stresses provided very much more than a summation of the effects of the separate stresses considered singly" (p. 15).

Rutter has also portrayed the cumulative effects of specific stressors, such as family breakup or hospitalization. He has found strong evidence, for example, that the longer the family disharmony lasts, the greater the risk to the children. Similar results emerge in studies of hospitalized children: While one hospital admission was found to do no long-term harm, two admissions were damaging.

The successful identification of those children who appear to be especially at risk would clearly satisfy the important goal of isolating high priority populations—in this case, the families and other key adults in the children's lives—as special targets for prevention programs (Goldston & Klein, 1976). In doing so, it would at the same time suggest key "targets of opportunity" for public education efforts.

Assuming that from the kind of data provided by Rutter and others, one could, indeed, identify critical target audiences, a second criterion remains to be satisfied: Are sufficient data available with which mental health communicators might develop appropriate messages to such audiences? In order to structure meaningful public education materials, one would need to know those attributes and conditions that seem to provide children with the capacities to resist the corrosive effects of stress. Here, too, a number of authors have begun to provide relevant data.

Garmezy in his chapter in this volume has summarized the results of a literature review of the attributes characteristic of competent children exposed to the stresses of parental poverty and prejudice (Garmezy, 1981; Garmezy & Nuechterlein, 1972). He writes:

> The intriguing point to be made about the findings of these studies is that despite the harshness of life that the families encounter, some parents appear to be able to foster or enhance in their children the confidence, self-control, determination, flexibility, and cognitive and social skills that accompany the development of competence and positive adaptation. These appear to be important precursors to the establishment of stress-resistance in children. (p. 211)

Although the characteristics he has described remain descriptive correlates of stress resistance rather than proven "causes," the question for mental health education purposes is, nevertheless, cogent: Can such characteristics and conditions be facilitated through mental health education efforts?

The task of doing so—of translating existing knowledge about both childhood stressors and the characteristics of "copers" into information of utility to broad consumer audiences—is not without its impediments. Two of these are discussed below.

Major Impediments to Effective Stress-and-Coping Public Education Programs

As noted earlier, a growing number of public education efforts are being devoted to informing the public about the stressors encountered by children, and to giving advice in regard to the development of effective coping responses. They provide suggestions for helping children to cope with such crises as divorce, bereavement, placement in foster care, and hospitalization, and, in terms of secondary prevention, to deal successfully with major developmental disorders such as dyslexia, delinquency, hyperactivity, and depression (Sobell, 1978; Wehrle, 1978; Sargent, 1978, 1979, 1980; Brenton, 1975; Bienvenu, 1967; Hill, 1973).

A number of such publications do take account of individual variability in children's coping responses. Most frequently, however, they are based on the assumption that, because certain childhood stressors are related to negative outcome, it can be concluded, therefore, that the guidance offered for improved coping is equally relevant to all intended recipients of the communications. The assumption may arise, in part, from what Kagan (1979) has described as "an obsession with finding absolute principles which declare that a particular set of external conditions is inevitably associated with a fixed set of consequences for all children" (p. 88).

Rarely acknowledged in the preparation of child-related public education materials is the notion that the ultimate consequences of stressful experiences depend heavily on a variety of personal and situational factors. There is an assumption of homogeneity when, in fact, responses of children to the challenge of a particular stressor may vary considerably. Elsewhere in this volume, for example, Rutter describes a number of the personal qualities that may affect the responses to stress—among them age, sex, genetic factors, temperament, intelligence, and other problem-solving skills.

Three specific childhood stress experiences—divorce, abuse, and maternal absence—may be cited. In the case of divorce, for example, Wallerstein and Kelly (1980) find that key factors in children's responses include not only age and developmental stage, but individual differences in lifestyle and culture; in the case of abuse, Starr (1979) emphasizes the need to take account of the total ecology of the family, and the social forces that impinge on it; and, as one more example, in the case of maternal absence, Hoffman (1979) underscores the variations in effects among boys and girls with different patterns of relationships operating between themselves and their mothers and fathers. The complexity of factors affecting the outcome of such stressful childhood experiences, although well documented, are rarely described or even acknowledged in typical public information materials available today.

The dangers inherent in attending to the nature of stressful situations, without regard to the characteristics of the "victims," may be dramatized by turning to studies other than those of children. The examples cited here deal with two populations of adults subjected to the stresses of captivity: American POWs captured in Korea and in North Vietnam.

The condition of those U.S. Army POWs who survived captivity in Korea was generally quite poor, especially so in psychological terms. They appeared bland, apathetic, almost retarded. Their talk was shallow and vague, and lacked affect. They seemed mildly confused and surprisingly unenthusiastic about their release. Lifton (1954) and others saw what they began to refer to as a "zombie reaction," much like that so often reported among concentration camp survivors; all this soon replaced by episodes of tension, anger, and agitation. There was no zest for returning home. Aboard ship on the homeward voyage, they made little attempt to interact with crew members, since they felt—as do many former captives—that no one could possibly understand who had not experienced incarceration.

The POWs incarcerated in Vietnam were subjected to even more prolonged and intense stresses than were those held in Korea: nutritional deprivation, long isolation from fellow prisoners, inadequate shelter, and chronic and severe cases of dysentery and parasitic infestations. Physical torture was common, and some men were manacled to their beds for months at a time. Solitary confinement periods ranged from several days up to four years, with a mean of 39 weeks. The average duration of captivity in Vietnam was considerably longer by several years than had been the case in previous wars. Based on data from Korean captivity and earlier POW episodes as well, there was reason to expect both acute and malignant sequelae among returnees from Vietnam; for them, serious and continuing physical and psychological problems were acknowledged in advance virtually as a given (Segal, 1973).

In fact, however, the results were surprising. While the blight of captivity was apparent in the appearance of the POWs, the "worst case" planning assumptions of the military turned out to be inappropriate; these men returned in relatively good health, surprising the psychiatrists and physicians arrayed to treat them. Moreover, although the expectation of long-term problems among the Vietnam returnees was surely warranted, the results of studies to date run contrary to expectation. From the latest five-year follow-up data (Richlin, Rahe, Shale, & Mitchell, 1980), it would appear that these men continue to be doing well by any standards, and particularly well when compared with American prisoners from other wars.

The reasons undoubtedly lie, in part, among several factors. The POWs returned from Vietnam to a benign and even worshipful society, whereas those who came back from Korea encountered harsh and judgmental attitudes. More important, however, was the contrasting nature of the two groups of POWs themselves. Those captured in Vietnam represented a select group: All were officers, older on the average than Korean War POWs, and enormously committed to fulfilling their military role in adverse circumstances; they had also received POW survival training prior to capture. In contrast, Americans captured in Korea were mostly young, poorly motivated, and poorly educated, and totally unprepared for the stresses they encountered.

Such data offer a reminder once again of the fragility of generalizations made only from the knowledge of a stressful episode without taking account of the characteristics of those subjected to that episode. Like many items of advice provided to parents, the education and orientation programs provided to wives and parents of POWs, prior to their return from Vietnam, were wide of the mark. They were based on a knowledge of the sequelae of captivity assumed to be typical, and did not take account of the nature of the individuals themselves.

A second and equally important impediment to the effective public education programs lies in the unwarranted assumption that children actually experience the degree and quality of responses to stressors that adults assume they do. Many of the public education interventions introduced on behalf of children are defined not necessarily by the child's perceptions and experiences, but by adult projections of them. Kagan (1979) has offered a note of caution regarding the tenuousness of such projections:

> Every interaction between adult and child is embedded in a matrix of implicit understandings created from past interactions. It is not possible to know the psychological significance or future consequences of a par-

> ticular set of encounters independent of the larger mural of which it is a part. . . . The child's private constructions are the critical consequences of familial experiences, but the transduction from external event to personal interpretation is not yet understood. (p. 887)

Kagan's observation is relevant not only to the child's encounters with acute stressors, but with everyday life experiences as well. Episodes apparently innocuous to the bystander, for example, may leave a wound in the child—a sudden and inexplicable harsh word, a diffident response of parents, the slight of a teacher or friend. In a letter to his father, Franz Kafka (1953) mourned the fact that the empathy and communication for which he searched was not forthcoming during his childhood.

> I cannot believe that a kindly word, a quiet taking by the hand, a friendly look, could not have got me to do anything that was wanted of me. Now you are, after all, at bottom a kindly and soft-hearted person . . . but not every child has the endurance and fearlessness to go on searching until it comes to the kindliness that lies beneath the surface. (p. 15)

We do not know from Kafka's words what his father was actually like, but it is at least possible that the child's response arose from an inner reality rather than an objective one. The assessment of a parent as hostile or accepting, Kagan (1979) contends, cannot be made simply by observing the parent's behavior; parental love or rejection arises from a belief held by the child rather than a set of actions by a parent.

Yamamoto (1979) attempted to ascertain whether children assess their experiences of stress in the same terms as adults perceive them. Fourth-, fifth-, and sixth-graders rated 20 life events on a seven-point scale. The children were found to make distinguishing judgments of perceived stressfulness that often differed from those of professionals. The arrival of a new baby sibling, for example, often regarded by adults as a "shocker" for youngsters, was not very highly rated. More traumatic was "a poor report card," "being sent to the principal," "getting lost," "being ridiculed in class," "a scary dream," "not making 100," or "being picked last on a team."

Such findings would not surprise E. B. White (1976) who has described a childhood in which, he claims, he was neither deprived nor unloved. Yet it would be inaccurate, he contends, to suggest that the period was untroubled.

> The normal fears and worries of every child were in me developed to a high degree; every day was an awesome prospect. I was uneasy about practically everything; the uncertainty of the future, the dark of the attic, the panoply and discipline of school, the transitoriness of life, the mystery of the church and of God, the frailty of the body, the sadness of

afternoon, the shadow of sex, the distant challenge of love and marriage, the far-off problem of a livelihood. I brooded about them all, lived with them day by day. (p. 1)

Mental health information personnel have depended primarily on adult judgments to describe the relative importance to children of various stresses. Few investigators have recognized, as Anthony (1974) puts it, that stress as experienced by the child and stress as estimated by the adult observing the impact of the stress on the child are frequently of very different orders of magnitude." The lack of that recognition defines a major limitation in the quality of public education materials available in the child development field.

Training Children to Cope with Stress

Stress management programs have been introduced in the recent past primarily as a therapeutic tool for treating patients suffering diagnosed problems rather than as a means of preventing problems before they arise. As a treatment technique, such programs have been used in attempts to help overcome a variety of conditions, among them phobias and anxiety, as well as to assist clients in confronting life crises such as bereavement, divorce, surgery, and even dental care (Nielsen, 1979; Siegel & Peterson 1980; Dart, 1980; Duthler, 1980; Bonkowski, 1979; Horowitz & Kaltreider, 1980; Horowitz, Krupnick, Kaltreider, Wilner, Leong, & Marmar, 1981). The techniques used vary with the population treated and with the problem, but generally include anti-anxiety approaches such as muscle relaxation, meditation, guided imagery, and biofeedback, as well as behavioral and cognitive approaches, including modeling, problem-solving, skills development, and assertiveness training.

Few stress management efforts have been developed specifically for children. While several "affective education" programs—among them the Magic Circle Program (Palomares & Rubini, 1974), and Primary Mental Health Project (Cowen & Lorion, 1975)—seek to "promote or enhance mental and emotional robustness," they do not specifically teach children to understand the nature and consequences of stress and to develop stress management skills.

One example of a study relevant to teaching children to deal with chronic stress was carried out with a group of school children in Lansing, Michigan (Stone, Hindz, & Schmidt, 1975). The study, conducted with third-, fourth-, and fifth-grade children, was based on the assumption that personal competence may be facilitated by training children in procedures and skills which allow them to deal independently with critical problems in living, and that problem-solving training represents an important preventive approach. Three hypotheses were tested: that teaching children problem-solving skills will increase the frequency of their seeking facts and information; that it will increase their development of choices or alternatives; and that it will enhance their selection of a solution when faced with a problem. Using videotapes showing children going through the process of solving problems—for example, reading difficulties, fighting with friends—the researchers showed that children can be trained to some degree to improve their ability to solve such problems when confronted by them.

A comparable competence-building approach was used by Spivack and Shure (1974), who developed a social problem curriculum for four-year-old Head Start children. Social problem-solving skills were built, using games and dialogues presented daily in 5- to 20-minute lessons over a 10-week period. Mental health personnel trained the teachers, who, in turn, instructed the children. At the end of the study, the experimentally trained children were shown to have made significant gains, especially initially maladjusted children who were shy and anxious. These gains were reinforced a year later in a follow-up kindergarten program.

While these and similar studies test individual techniques in the prevention area, and suggest the feasibility of teaching children coping skills, the relevant literature does not presently yield a tested program directed at meeting a broader criterion—that is, at helping children to understand the concept of stress, how it can effect them, and how they might control its effects. Theoretically, such a program, if successful, could produce a generation better educated about stress, and better able to control or manage its sequelae.

A model for such a program—at this writing still to be evaluated—has been developed by Pfohl (1979). The Children's Anxiety Management Program (CAMP) has as its ultimate goals to help children improve both academically and socially. The specific objectives of the program are, among others, to sensitize teachers to children's vulnerability to stress and anxiety, and to teach children strategies for coping with stress and anxiety encountered by them. The CAMP program is designed to be implemented in the fourth through the sixth grades by the classroom teacher, school psychologist, or other professional on the school staff. The program children are monitored in their application of their newly learned skills throughout the school year.

Techniques utilized in CAMP are drawn from those used therapeutically with both adults and children, including muscle relaxation, cognitive restructuring, problem-solving, guided imagery, modeling, and assertiveness and self-control training. Activities also include exposure of the children to stressors—among them classroom presentations and rehearsing anxiety-provoking situations—as stimuli for practicing stress inoculation procedures.

The basic program consumes 30 weeks, each 15 to 20 minute lesson being given 2 to 3 times a week. Outcome evaluation involves comparison of the program group with controls, with respect to such criteria as test scores, attendance, and report card grades. Each child also serves as his or her own control in a pre- and post-test design.

Until CAMP is evaluated in practice—the program is currently being implemented in several Kentucky school districts—no data are available describing the effectiveness of this broad programmatic approach. Indeed, the project itself does not provide for the assessment of the durability of stress management training over the long term. Nonetheless, the program does suggest the potential for introducing mental health education initiatives intended to train children themselves to cope with the stressful experiences they may encounter.

Evaluating Public Education Programs in Stress and Coping

Mental health education programs in child development—indeed, mental health education programs in general—have rarely been subjected to rigorous evaluation. A number of factors account for the gap, among them the following ones identified by Hall (1977): evaluative studies require research expertise that generally is not among the major strengths or interests of those who actually plan and direct information and education programs; the conduct of evaluation studies requires a difficult administrative coordination of research interests and talents with communications skills; evaluation studies are costly, since they typically must be longitudinal in scope, requiring long-term investments of energy and resources; and those devoted to information and education programs, faced with a choice between funding new programs or funding the evaluation of existing ones, typically perceive greater advantage in initiating new programs.

The major impediment in the pursuit of evaluation studies, however, has been methodological. Although precise evaluation methodologies do exist for the assessment of mental health education programs, they are typically applied to small projects in which the outcome measures are narrow, and the results cannot be generalized usefully. The studies, therefore, appear to be trivial in the light of the serious questions being asked about public education initiatives.

Even in the case of direct parent education programs in which the target audience is known and available to the researcher, evaluation studies have been inadequate in both number and quality. The numerous publications existing on the subject provide, for the most part, only programmatic descriptions, not the outcome of attempts to measure results. When pre- and post-measurements have been made, changes have typically been attributed to the program, without benefit of evidence from a comparison or control group. Moreover, evaluation is most often accomplished by the same individual who communicates the information, and, in many cases, comments by participants are cited as the only evidence of positive results (Croake & Glover, 1977).

Most successful evaluations have been made primarily of experimental parent education programs in which the content is carefully programmed and the information delivered directly to a target audience available for study. Training procedures for families intended to help them deal with extremely aggressive youngsters, for example, provide a model for carefully crafted education programs relatively amenable to evaluation (Patterson, 1980).

In contrast, most mental health education programs do not involve a direct relationship between the intervener (in this case, the mental health educator) and the client. They depend on the input of either printed or electronic media, or what Cowen (1980) describes as the "indirect technologies" of community psychology—specifically, the consultation and education functions of community mental health programs. For such programs to be considered as effective initiatives in primary prevention, the outcomes for the ultimate beneficiaries must be assessed, and evidence of benefits for the target audience shown. In the view of Cowen (1980), "Much of what has gone on, and is still going on, in parent education . . . should be seen, at best, as preliminary flirtations with models that may, or may not, prove to be true primary prevention in mental health" (p. 269).

It should be acknowledged that the absence of evaluation data does not necessarily mean that mental health education programs are without impact. Leon Eisenberg's (1981) cautionary note regarding the difficulty encountered in the measurement of distant outcomes is as relevant here as in the case of more traditional interventions in the child mental health field. Childhood interventions, he points out, must be powerful, indeed, to be able to show a clear effect, despite the vicissitudes of subsequent life experience. Although overwhelming evidence exists on the importance of infant nutrition, even the best-fed baby will not grow to healthy adolescence if it is starved in later childhood. That fact, Eisenberg contends, does not demonstrate, however, that feeding infants well is not worthwhile.

Public education programs in child development carry a potentially significant impact, but there is a pressing need to structure sound evaluation programs to demonstrate such an impact. Unfortunately, sound evaluation models do not abound in child development education, but those in other health fields reveal potentially useful approaches.

One such study worthy of scrutiny—an element of the Stanford Heart Disease Prevention Program—is described by Maccoby and Alexander

(1979). The study measured the results over the three-year period (1972–1975) of a public education program aimed at reducing cardiovascular disease risk factors among randomly selected men and women, aged 35 to 49, in three northern California communities. The study measured, as well, the comparative effectiveness of the two strategies used—mass media and face-to-face, intensive instruction.

The risk reduction program recommended dietary habits which, if followed, would lead to reduced intake of saturated fat, cholesterol, salt, sugar, and alcohol; it also focused on reducing weight by lessening caloric intake and increasing physical activity, and on reducing or stopping cigarette smoking. Mass media messages were developed in English and Spanish in various formats—including TV and radio spots, brochures, direct mail pieces, and newspaper columns—and applied in the two treatment communities. In addition, a subgroup of high-risk individuals in the second treatment community received intensive instruction on a personal basis as well. A third community was used as a control.

To measure the program's effectiveness, an initial baseline survey was conducted of the participants in the three communities, using interviews and medical examinations. Interviewers recorded individuals' levels of knowledge about cardiovascular risk, attitudes, and associated behaviors, such as smoking and eating habits. A risk score, derived from the Framingham Study (Department of Health, Education, and Welfare, 1968), was assigned to all participants.

Surveys were conducted of the mass media only, of mass media plus intensive instruction, and of control communities at the end of the first, second, and third years of the program. These annual surveys were supplemented by a series of mini-surveys designed to provide the media planners with immediate feedback on the public's awareness and acceptance of specific communications, and their responses to them.

At the end of the program's second year, the level of estimated coronary risk (reduction in systolic blood pressure, reduction in cigarette consumption, and improvements in dietary practices) in the two treatment communities was found to have decreased by roughly 18%, a significant improvement compared to the control community. Information levels, attitudes, and behaviors changed more in the treatment communities. In comparing the two public education methods, intensive instruction combined with mass media was shown to produce more dramatic results initially than mass media alone, but by the end of the third year this advantage had disappeared. Both methods produced roughly equal results, except in the case of cigarette consumption, which decreased more in the combined strategy group.

There are some drawbacks to the study: only two-thirds of the 35–49 year olds in the three communities participated in or completed the program, thereby possibly restricting the generalizability of the results. Moreover, the program was not successful in one of its goals—helping people manage a sustained weight loss. Nor were the researchers able to measure accurately increases in physical activity—another program goal.

In the view of McAlister and his co-workers (1980), the use of a single medium in education programs does not offer promise of lasting results. In the case of smoking cessation programs, for example, viewers of televised group counseling sessions tend not to apply to themselves what they learn. The missing ingredient is personal involvement, or as Bandura (1977) terms it, "performance modeled behavior" as contrasted with "acquisition behavior." Another way of stating it may be "active involvement" as opposed to "passive involvement." Effective public education programs would appear to require incorporation of two essential components: expert instruction provided through mass media; and social support, which can be provided through volunteer-led self-help groups.

This approach was tested in Finland (McAlister, Puska, Koskela, Pallonen, & Maccoby, 1980), where a smoking cessation program emphasizing relapse prevention was televised nationwide, and where community self-help groups were organized in one province. Programs consisted of group discussions, and were led by two leading experts who addressed both the group and the viewers. Program content included individual analysis of the probable causes of relapse, the development of coping plans, the practice of such coping skills as stress management, and dietary self-control instruction.

Results were measured after one month and after six months. They failed to reveal any clear differentiation between the "television viewing only" and the "television viewing plus discussion" groups—in part, the program designers feel, because of inadequate data collection. Results did, however, show much higher viewing in the province in which self-help groups were organized. This leads McAlister to conclude that "the creation of a supportive social environment is an essential accompaniment for any counseling that might be delivered through the mass media" (p. 378).

The methods incorporated into the studies described here clearly can be extended beyond smoking to other behavioral issues. Given the audience participation innovations that cable TV technology and other anticipated communication developments permit, public education vehicles could no doubt be refined for potential application to child-development education programs.

While decreases in systolic blood pressure and reduced consumption of cigarettes are more readily measured than the less tangible results aimed for by mental health educators, the strength of consumerism today makes it imperative for mental health education practitioners to be accountable for their efforts. If evidence of effectiveness cannot be shown, existing programs will be discarded and new ones will go unsupported. Moreover, with the increased current pressure to conceptualize how preventive methods in mental health may be reimbursable through third-party agreements, mental health educators will have to prove that their work actually prevents costly treatment, or education programs will find fewer sources of support.

Evaluative studies need to be addressed first to programs of limited scope and with modest goals—i.e., programs with potential for yielding precise but generalizable results. Next, it is important to develop large-scale evaluation systems to make possible the study of broadly based communication programs. The design of such systems continues to be of concern to a number of investigators, some of whose efforts have been described earlier. Others include Mielke and Swinehart (1976), Haskins (1978), Robertson (1976), Green (1975), Kline (1972), Blane and Hewitt (1973), and Sundale and Schanie (1978) who have directed their attention to such areas as health promotion, auto safety, alcohol and drug use reduction, and mental health practices. The repeated implication drawn from such efforts is that the successful solution of methodological problems in evaluation will require the combined attention and skills of clinicians, behavioral scientists, and communication experts. Given the potential for effective prevention initiatives through public education in the arena of child mental health, continued efforts to overcome existing problems in the design of evaluation research are surely warranted.

Ethical Issues in Stress and Coping Education

Recent years have brought a crescendo of activity in the field of behavioral medicine, and an increasingly widespread acceptance of the notion that major alterations in behavior and lifestyle provide one of the strongest weapons in the armamentarium of prevention. A host of factors underlie this trend, among them the increasing interest among researchers and clinicians in data that relates disease and poor health to living styles and habits, and a growing wave of therapeutic nihilism—an attitude that "questions medical intervention and is more friendly to health efforts that begin and end at home" (Wikler, 1978). The practical implications of behavioral medicine have been expressed by many writers, among them, for example, Fuchs (1974) who concludes that "the greatest current potential for improving the health of the American people is to be found in what they do and don't do for themselves."

Not all citizens, however, readily accept the notion that they should be urged to alter their style of life in order to win good health and long life. Many patients recoil at their doctors' preaching to them about the ravages of smoking, eating foods that will reduce their cholesterol level, or—moving more closely to the mental health field—working too long hours, being too achievement-oriented, or using corporal punishment in rearing their children. The following observation by Mencken (1977) epitomizes the revulsion some feel at the contraceptive, preventive, or—as the author calls it—the "hygienic" approach to medicine and mental health:

> Hygiene is the corruption of medicine by morality. It is impossible to find a hygienist who does not debase this theory of the healthful with a theory of the virtuous. The whole hygienic art, indeed, resolves itself into an ethical exhortation. This brings it, at the end, into diametrical conflict with medicine proper. The true aim of medicine is not to make men virtuous; it is to safeguard and rescue them from the consequences of their vices. The physician does not preach repentance; he offers absolution. (p. 269)

The issue sardonically highlighted by Mencken cannot be dismissed, especially by those in the mental health field—and particularly by those working in the twin fields of child development and family life. In the latter areas, a great deal of what experts have to offer does, indeed, comprise "ethical exhortations." Moreover, there are those who argue that preventive interventions, however well intentioned, may have unfortunate consequences. Although they may right one "wrong," they frequently cause yet another to develop; this becomes likely when we do not fully understand all of the mechanisms involved in the item of behavior at issue.

Thomas (1974) has made the point effectively:

> You cannot meddle with one part of a complex system from the outside without the almost certain risk of setting off disastrous events that you hadn't counted on in other, remote parts. If you want to fix something you are first obliged to understand, in detail, the whole system. . . . Intervening is a way of causing trouble.

Thomas cites the case of syphilis as an example, in that

> before the recognition of microbial disease mechanisms, a patient with advanced syphilis was a complex system gone wrong without any single, isolatable cause, and medicine's approach was, essentially, to meddle. The analogy becomes more spectacular if you begin imagining what would happen if we knew everything else about modern medicine with the single exception of microbial infection and the spirochete. We would be doing all sorts of things to intervene: inventing new modifications of group psychotherapy to correct the flawed thinking of general paresis, transplanting hearts with aortas attached for cardiovascular lues, administering immunosuppressant drugs to reverse the autoimmune reactions in tabes, enucleating gummas from the liver. . . . We might even be wondering about the role of stress in this peculiar, "multi-

factorial," chronic disease, and there would be all kinds of suggestions for "holistic" approaches, ranging from changes in the home environment to White House commissions on the role of air pollution. At an earlier time we would have been busy with bleeding, cupping, and purging, as indeed we once were. Or incantations, or shamanist fits of public ecstasy. Anything, in the hope of bringing about a change for the better in the whole body. (pp. 111–112)

As Thomas points out, it is even more complicated to intervene in pathological social systems. Certainly this is the case where interventions in the child-and-family system are concerned; these need to be assessed carefully in terms of unforeseen consequences that may flow from the intervention itself. One example arises from efforts to improve the quality of housing in the West End of Boston (Fried, 1973). New housing developments providing increased living space for family members reduced some tensions by day but had the effect of causing insomnia problems among children who had grown accustomed to the comfort of going to sleep in close quarters with their siblings.

Especially problematic is the involvement of the government in attempts to alter individual and group behavior. Such governmental efforts to promote patterns of living thought to be healthful is not wholly new; public health and labor laws have existed for a long time. In recent years, however, the government has steadily increased its investment in programs to reform lifestyles as a vehicle for promoting health and preventing the onset of illness. Major health policy documents both in the United States (DHEW, 1979) and Canada (Lalonde Report, 1974) herald a change of emphasis from "attempts to rescue us from the consequences of our vices" to making us "virtuous."

Given the fact that, in many areas of child development and family life, a need exists for providing guidance on childrearing and family functioning, what is the proper role of a government agency? The issue deserves scrutiny, especially considering the apparent fragility of the guidance that has been provided over time. It would appear that the "behavioral medicine" offered to the public shifts dramatically, in part, with alterations in the values and mores of the culture. Today's "best" guidance on childrearing and family life may be tomorrow's anathema.

Consider the 1914 publication, *Infant Care*, of the U.S. Children's Bureau, which suggested that "the rule that parents should not play with their children may seem hard but it is without doubt a safe one." That same publication carried a picture of a recommended patient cuff which would hold the child's arm stiff at the elbow and thus prevent him from sucking his thumb—an act considered a great evil requiring the mother's repressive interference since it expressed a child's dark and dangerous impulses.

In stark contrast, a report by NIMH 60 years later (Krasner & Ullman, 1975) describing the research of Catherine J. Garvey, emphasized that "children learn a great deal from play." Garvey is quoted as observing:

> What we see going together in play are not just wagons and horses, tea cups and saucers, a spoon and feeding, but attitudes with sex-typing, typical desires and behaviors with age and sex distinctions, steps in action or event sequences. (p. 22)

Still another recent NIMH publication, *The Importance of Play*, informs the reader that "to most children, play is life. It is . . . an important part of physical and mental development" (Stapleton & Yahraes, 1980).

The variability of childrearing advice offered to parents is even more marked in commercial publications. It is instructive in this connection to compare yesterday's stringent and forbidding approaches to childrearing with today's avalanche of parenting guides that suggest virtually unlimited freedom of expression as the birthright of every child, and the optimum avenue for development. Contrast, for example, the advice offered not too long ago to avoid picking up a crying infant with that of a prominent contemporary child development advisor:

> I feel it is impossible to spoil an infant. The concept of spoiling (by excessive attention) does not apply to babies under the age of nine or ten months, since they are utterly dependent, completely incapable of satisfying their own needs, and absolutely unable to put off any gratification without some sense of frustration (Salk, 1973).

The shift in American childrearing approaches over the past century is perhaps most dramatically exposed in the matter of sexual development. *Godey's Lady's Book*, a nineteenth-century woman's magazine long before *Redbook*, offered this advice by a writer holding both M.D. and Ph.D degrees:

> Teach (the child) that (his genital) organs are given as a sacred trust. . . .
>
> Impress upon him that if these organs are abused, or if they are put to any use besides that for which God made them, they will bring disease or ruin. . . .
>
> Teach him that when he handles or excites the sexual organs, all parts of the body suffer because they are connected by nerves that run throughout the system. That is why it is called "self-abuse." The whole body is abused when this part of the body is handled or excited in any manner whatever.

One of the leading advisors on children of the day, Dr. Dewees, offered the following warning on spontaneous auto-eroticism: "Children should not be permitted to indulge in bed long after daylight; as its warmth, the accumulation of urine and faeces; and the exercise of the imagination, but too often leads to the precocious development of the sexual instinct."

It would be difficult, indeed, to offer such advice today to parents who now keep at their own bedside a supply of manuals and magazines that teach them in clinical detail how to engineer the optimum sexual thrill from their self-manipulation efforts. Instructing children about sex today often means teaching them not how to protect themselves from satanic sexual impulses through prayer and self-denial, but how to keep from becoming pregnant through judicious use of condoms and diaphragms. Science does not provide us with concrete evidence regarding the advisability of inhibiting or facilitating a young child's sexual fantasies. There can be no officially sanctioned parental "policy" on the matter. Current wisdom, however, reflects cultural attitudes, and it would be difficult for a parent to inhibit a child's erotic fantasies after devouring, for example, Nancy Friday's (1973) graphic compilations of what are now widely regarded as the natural and totally acceptable, if not necessarily model, sexual fantasies of adult men and women.

Previous generations of parents at least had the advantage of living in a simpler time and, therefore, in a homogeneous culture in which there were fewer contradictory currents of thought. Today, in contrast, parents are often victims of conflicting philosophies and theories. The pluralism of American society has led to a bewildering range of approaches and techniques in childrearing. Because "parenting" guides available today are rarely based on rigorous data, the programs offered by their authors differ wildly. Some recommend punitive reprisals for acts of childishness that would have delighted a Calvinist schoolmaster, while others urge parents always to accept rather than to judge their children, no matter how intolerable their behavior.

One can readily sympathize with the complaint of the late Sam Levenson (1966):

> My wife and I were blessed with two kids and eight hundred theories beamed at us every day, all day, from magazines, radio and TV programs, diaper-service bulletins, books, pamphlets, checklists, progress charts, authorities, authorities.

In the view of Kessen (1979), children have been catalogued in so many wildly different forms that "a perceptive extraterrestrial could never see them as reflecting the same organism."

However varied their approach, all programmed guides to childrearing carry a similar, self-defeating message: that parents can engineer a generation of trouble-free children simply by using the "right" techniques. Mothers and fathers, we are told, can shape their young at will if only they will follow simple instructions.

While not all parents rely on the "experts" to tell them how to raise their children, for many others, childrearing manuals often leave a cruel residue of unwarranted anxiety and guilt. Not being able to get the nuts and bolts of Junior's personality put together quite right, they see themselves as failures, behaving as if each of their acts is being critically scrutinized by a psychiatrist.

The readiness of many parents to accept the seductive message that their children can be made trouble-free is hardly surprising. Psychologists have richly prepared the way by suggesting repeatedly the existence of a simple relationship between childrearing techniques and the course of a child's development. We have been convinced for decades that, if only we would look diligently enough, we would readily find the causal chain that links *this* parental intervention with *that* outcome in every child. Few parents are aware of the reality: "There is reason to question the expectation of universal behavioral outcomes from particular rearing regimens" (Kagan, 1979).

Despite such honest reappraisals, hordes of pundits and armchair psychologists continue to peddle "quick fixes" for the pains and perplexities of childrearing. Millions of mothers and fathers, hungry for approaches that might reduce the tensions and the burdens of rearing the young, continue to be willing customers for the avalanche of parenting manuals that roll off the nation's presses. The result is a generation of adults persisting in the belief that they can reshape their children—make them energetic or relaxed, social or studious, sensitive or thick-skinned—if only an expert would give them the key, tell them what strings to pull to produce the desired changes. Encouraged by the advice of a phalanx of childrearing gurus, parents have come to expect miracles of themselves, and of their children.

But virtually ignored by the writers of parenting guides is a recognition of the clear message from child development: the destiny of a child is determined not by one factor but by a mosaic of forces, all of them interacting. Parents and caretakers are rarely informed that a child's emotional health and personality development is a complex product of many forces—the information contained in each unique genetic configuration, prenatal experiences, parental attitudes, familial dynamics, the influence of peers, teachers, and major social forces.

The greatest potential damage arising from programmed childrearing approaches lies in the tendency provoked among parents to abdicate the responsibility for understanding the uniqueness of *their* child. Parenting by the book is possible only if one assumes that all children are miraculously identical—if, in effect, one denies a central fact of child development: the extraordinary range of individual differences that characterize children from the moment of birth.

Simple and unequivocal answers to complex questions adults ask about their children's mental health do little service to either the parents or their children. Researchers have learned a great deal about the subject, but despite the glib pronouncements emanating from both governmental and private sources, many questions remain to which answers from science continue to be either ambiguous or altogether unavailable. It would appear important for mental health educators to communicate what is *not* known for certain, as well as what seems clear in the light of research.

Even were more certainty possible regarding the outcome of particular childrearing approaches, the use of public education vehicles to alter behavior would still not be without its hazards. Recipients of mental health education materials comprise an unseen audience whose response to the messages directed to them remains unknown. No opportunity exists, as it does in a therapeutic setting, for the service provider—in this case, the information expert—to observe and react to the recipients' responses. Only improved evaluation studies, discussed earlier in this chapter, might begin to overcome this limitation.

Issues of Policy Implementation

As stated previously in this chapter, while not all agree on the degree of guidance and direction found in the considerable body of child-development research data that now exists, many feel that these have not been adequately utilized in setting public policy because policy and lawmakers have been remiss in ignoring directions for social change inherent in the data. Indeed, few subjects in the behavioral sciences have been the subject of more intense exhortations and emotional appeals. Sermons abound, many of them convincing in their rhetoric, suggesting, as stated earlier, that it is only the inability or unwillingness of political figures to act on existing information that blocks children from succeeding in their developmental tasks (Zigler, 1973; Fraiberg, 1977; Keniston, 1977; Brim, 1975).

While these points of view may be fairly regarded as extreme, it seems clear enough that needs of children, in fact, have not figured prominently in the priority-setting processes of the government. Federal programs appear to continue to be weighted for their impact on the nation's budget, on foreign policy, on energy supplies, and on the quality of the environment—but not on the lives of children. "Today," reports the Carnegie Council on Children, "virtually the last question we ask of any public policy is how it will affect children. It should be the first question" (Keniston, 1977).

A number of examples of gaps in the implementation of federal child welfare policies were identified by Segal and Yahraes (1978). For instance, despite evidence that adequate substitute care for children of working mothers is critical to the child's well-being, a coherent day-care program is still unavailable to needy parents. Also, although the father's presence appears to be an important ingredient in the child's development, an unemployed father who stays home can adversely affect his family's welfare benefits under federal law. Another example is that, in spite of evidence that early, sustained contacts between a child and his parents help establish important emotional bonds, U.S. laws insist that Social Security credits toward later retirement may be earned only by working outside the home, but not by staying home and caring for one's children. Finally, although members of the extended family can serve as emotional lifelines for troubled children, laws permit the tax-deductible payment of costs for care for the elderly only in an outside nursing home—but not if they live in their own homes with their own children and grandchildren.

Thus, what may seem to be the solution to a social problem, often meets serious obstacles, frequently political or financial in nature. But the problem of the adequacy of the knowledge base is also one that elicits concern among many researchers.

In many cases, the gaps between apparent needs and policy implementation arise because of inadequate knowledge on the part of researchers regarding specific directions for change. Rutter (1981) points out that "while political inertia or competing priorities may serve to block policy implementation initiatives in many instances, it is not true, as many assume, that the directions for implementation are entirely clear and well laid out." He reminds us that, although many think that answers are available to implement broad preventive measures "likely to raise the general level of children's intellectual, educational, social and emotional development," the specific measures are far from clear, in that

> there is a disparity between our knowledge of what is important and our ignorance of what to do about it. Preschool intervention is worthwhile, but do we know what sort is most effective in aiding children's social and emotional development? One-parent families frequently experience poverty and the children suffer thereby. However, remarriage is one effective means of raising economic status and yet there is evidence that sometimes this makes things worse for children. Certainly, the families of handicapped children need better support services but how confident are we that we know the best way of providing them? Children in residential care do indeed need continuity of relationships but this calls in question our whole pattern of residential services. The point is *not* that we know nothing. There are many instances where knowledge is available but it is just not acted on. However, the translation of general

principles of child rearing into effective policies of preventive action poses many unresolved problems, and we delude ourselves if we think that we already have the answers.

In cases where sufficient knowledge is apparently available, but implementation is slow, there may be a variety of factors at play. It is instructive, therefore, to examine some of the possible reasons why the path between research and policy continues to be such a tortuous one. These are: (1) the politicization of research evidence; (2) the staying power of popular beliefs; (3) the ambiguity of research data; and (4) the lack of central organization.

The Politicization of Research Evidence

The acceptance and implementation of research findings by policymakers are often blocked by virtue of the fact that the data produced run counter to strongly entrenched political convictions. Rein (1976) has summarized the dilemma succinctly: "A study may be valid by internal criteria and still arouse violent opposition from people against whose interest it goes."

A classic instance emerged following the Korean War during my own studies of the behavior of prisoners in captivity (Segal, 1956, 1976). The central question for the U.S. Army-sponsored research was straight-forward: What led some of our men in captivity to yield under stress to the enemy's demands, while others resisted?

The Korean POW episode, with its new and painful lexicon of human behavior—"brainwashing," "collaboration," "give-up-itis"—evoked strong political currents, and the result was that carefully analyzed data were ignored in the face of passionately held convictions. As in the case of many personal and social crises, the event became less important than the response to it.

The results of the research showed that collaborative behavior in the Korean compounds could be understood in very pragmatic, everyday terms. The Chinese Communists viewed their prisoners primarily as a rich source of potent propaganda materials. In exchange for petitions, confessions, or radio broadcasts (to name just a few of the propaganda "bullets" our men were put upon to manufacture), the enemy offered the type of material rewards most people can understand and appreciate: creature comforts, and freedom from fear and the threat of pain.

The results showed that in a world of barbed wire, blanketed by fear, in which the enemy's goals were obscure and difficult to comprehend, it was susceptibility to material inducements—not ideological persuasions—that best explained the behavior of that very small proportion of U.S. Army troops who "collapsed" before the enemy's psychological onslaughts.

This finding, however, ran directly counter to the popular political stance of the time. It soon became apparent that the latter was too well-entrenched to be shaken by contrary evidence drawn from research data. The politically attractive conviction that large numbers of captives were ideologically converted by exotic communist brainwashing techniques was nowhere supported by the data; yet the "brainwashing" myth gained ever-increasing momentum during the post-Korean decade.

Collaborative activity, it was argued, *must* have been ideologically inspired and there were many who, sharing this belief, maintained that we could best strengthen the fiber of U.S. warriors (in Korea, their average education was ninth grade) only by teaching them the virtues of Jeffersonian democracy as against the dialectic errors of Marxist communism. The fact that the results of the study clearly suggested that ideological training would have a limited value as a vehicle for preventing breakdown under the stresses of captivity was either ignored or challenged openly. Indeed, on a number of occasions, the validity of the research findings (and even the author's loyalty) were challenged by military and political leaders of the time.

The ultimate test of the acceptability of data is political, concludes Caplan (1977) from his study of the utilization of research by policymakers. This is particularly true in the area of domestic social policy, and the rationale most often advanced for rejecting relevant social science information is that its implications are politically unfeasible. It is rare for data to be so compelling as to take precedence over political significance.

The Staying Power of Popular Beliefs

The second issue is produced by the tendency of policymakers, and the public at large, to accept minimal or negligible evidence that supports a popular and emotionally entrenched belief, and to ignore data that do not. The likely result is that the gap between scientific knowledge and practical implementation is further widened.

Kagan (1979) cites, as an example, existing convictions about the superordinate importance of the mother-infant bond, stating that

> the findings of future empirical inquiry may affirm the popular belief that surrogate care of infants has psychological dangers (but) even the most traditional student of child development would admit that these beliefs remain largely unproven. . . . A combination of emotional conviction and frail evidence often betrays the fact that a deep value is being threatened. In the present case, I believe that the possibility that the biological mother might be partially replaced bothers a great many citizens. (p. 890)

Caplan (1977) found that many respondents who rejected policy-relevant information did so because the result contradicted what they considered to be true. For example, they were impressed with the concepts of democratic leadership in organization management, and the data supporting these ideas, but given the nature and pressures of their situation, many upper-level officials were convinced that such approaches to management would probably fail. To illustrate further: Although the evaluation of some governmental programs showed failure, program administrators and sponsors remained convinced that the programs had succeeded. Similar examples in research on criminal justice, welfare, work satisfaction, and education could be cited to illustrate the notion that officials are willing to accept findings which coincide with their beliefs, but not those which are counterintuitive to their beliefs, quite apart from issues of scientific objectivity and political feasibility.

The Ambiguity of Research Data

The crucial issues in a policy debate are not so much matters of fact, as questions of interpretation. In this connection, Rein (1976) points out that research findings can sharpen the areas of disagreement, and make the issues more uncertain, complex, and technical; as a result, the contribution of social science to policy becomes more remote. He cites the debate about the heritability of I.Q., or the relationship between education and income as two examples: "Social science does contribute to policy and practice, but the link is neither consensual, graceful nor self-evident" (p. 12).

Information increases power, and as people who hold different views acquire knowledge, they tend to argue their positions more cogently; they attempt to influence others by virtue of the fact that their data may now be described as "objective." Thus, Rein maintains, "more knowledge, more equitably distributed, may produce more disagreement and make it more difficult for a government to act" (p. 12).

Rein's perceptive analysis of the failure of research to provide a sure method for selecting among social policy alternatives is especially relevent to the child development field:

> Data are seldom convincing enough . . . to settle questions about contrasting world views. More factual information alone will not settle the question of how the world works and how to intervene in it. When there are many causes for a single event, and the causes are interdependent, we may truthfully say that everything is in some sense causally linked to everything else. However, it is extremely difficult to isolate the independent contribution of these interrelated events. Even if this task could be accomplished, it does not necessarily follow that by altering the isolated factor we will bring about the desired state of affairs. Social science fails in practice to provide a single synthetic sophisticated regression model which parcels out the independent contribution of each variable and assigns a rating to each which can be accepted as a general law, faith-

> fully capturing reality as it is, and predicting future outcomes as well. But since the ideal is still accepted in principle, each disappointment leads to a renewed call for further inquiry which can rescue the earlier studies from their methodological weakness. (pp. 211–212)

In many instances, the methods utilized to test the effects of a given policy are far from perfect, partly because of the complexity of the research required. In other instances, the choice of dependent variable becomes problematic. Rutter (1981) points out, for example, that the Head Start Program was largely evaluated in terms of IQ gains, but actually that constituted only a small part of the objectives of the program. When this state of affairs occurs, Rutter believes, there is the danger that unevaluated benefits will be unknown and ignored, and that policies effective in some respects may be rejected simply because the wrong dependent variables were chosen. Even accepting this, Rutter maintains, there is the great difficulty of deciding what are the most appropriate outcome variables. For example, what is the appropriate outcome variable with respect to the use of day-care; the immediate mental health of the child; the mental health of the mother; the child's ability to make adequate family relationships when grown up; or the child's abilities to be an effective parent himself? Is it necessary that children and/or mothers should be better off in some measure of health as a result of day-care, or is it sufficient that they be more contented? And if one is made more content and the other less so, how do you decide which should be given the greater weight?

The Lack of Central Organization

A fourth impediment to the acceptance and utilization of scientific data lies in the lack of coherent vehicles within the governing structure to act on the data at hand.

As described by Steiner (1976), a broad and well-defined national policy on children has never been clearly formulated; few tested ideas have been translated from researchers' journals to legal statutes; the nation's child advocates have failed to join in common cause; and the awesome responsibilities for children's programs have been scattered haphazardly throughout the Congress and federal bureaucracy.

Caplan (1977) studied 575 instances of the utilization of social science information by upper-level officials in the United States government. While many occurred in instances without an identifiable set of conditions present (i.e., as a result of chance factors), Caplan did find a cluster of interrelated conditions which help increase the probability for what he calls "the creative systematic and creative application of social science knowledge in the formulation of public policy" (p. 183). He concludes that research utilization is most likely to occur when six conditions are present: (1) the decision-making orientation of the policymaker is characterized by a reasoned appreciation of both the scientific and the extrascientific aspects of the policy issue; (2) the ethical-scientific values of the policymaker embody a conscious sense of social direction and responsibility; (3) the policy issue is well defined and of such a nature that a "best" solution requires research knowledge; (4) the research findings are not counterintuitive, but rather they are believable on grounds of objectivity; (5) their action implications are politically feasible; and (6) the policymaker and knowledge producers are linked by information specialists capable of coupling scientific inputs to policy goals. Such conditions rarely coexist in the terrain shared by child-development researchers and policy personnel.

Despite existing barriers to the development of broadly based stress-and-coping education programs on behalf of children, the pursuit of such efforts continues to be warranted. Required will be ingeniously designed programs and, equally important, long-range evaluation studies. Only by meeting both criteria are both the public and professionals likely to be persuaded of the benefits to be derived from translating knowledge in the field into pragmatic action.

REFERENCES

Anthony, E. J., & Koupernik, C. (Eds.). *The child in his family: Children at psychiatric risk.* New York: Wiley-Interscience, 1974.

Bandura, A. *Social learning theory*. Englewood Cliffs, N.J.: Prentice-Hall, Inc., 1977.

Bienvenu, M. *Helping the slow learner.* New York: Public Affairs Committee, No. 405, 1967.

Blane, H. T., & Hewitt, L. C. *Mass media, public education and alcohol: A state-of-art review.* Rockville, Md.: National Institute of Alcohol Abuse and Alcoholism; Alcohol, Drug Abuse, and Mental Health Administration (ADAMHA), 1973.

Bonkowski, S., & Wanner-Westly, B. The divorce group: A new treatment modality. *Social Casework*, 1979, *60*, 552–557.

Brenton, M. *Playmates: The importance of childhood friendships*. New York: Public Affairs Committee, No. 525, 1975.

Brim, O. G., Jr. Macro-structural influences on child development and the need for childhood social indicators. *American Journal of Orthopsychiatry*, 1975, *45*, 516–524.

Caplan, N. A minimal set of conditions necessary for the utilization of social science knowledge in policy formulations at the national level. In C. H. Weiss (Ed.), *Using social research in public policymaking*. Lexington, Mass: D. C. Heath & Co., 1977.

Cowen, E. L. The wooing of primary prevention. *American Journal of Community Psychology*, 1980, *8*, 258–284.

Cowen, E. L., & Lorion, R. P. New directions in school mental health: A secondary preventive approach. In L. Bellak, & H. H. Barten (Eds.), *Progress in community mental health* (Vol. 3). New York: Brunner/Mazel, 1975.

Croake, J. W., & Glover, K. W. A history and evaluation of parent education. *The Family Coordinator*, 1977, 153–154.

Dart, R. J. Reducing stress in young children: Effects of mother's picture and voice recordings on response to hospitalization (Doctoral dissertation, University of Waterloo, Canada, 1980). *Dissertation Abstracts International*, 1980, *41*, 1104-B. (Not available from University Microfilms.)

Davis, J. A. *Education for positive mental health*. Chicago: Aldine, 1965.

Department of Health, Education, and Welfare. *The Framingham study: An epidemiological investigation of cardiovascular disease* (DHEW Publication No. NIH 74-478). Washington, D.C.: U.S. Government Printing Office, 1968.

Department of Health, Education, and Welfare. *Healthy people: The Surgeon General's report on health promotion and disease prevention* (DHEW Publication No. PHS 79-55071). Washington, D.C.: U.S. Government Printing Office, 1979.

Dobson, J. *Dare to discipline*. Wheaton, Ill.: Tyndale House Publications, 1970.

Duthler, T. B. An investigation of the reduction of psychological stress in patients facing surgical removal of tumors (Doctoral dissertation, University of Missouri-Columbia, 1979). *Dissertation Abstracts International*, 1980, *40*, 4477-B (University Microfilms No. 8007144, 133).

Eisenberg, L. A research framework for evaluating the promotion of mental health and prevention of mental illness. *Public Health Reports*, 1981, *96*, 3–19.

Fishman, M. E. *The child and youth activities of the National Institute of Mental Health: October 1, 1979–September 30, 1980*. Unpublished paper presented at the meeting of the National Advisory Mental Health Council, Washington, D.C., 1980.

Fraiberg, S. *Every child's birthright: In defense of mothering*. New York: Basic Books, 1977.

Friday, N. *My secret garden: Women's sexual fantasies*. New York: Trident, 1973.

Fried, M. *The world of the urban working class*. Cambridge, Mass.: Harvard University Press, 1973.

Fuchs, V. R. *Who shall live?* New York: Basic Books, 1974.

Garmezy, N. Children under stress: Perspectives on antecedents and correlates of vulnerability and resistance to psychopathology. In A. I. Rabin, J. Aronoff, A. M. Barclay, & R. A. Zucker (Eds.), *Further explorations on personality*. New York: Wiley-Interscience, 1981.

Garmezy, N., & Nuechterlein, K. H. Invulnerable children: The fact and fiction of competence and disadvantage. *American Journal of Orthopsychiatry*, 1972, *42*, 328–329. (Abstract)

Ginott, H. G. *Between parent and child*. New York: Macmillan Publishing Co., 1965.

Goldston, S., & Klein, D. C. (Eds.). *Primary prevention: An idea whose time has come* (DHEW Publication No. ADM 77-4477). Washington, D.C.: U.S. Government Printing Office, 1976.

Green, P. The mass media anti-smoking campaign around the world. *Proceedings of Third World Conference on Smoking and Health* (Vol. 2), 1975, 245–253.

Hall, J. J. *Evaluation of mental health education programs*. Unpublished manuscript, 1977.

Haskins, J. B. Evaluative research on the effects of mass communication safety campaigns: A methodological critique. *Journal of Safety Research*, 1978, *2*, 86–90.

Hill, M. *Parents and teenagers*. New York: Public Affairs Committee, No. 490, 1973.

Hoffman, L. W. Maternal employment, 1979. *American Psychologist*, 1979, *34*, 859–865.

Horowitz, M. J., & Kaltreider, N. B. Brief treatment of post-traumatic stress disorders. *New Directions for Mental Health Services*, 1980, *6*, 67–79.

Horowitz, M. J., Krupnick, J., Kaltreider, N., Wilner, N., Leong, A., & Marmar, C. Initial psychological response to parental death. *Archives of General Psychiatry*, 1981, *38*, 316–323.

Kafka, F. *Letter to his father*. New York: Schocken Books, 1953.

Kagan, J. Family experience and the child's development. *American Psychologist*, 1979, *34*, 886–891.

Keniston, K., & the Carnegie Council on Children. *All our children*. New York: Harcourt Brace Jovanovich, 1977.

Kessen, W. *Psychological development from infancy: Image to intention*. Hillsdale, N.J.: Lawrence Erlbaum Associates, 1979.

Kline, F. G. Evaluation of a multimedia drug education program. *Journal of Drug Education*, 1972, 2, 229–239.

Krasner, L., & Ullman, L. A *psychological approach to abnormal behavior*. Englewood Cliffs, N.J.: Prentice-Hall, 1975.

Lalonde, M. A *new perspective on the health of Canadians: A working document*. Ottawa: The Government of Canada, 1974.

Levenson, S. *Everything but money*. New York: Simon & Schuster, 1966.

Lifton, R. J. Home by ship: Reaction patterns of American POWs repatriated from North Korea. *American Journal of Psychiatry*, 1954, *110*, 732–738.

Lynn, L. E. (Ed.), *Knowledge and policy: The uncertain connection*. Washington, D.C.: National Academy of Sciences, 1978.

Maccoby, N., & Alexander, J. Reducing heart disease risk using the mass media: Comparing the effects on three communities. In R. F. Munoz, L. R. Snowden, & J. G. Kelly (Eds.), *Social and psychological research in community settings*. San Francisco: Jossey-Bass, 1979.

McAlister, A., Puska, P., Koskela, K., Pallonen, U., & Maccoby, N. Psychology in action: Mass communication and community organization for public health education. *American Psychologist*, 1980, 35, 375–379.

Mencken, H. L. *Prejudices. Third series*. New York: Octagon Books, 1977.

Mielke, K. W., & Swinehart, J. W. *Evaluation of the "Feeling Good" television series*. New York: Children's Television Workshop, 1976.

Nielsen, E. S. The effects of training children to cope with stress: A comparison of procedures for preparing children to control stress response during a dental examination (Doctoral dissertation, University of Nevada, Reno, 1979). *Dissertation Abstracts International*, 1980, *40*, 5013-B (University Microfilms No. 8008366, 125).

Palomares, U. H., & Rubini, T. *Magic circle*. La Mesa, Calif.: Human Development Training Institute, 1974.

Patterson, G. R. Mothers: The unacknowledged victims. *Monographs of the Society for Research in Child Development*, 1980, 45, (0.5, Serial No. 186).

Pfohl, W., Jr. Children's anxiety management program: A broad-based behavioral program teaching children to cope with stress and anxiety (Doctoral dissertation, Rutgers University, 1979). *Dissertation Abstracts International*, 1980, *41*, 3424-A (University Microfilms No. 8103414, 148).

Rein, M. *Social science and public policy*. Harmondsworth, England: Penguin Books, 1976.

Richlin, M., Rahe, R. H., Shale, J. H., Jr., & Mitchell, R. E. Five-year medical followup of Vietnam POWs: Preliminary results. *U.S. Navy Medicine*, 1980, *71*, 18–26.

Robertson, L. S. The great seat belt campaign flop. *Journal of Communications*, 1976, 4, 41–45.

Rutter, M. Private correspondence, 1981.

Rutter, M. Protective factors in children's responses to stress and disadvantage. In M. W. Kent, & J. E. Rolf (Eds.), *Social competence in children: Primary prevention of psychopathology* (Vol. 3). Hanover, N.H.: University Press of New England, 1979.

Salk, L. *What every child would like his parents to know*. New York: Warner Books, 1973.

Sargent, M. *Caring about kids: Stimulating baby senses* (DHEW Publication No. ADM 77-481). Washington, D.C.: U.S. Government Printing Office, 1978.

Sargent, M. *Caring about kids: Talking to children about death* (DHEW Publication No. ADM 80-838). Washington, D.C.: U.S. Government Printing Office, 1979.

Sargent, M. *Caring about kids: Pre-term babies* (DHHS Publication No. ADM 80-972). Washington, D.C.: U.S. Government Printing Office, 1980.

Segal, J. *Correlates of collaboration and resistance of U.S. Army POWs in Korea* (HumRRO Tech. Rep. 33). Alexandria, Va.: Human Resources Research Organization, 1956.

Segal, J. Therapeutic considerations in planning the return of American POWs to continental U.S. *Military Medicine*, 1973, *138*, 73–77.

Segal, J. (Ed.). *Research in the service of mental health, report of the research task force of the National Institute of Mental Health* (DHEW Publication No. ADM 75-236). Washington, D.C.: U.S. Government Printing Office, 1975.

Segal, J. Universal consequences of captivity: Stress reactions among divergent populations of prisoners of war and their families. *International Social Science Journal*, 1976, *28*, 593–609.

Segal, J., & Yahraes, H. A *child's journey: Forces that shape the lives of our young*. New York: McGraw-Hill, 1978.

Siegel, L. J., & Peterson, L. Stress reduction in young dental patients through coping skills and sensory information. *Journal of Consulting and Clinical Psychology*, 1980, *48*, 785–787.

Sobell, S. *Caring about kids: Helping the hyperactive child* (DHEW Publication No. ADM 80-561). Washington, D.C.: U.S. Government Printing Office, 1978.

Spivack, G., & Shure, M. B. *Social adjustment of young children*. San Francisco: Jossey-Bass, 1974.

Stapleton, C., & Yahraes, H. *The importance of play* (DHHS Publication No. ADM 80-969). Washington, D.C.: U.S. Government Printing Office, 1980.

Starr, R. H. Child abuse. *American Psychologist*, 1979, *34*, 872–878.

Steiner, G. Y. *The children's cause*. Washington, D.C.: The Brookings Institution, 1976.

Stone, G., Hindz, W. C., & Schmidt, G. W. Teaching mental health behaviors to elementary school children. *Professional Psychology*, 1975, *6*, 34–40.

Sundale, M., & Schanie, C. F. Community mental health and mass media preventive education: The alternatives project. *Social Science Review*, June 1978, 297–306.

Sunley, R. Early nineteenth-century American literature on childrearing. In M. Mead, & M. Wolfenstein (Eds.), *Childhood in contemporary cultures*. Chicago: University of Chicago Press, 1955.

Thomas, L. *The medusa and the snail*. New York: Viking Press, 1974.

Wallerstein, J., & Kelly, J. B. *Surviving the breakup: How children and parents cope with divorce*. New York: Basic Books, 1980.

Wehrle, S. *Caring about kids: Dyslexia* (DHHS Publication No. ADM 80-616). Washington, D.C.: U.S. Government Printing Office, 1978.

White, E. B. *Letters of E. B. White*. New York: Harper & Row, 1976.

Wikler, D. I. Persuasion and coercion for health: Ethical issues in government efforts to change lifestyles. *Health and Society*, 1978, *56*, 303–338.

Yamamoto, K. Children's ratings of the stressfulness of experiences. *Developmental Psychology*, 1979, *15*, 581–582.

Zigler, E. The future of social policy for children. *Notes from the Center* (No. 5). Syracuse, N.Y.: The Center on Human Policy, 1973.

CHAPTER 12

SOME METHODOLOGICAL PROBLEMS AND RESEARCH DIRECTIONS IN THE STUDY OF THE EFFECTS OF STRESS ON CHILDREN

LEE N. ROBINS
PROFESSOR OF SOCIOLOGY IN PSYCHIATRY
DEPARTMENT OF PSYCHIATRY
WASHINGTON UNIVERSITY SCHOOL OF MEDICINE

STRESS AND OUTCOME RESEARCH

How does stress research differ from the study of other environmental predictors of outcomes? The traditional difference lies in the fact that the independent variable in stress research is often a single dramatic event, like death or divorce. The question then asked is what effect does this event have on the individual's subsequent mental health? This singling out of a specific presumed etiological factor occurring at a specific moment in time avoids the vagueness that has plagued research findings of the association between demographic factors, such as low social status, female gender, or advanced age, and an increased risk of psychiatric disorder. These demographic variables are seen as vague causal factors, since we do not know what are the underlying processes that make them harmful. For example, there are many possible mechanisms whereby low social status might affect mental health: inadequate nutrition, low self-esteem, overcrowding in the home, worry over money, lack of education, exposure to physical hazards, inadequate medical care, etc. When one wants to advance from noting correlations between poverty and disorder to recommending policy for reducing such a relationship, these multiple possibilities make it difficult to decide what is the most promising intervention to initiate. Clearly, this problem is reduced when one deals with a specific event. However, the gain in specificity is accompanied by a sacrifice in the predictive power that a variable such as social status has demonstrated in many studies. Because demographic statuses are long lasting, and perhaps because they implicate many different types of stressors, they often prove to be reasonably powerful predictors of psychiatric outcomes. Single dramatic life events are, by definition, time-limited and differ from one's typical living situation; therefore, they often fail to provide very strong correlations between specific events and the mental health of persons exposed to them (Tennant, Bebbington, & Hurry, 1981).

THE IMPUTATION OF CAUSALITY

Even the assets of clarity and simplicity implicit in studying a single life event as a cause of mental disorder may be more apparent than real. The difficulty is that both the event and the subsequent behavioral difficulty we seek to interpret as its consequence may be the result of other events that preceded both of these. If this is so, any imputation of a causal connection between the two may be spurious, even though they may be highly correlated, and despite the fact that the event clearly preceded the onset of the person's psychological problem. Unfortunately, the need to search for possible common antecedents is often overlooked in stress research. Only rarely is the explanation that a specific stressor is responsible for a subsequent disorder forced to compete with other equally plausible explanations for such an association.

Divorce

Divorce can provide an example of this methodological issue. Wallerstein, in her fascinating chapter in this volume, has observed that parental divorce is often associated with subsequent maladjustment in the child. However, we know from a host of studies (e.g., Briscoe, Smith, & Robins, 1973) that adults with certain psychiatric disorders, such as alcoholism, have an increased likelihood of being divorced. Children of alcoholics are known to have an excess of antisocial behavior irrespective of whether or not their parents divorce. Depression tends to run in families. Thus, the children of depressives can be expected to have an elevated rate of depression without regard to parental divorce status. We must wonder, then, whether the high rate of antisocial activity and depression in the children of divorce is necessarily accounted for by the divorce per se. Rather, the relationship may be the result of having alcoholic or depressive parents whose disorders can account both for heightened incidence of divorce and for the children's tendencies toward antisocial or depressed behaviors.

Does this search for alternative explanations become trivial once the life events under study become as commonplace as divorce has become in the last 15 years? How can one continue to associate parental divorce status with parents' psychiatric disorder when such a large number of married couples now separate and seek divorces? Of course, were it literally the case that *every* parent ultimately was divorced, one could not do so. But so long as some do and some do not, even if the percentage of doers increases, an association between preexisting psychiatric problems and divorce can remain a significant factor.

Examples of continued predictive power when outcome becomes common:

Childhood Deviance Predicts Adult Arrests

Our research at Washington University has provided several examples in which the commonsense expectation that correlations will be attenuated when a behavior becomes more commonplace has been proved wrong. For example, we first studied predictors of adult antisocial behavior by a follow-up study of white former child guidance clinic patients who were in their 40s (Robins, 1966), and then replicated that study by a follow-up of black men in their 30s who had not been patients (Robins, Murphy, Woodruff, & King, 1971). In the initial child guidance clinic study, we found a strong correlation between early school failure, truancy, and misbehavior and various measures of adult antisocial behavior, particularly arrests. At the time the second study was underway, in the late 1960s, it was commonly believed that arrests of black men were as frequent as they were due to police prejudice and the pressures of poverty and racism on *adult* behavior. If so, the relationship between adult arrests and childhood behavior found for whites should not be evident in studies of black persons. Actually, we found the strength of the correlation between early childhood deviance and adult arrests to be as high for blacks as it had been for whites, although the *prevalence* of arrests was considerably higher for blacks. While we were able to state that almost the *only* whites who would be arrested as adults were those who had exhibited deviant behavior in childhood, for blacks the data indicated that similarly highly deviant boys were almost certain to be arrested as adults, while others without such histories were at a reduced, albeit not negligible, level of risk. The degree of certainty with which these two statements could be made proved to be quite similar.

Childhood History Predicts Drug Usage

A further example is provided by our follow-up study of army enlisted men who had served in Vietnam in 1971 and who had typically entered the service at about age 19. At the time of entry, about 50% of the group had already tried marijuana, 25% had tried amphetamines, 5% had tried codeine, and only 2% had tried heroin. The year in which they reached their twentieth birthday was spent in service in Vietnam, where the use of drugs was commonplace. In that year, 75% used marijuana, and 43% used heroin. Initially, we looked for correlates of drug use prior to service and found substantial correlations for preservice drug use with various forms of preservice behavioral deviance, such as school truancy, fighting, dropout, and early drunkenness, and with the demographic variables of being black and residing in a large city. We doubted that these same variables would correlate strongly with drug use in Vietnam for a number of reasons: usage there was so common; the setting was so different from the setting in which the preservice drug use had occurred; and even the particular drugs used were different. In Vietnam, heroin and opium replaced amphetamines and codeine as the popular "hard" drugs. We found, however, that those very preservice variables that had been associated with preservice drug use were even *more* strongly correlated with the use of drugs in Vietnam than with earlier drug use (Robins, 1974). Apparently the ready availability of drugs in Vietnam allowed differences in the propensity to use them to be more fully expressed than they had been at home where opportunities, even for those predisposed, were more limited. Thus, rather than the commonness of the phenomenon damping the power of the predictor variables, it actually enhanced their power.

Were the effects of an increase in levels of crime and drug use to hold for divorce as well, the rise in the divorce rate might well mean that psychiatric disorder in marriage partners, rather than losing its power to predict divorce, may have as much or even more impact in the present climate than it had previously. Now, however, we may expect to find that married psychiatrically disturbed persons are almost *certain* to divorce, while only a fraction of the psychiatrically healthy do so, whereas when divorce was less common, it tended to occur chiefly among those who were psychiatrically disturbed.

Choosing the Appropriate Control Group

What can we do to overcome the danger of falsely attributing causal power to a life event when its correlation with the subsequent onset of disordered behavior may be spurious? A typical answer is to use a control group. But choosing the appropriate control group requires knowledge about the confounding variable that may be operative. In the case of divorce, if psychiatric disorder in the parent causes both divorce and maladjustment in children, comparing the adjustment of offspring of divorced parents with the adjustment of a control group made up of a random selection of offspring of intact marriages does not solve the problem. Instead, one has to compare children of broken marriages with children of intact marriages *whose parents have the same type and severity of psychiatric disorders that are present in divorcing parents*. Only then could one argue effectively that divorce has either good or bad consequences for the offspring, independent of the effect of the parents' mental health status.

The same design is necessary for studying the impact of any event in the child's life that is directly or indirectly caused by the personal characteristics of a parent. For example, children reared in large impersonal institutions with many caretakers have been found later to show more antisocial behavior than noninstitutionalized children, regardless of whether they were eventually returned to their own homes or placed for adoption (Tizard & Hodges, 1978). Is this finding due to the experience of institutionalization, or can it be explained by characteristics of parents that led to the institutionalization of the offspring? The placement of children in institutions often occurs because of reasons associated with parental behavior: parents have been hospitalized or jailed; or they have died either by suicide, homicide, or accident; or they have borne children out of wedlock who are unwanted; or they have been found guilty of child neglect. The psychiatric disorders of antisocial personality and alcoholism in parents heighten the probability of such events; these parental disorders are also associated with high rates of antisocial behavior in the offspring, even if the children are not institutionalized (Robins, 1966).

It is worth noting that even a parent's death is not immune from this possibility of spuriousness. Death of a parent has been one of the most studied of life events, particularly as it relates to depression in offspring, either during childhood (Caplan & Douglas, 1969) or adulthood (Brown & Harris, 1978). Parental death has been a popular object of study because it is rarely caused by the offspring's own behavior, as can be the case in a decision to institutionalize a child, since a child may be given up to an institution because he or she is very difficult for the mother or foster mother to control. In addition, the temporal order is reasonably certain. Death of a parent during childhood can generally be assumed to be antecedent to depressive disorder in the offspring since depression is rare prior to adulthood. However, to experience the death of a parent in childhood means that the parent must have died, on the average, by his or her mid-40s. The leading cause of death in young adults twenty-five to forty-four is accidents, with suicide and homicide ranking fourth and fifth respectively (National Center for Health Statistics, 1978). Accidents, suicide, and homicide, in turn, are predicted by several psychiatric disorders: alcoholism, depression, drug dependence, and antisocial personality. In the light of these relationships, wherein lies the causal relationship? Was it that the death of the parent caused the child's illness? Or can a parent's psychiatric disorder account both for his or her own death, as well as for the offspring's subsequent disorder?

The Stress of Combat

To realize how pervasive is the problem that antecedents may explain both the life event and its presumed consequence, consider a final example—combat—which seems to be a stressful life event almost immune from confounders. While death and divorce are familial events, and therefore possible signs of familial psychiatric disorders which could be the true causes of the child's later disorder, combat occurs during wartime, an event over which neither family members nor the soldier at risk has any control. During the Vietnam era, there was even a draft lottery, which was intended to leave completely to chance whether one was drafted or not drafted for military service. Combat in Vietnam, then, might seem to provide the ideal "natural" experiment by which to show the impact of a dramatic and important life experience on later psychiatric status.

To ascertain the long-term effect of combat on mental health, we evaluated the adjustment of veterans during the second and third years following their return from Vietnam. We used a variety of measures to assess their post-Vietnam adjustment, including the presence or absence of a depressive syndrome, alcohol problems, drug abuse, violence, an arrest record, vagrancy, a marital breakup, job instability, and credit problems. We compared the number of these problems per veteran to the number per member of a control group of nonveterans chosen from Selective Service records and matched with the veteran group for age, education, geographic location, and eligibility to serve in the military. As expected, we found more problems in this two-year period for veterans than for nonveterans; and among the veterans, we found that those who reported more exposure to combat had more post-Vietnam problems.

If we had looked no further, we would have considered these results to be a clear demonstration of the adverse effect of a major life event on later adjustment. However, things proved to be more complex. First, we noted that although the control group of nonveterans resembled the *draftees* in the variety of their deviant behaviors prior to the date of the veterans' induction, they were much less deviant than soldiers who had *volunteered* to serve. The draft lottery, which we had hoped would insure that soldiers and civilians would be alike in those individual characteristics known to forecast later adjustment, did not operate for the volunteers, who constituted 40% of the enlisted army in Vietnam. When we controlled for degree of deviance prior to service, differences between veterans and nonveterans, with respect to each of these forms of adjustment problems manifested in the post-Vietnam period, either diminished or disappeared (Robins & Helzer, in preparation). Having found that preservice behavioral history largely accounted for the differences in postservice adjustment between veterans and nonveterans, how could the association between amount of combat exposure and degree of later maladjustment be explained?

The results indicated that exposure to combat was *also* predicted by preservice deviant behavior: once this factor was controlled for, we no longer found a relationship between combat and later adjustment. That preservice deviance would predict the extent of combat exposure was not surprising once we considered the following finding. Men in service are given assignments on the basis of skills acquired before entering service. Soldiers with behavior problems prior to service had often volunteered for military service, in part because they were not qualified for good civilian jobs or were chronically unemployed. They generally had acquired none of the skills that might have resulted in their assignment in the military to jobs as clerks or cooks, or to other specialty occupations that would have kept them out of combat. Thus, preservice deviance proved to be the confounding variable. Not only did it predict both postservice problems and entry into the military, but it also predicted the exposure of soldiers to combat experiences. Thus, despite a "natural experiment" with initially positive findings, we were not able to demonstrate definitively that the stress of combat explained the higher rate of postservice maladjustment in veterans when compared with nonveteran controls.

The Use of Epidemiological Data

In addition to the search for a predictor that accounts both for the experience of stress and a negative outcome, there is another test that can be applied before assuming that life events explain such outcomes. This test involves consideration as to whether epidemiological changes in rates of disorder have occurred that are commensurate with expectations based on dramatic changes in the events presumed to be a causal factor. Death rates of young adults born into different historical cohorts have varied considerably, depending on their exposure to wars, epidemics, and to advances in public health measures. If parental deaths experienced in childhood are important causes of psychiatric disorder, one should expect to find more psychiatric disorder in those cohorts who were children during eras of high young-adult death rates in comparison with children born in other eras. If maternal death experienced prior to age 11 creates vulnerability to depression in daughters, as Brown and Harris' work suggests (1978), then the excess of maternal deaths caused by the flu epidemic of 1918 should have been reflected in an excess of depression in women born between 1907 and 1917. On the other hand, rates of depression in women should have shown a general decline over time, with the decline in their mothers' risk of perinatal death associated with the birth of the younger siblings. Similarly, if divorce is an important cause of adjustment problems in children, one would expect to see a steady increase in the case loads of childrens' psychiatric services during the past 15 years, in phase with the rapidly rising divorce rate. If these historical fluctuations in population rates are *not* found, one can begin to suspect that the high level of problems noted in the children of deceased and divorced parents may have some alternative explanation, such as those that have been suggested.

IMPLICATIONS FOR INTERVENTION

If we fail to subject those stressful experiences that are presumed to be causes of children's disturbed and disordered behavior to tests for spuriousness and epidemiological change, we may recommend social policies that, although they sound reasonable, may not be focused on the true causes of the disorders we seek to alleviate. Yet, even after a causal event is correctly identified (having survived these tests), the programs we introduce to reduce the stress may not prove helpful. We must choose interventions which will effectively prevent the occurrence of the cause or reduce its impact without creating new problems worse than those we are attempting to solve. Proposed interventions should be tested to compare their feasibility and effectiveness against other possible alternatives. While such a recommendation seems self-evident, history reveals that small-scale tests of new policies prior to their adoption tend to be rare.

For example, failing in school has been observed to be painful for children. This observation has led to a general policy of social promotions for children who fail to meet grade standards—a policy that seems more humane. But there was no preliminary experiment to compare the long-term consequences of social promotions versus repeating a grade either in terms of eventual achievement levels, preparation for future employment, or later psychological health. We still do not know which would have been the wiser choice; social promotion or grade repetition with an emphasis on needed skills acquisition.

It has been difficult to persuade granting agencies to support a slow, painstaking demonstration of efficacy when a pressing problem exists and a solution seems relevant and attractive. There are also ethical hurdles to experimentation before instituting new policies. Some claim that it is unfair to deny help to a control group used as the basis for comparison with a treated group. The response to such a claim, of course, is that we do not know whether the intervention denied to the control group truly constitutes help until after the experiment has been completed.

The Need for Baseline Measures

Perhaps an even greater obstacle to implementing policies related to stress prevention has been the lack of research instruments necessary to measure the baseline status of those children who will be affected by the intervention. Yet, such baseline equivalence between the experimental and control groups should be demonstrated prior to any intervention effort. Similarly, instruments are needed to measure the childrens' behavioral status at the completion of the experimental intervention, and at follow-up, to discover the extent to which favorable change has been achieved. Unfortunately, among other shortcomings we have also lacked statistical methods sensitive and efficient enough to detect treatment effects in small groups.

The need for baseline measures is often finessed by using random assignments to experimental and control groups on the assumption that the groups will be alike or only minimally different, and that chance differences that occur can be corrected subsequently by using covariance analysis. Experiments, however, are expensive, and groups are usually kept so small that random assignment is unlikely to result in well-matched groups. With small groups, one needs baseline measures to allow stratification at the time of random selection. This would permit the separation of children into high-, medium-, and low-risk groups, with half of each group being assigned subsequently to the control and half to the experimental conditions, thus insuring intergroup similarity. It may still prove necessary to use analysis of covariance, since even well-matched initial groups can become ill-matched over time, as a result of differential attrition rates. However, such an experimental design will tend to reduce the amount of adjustment required, compared with a design calling for simple random assignment initially.

It is not uncommon to make a "Type B" error (i.e., to fail to recognize the experiment has been successful) in evaluation research, because samples tend to be small. With small samples, we are better protected against wrongly claiming effectiveness than against missing a relatively small positive effect of intervention. Because a brief intervention is unlikely to have nearly so large an effect as do preexisting personality attributes, familial factors, and situational context, it is easy to interpret its contribution as trivial or nonexistent. There is a need to develop statistical methods that do not lead to premature nihilistic conclusions when in actuality an intervention has proved helpful.

Needed Research Tools

To study the efficacy of policies designed to prevent adverse effects of life stressors on childrens' mental health, we need at least the following tools: (1) methods whereby we can measure the psychiatric status of children prior to an intervention, at its conclusion, and following a subsequent untreated time span. That tool must assess not only the child's overall status, but those particular symptoms the intervention is supposed to relieve; (2) a method must be developed for assessing the psychiatric status of parents and siblings, so that the effect of an intervention can be distinguished from the influence of family pathology; (3) efficient methods must be devised for measuring the quality of the home environment, since this factor has been shown to be related to the outcome of the child, independent of both parental psychiatric diagnosis and the children's own psychopathology (Robins, West, Ratcliff, & Herjanic, 1978; Robins & Ratcliff, 1979); and (4) adequate methods must be developed to describe and quantify the attempted intervention.

We have been working intensively in the Department of Psychiatry at Washington University over the past few years to develop some of these requisite tools in the form of standardized interviews. There now exist interview schedules for adults and children that provide diagnoses consistent with the diagnostic criteria of the American Psychiatric Associations' *Diagnostic and Statistical Manual, Third Edition* (*DSM III*). These procedures, which can be used by lay interviewers or trained clinicians, provide for detailing whether any or all symptoms used in such diagnoses are: (1) absent; (2) of no clinical significance; (3) accounted for by substance ingestion; (4) accounted for by physical disorder; or (5) of possible psychiatric relevance. The diagnostic instruments are known as the *Diagnostic Interview Schedule* (DIS) (Robins, Helzer, Croughan, Williams, & Spitzer, 1981b) for adults, and the *Diagnostic Interview Schedule for Children* (DISC) (Conners, Herjanic, & Puig-Antich, in preparation). The DIS has been shown to be valid and reliable by test-retest comparisons of diagnoses achieved by lay interviewers with those achieved by psychiatrists administering the same schedule or supplementing the schedule with a clinical interview (Robins, Helzer, Croughan, & Ratcliff, 1981a). The DISC is in the process of being tested for its validity and reliability. We have also created an interview designed to assess the rearing environment of the child when he or she was between the ages of 6 and 13. Validity of the *Home Environment Interview* (HEI) has been tested by comparing responses of pairs of adult siblings reared together to learn how well they agree in their evaluation of the home they shared. The reliability of the instrument has been measured by test-retest comparisons based upon reinterviews of the same persons a week or two apart.

These and similar instruments serve two important purposes: first, they enable us to decide whether unwanted outcomes can be attributed to the effect of a specific stress, rather than to differences in family background and/or preexisting pathology in the child; second, they facilitate ascertainment of whether experimental interventions (that hope to prevent stress or ameliorate its effect) are comparing treated children with control children drawn from similar backgrounds and with similar initial psychiatric statuses. Additional instruments are also needed that will be sensitive indicators of short-term changes in symptoms. Finally, improved design and statistical techniques must be developed to evaluate the degree of change in symptom levels attributable to the stress or to the intervention, and to learn what aspects of the intervention are responsible for its effects.

We appear to be on the threshold of being able to measure our ability to intervene in an effort to attenuate a prospective stress experience or to generate effective treatments after a stressor has occurred. We will make more rapid strides in developing successful preventive strategies if we recognize that the development of methods to make correct assessments is as important as the accumulation of empirical data. If we can evaluate such data critically, while recognizing that our limitations in technique now hamper our ability to attribute definitively specific adverse outcomes to specific stress experiences, the experimental study of stress and coping in children can be expected to show marked advances in the decade ahead.

REFERENCES

Briscoe, D. W., Smith, J. B., & Robins, E. Divorce and psychiatric disease. *Archives of General Psychiatry*, 1973, 29, 119–125.

Brown, G. W., & Harris, T. *Social origins of depression: A study of psychiatric disorder in women*. New York: The Free Press, 1978.

Caplan, M. G., & Douglas, V. I. Incidence of parental loss in children with depressed mood. *Journal of Child Psychology and Psychiatry*, 1969, *10*, 225–232.

Conners, K., Herjanic, B., & Puig-Antich, J. *The diagnostic interview schedule for children (DISC)*. National Institute of Mental Health, in preparation.

National Center for Health Statistics. *Facts of life and death*. Washington, D.C. DHEW Pub. No (PHS), 79-1222, 1978.

Robins, L. *Deviant children grown up: A sociological and psychiatric study of sociopathic personality*. Baltimore: Williams & Wilkins, 1966. Reprinted by Robert E. Krieger, Huntington, New York, 1974.

Robins, L. Interaction of setting and predisposition in explaining novel behavior: Drug initiations before, in, and after Vietnam. In Denise Kandel (Ed.), *Longitudinal research in drug use: Empirical findings and methodological issues*. Washington: Hemisphere, 1978.

Robins, L., & Helzer, J. E. What effect did Vietnam have on veteran's mental health? In preparation.

Robins, L., Helzer, L. E., Croughan, J., & Ratcliff, K. S. The NIMH diagnostic interview schedule: Its history, characteristics, and validity. *Archives of General Psychiatry*, 1981a, *38*, 381–389.

Robins, L., Helzer, J. E., Croughan, J., Williams, J. B. W., & Spitzer, R. L. *The NIMH diagnostic interview schedule: Version III*. Public Health Service (HSS) Adm-T-42-3 (5-81, 8-81). Washington, D.C., 1981b.

Robins, L., Murphy, G. E., Woodruff, R. A., Jr., & King, L. J. The adult psychiatric status of black school boys. *Archives of General Psychiatry*, 1971, *24*, 338–345.

Robins, L., & Ratcliff, K. Risk factors in the continuation of child antisocial behaviors into adulthood. *International Journal of Mental Health*, 1979, *7*, 96–116.

Robins, L., West, P. A., Ratcliff, K. S., & Herjanic, B. M. Father's alcoholism and children's outcomes. In F. X. Seixas (Ed.), *Currents in alcoholism, Vol. IV, Psychiatric, psychological, social, and epidemiological studies*. New York: Grune & Stratton, 1978.

Tennant, C., Bebbington, P., & Hurry, J. The role of life events in depressive illness: Is there a substantial causal relation? *Psychological Medicine*, 1981, *11*, 379–389.

Tizard, B., & Hodges, J. The effect of early institutional rearing on the development of eight year old children. *Journal of Child Psychology and Psychiatry*, 1978, *19*, 99–118.

CONTRIBUTORS

Roland D. Ciaranello is professor of psychiatry and chief of the Division of Child Psychiatry and Child Development at Stanford University Medical Center. His books include *Genetic Strategies in Psychobiology and Psychiatry* (1981), and he has been published in many journals, including *Journal of Pharmacology and Experimental Therapeutics* and *Brain Research.* He has been honored with the John Merck Faculty Fellowship Award for Research in Autism and the A. E. Bennett Neuropsychiatry Award.

Norman Garmezy is professor of psychology at the University of Minnesota where he is also associated with the Institute of Child Development. He holds a Lifetime Research Career Award from the National Institute of Mental Health to continue his studies of stress-resistance in children and of children vulnerable to psychopathology. Dr. Garmezy is a member of the Institute of Medicine, National Academy of Sciences, and a Fellow of the American Academy of Arts and Sciences. He has been appointed an associate editor of the forthcoming *Journal of Development and Psychopathology* and currently serves as chair of the MacArthur Foundation's Research Network on Risk and Protective Factors in the Major Mental Disorders. In 1986 he received the Ittleson Award of the American Orthopsychiatric Association for his research with children.

Jerome Kagan is professor of human development at Harvard University. He has authored or co-authored many books, including *The Second Year* and *Infancy: Its Place in Human Development;* he co-edited *Constancy and Change in Human Development* and has been a contributing author to many volumes, including *Psychophysiological Perspectives* (1984), and *Handbook of Infant Development* (1979, 1987). Dr. Kagan has received many distinguished awards including the Hofheimer Prize for Research of the American Psychiatric Association and, in 1987, the Distinguished Scientist Award of the American Psychological Association. He is a member of the Institute of Medicine, National Academy of Sciences.

P. Herbert Leiderman is professor of psychiatry and behavioral sciences at Stanford University Medical School. He is a contributing author to *Behavioral Development*

(1981) and *Culture and Early Interactions* (1981) and has had many articles published in distinguished journals, among them, *International Journal of Behavioral Development* and *Sociological Perspectives.* He is a member of the Center for the Study of Youth and Families at Stanford University.

Seymour Levine is professor of psychiatry in the Department of Psychiatry and Behavioral Sciences at the Stanford University School of Medicine. He is the director of the Laboratory of Developmental Psychobiology. He has edited several books, including *Hormones and Behavior, Psychology of Stress,* and *Coping and Health.* He is on the editorial boards of *Behavioral Neuroscience, Psychology and Behavior,* and *Experimental and Clinical Psychiatry.* Dr. Levine received the Hofheimer Prize for Research in Psychiatry in 1961 and has been a recipient of an NIMH Career Scientist Award since 1967. He is a member of numerous societies, including the Society of Neurosciences, the Endocrine Society, and the Society for Experimental Psychology and is a Fellow of the American Psychological Association. He is a past president of the International Society of Developmental Psychobiology and is currently president-elect of the International Society for Psychoneuroendocrinology.

Lewis P. Lipsitt is professor of psychology and medical science and director of the Child Study Center at Brown University, was the founding editor of *Infant Behavior and Development,* and now co-edits the *Advances in Infancy Research* series. He is the author of numerous scientific articles on sensory and learning processes in infants and young children and on conditions that impede development or threaten the lives of children, including prenatal risk, crib death, and adolescent suicide. Dr. Lipsitt has been a Guggenheim Fellow and a Fellow at the Tavistock Institute of Human Relations and at St. Mary's Hospital, London. In 1979–80 he was a Fellow at the Center for Advanced Study in the Behavioral Sciences, Stanford, California, for which he received a James McKeen Cattell Foundation fellowship award.

Eleanor E. Maccoby is professor of psychology at Stanford University. She is author of *Social Development: Psychological Growth and the Parent-Child Relationship,* has co-authored or co-edited several other books, and has contributed to many, including *Development of Antisocial and Prosocial Behavior* and *Development during Middle Childhood: The Years from Six to Twelve.* Dr. Maccoby was awarded the Walter J. Gores Award for Excellence in Teaching in 1981, the American Educational Research Association Award for Distinguished Contributions in Educational Research in 1984, and the Award for Distinguished Scientific Contributions to Child Development, from the Society for Research in Child Development, in 1987.

Gerald R. Patterson is director and a research scientist at the Oregon Social Learning Center. His recent publications include chapters in *Development of Antisocial and Prosocial Behavior* (1986) and *Anger and Hostility in Behavioral and Cardiovascular Medicine* (1985). He has been published in distinguished journals such as

Child Development, Journal of Abnormal Child Psychology, and *Criminology.* Among his awards are the Cumulative Contribution to Research in Family Therapy Award of the American Association for Marriage and Family Therapy in 1986 and the Award for Distinguished Contributions to Family Therapy of the American Family Therapy Association in 1984. He has served on the editorial boards of the *American Journal of Family Therapy, Behavioral Assessment, International Journal of Family Counseling, Journal of Consulting and Clinical Psychology, Journal of Applied Behavior Analysis,* and *Child Development.*

Lee N. Robins is professor of psychiatry at Washington University School of Medicine. Her books include *Nature and Extent of Alcohol Problems among the Elderly* (1984), *Studying Drug Abuse* (1985), and *The Social Consequences of Psychiatric Illness* (1980). She serves on the editorial boards of *Development and Psychopathology, Advances in Adolescent Mental Health, Alcohol, Journal of Child Psychology and Psychiatry, Children and Youth Services Review,* and *Social Psychiatry.* Dr. Robins has been honored with numerous awards, among them the Rema Lapouse Award of the American Public Health Association and the Paul Hoch Award of the American Psychopathological Association.

Michael Rutter is professor of child psychiatry and honorary director, M.R.C. Child Psychiatry Unit, Institute of Psychiatry, and Honorary Consultant at Bethlem Royal and Maudsley Hospitals, London. His publications include some 27 books, 67 chapters, and 180 scientific papers. He is the European editor of the *Journal of Autism and Developmental Disorders* and is on the editorial boards of another nine journals. Dr. Rutter has been a Fellow at the Center for Advanced Study in the Behavioral Sciences at Stanford, California, a Fellow of the Royal Society, London, an Honorary Fellow of the British Psychological Society and of the American Academy of Pediatrics, and an honorary member of the American Academy of Child Psychiatry.

Julius Segal is a psychologist, author, and lecturer. At the National Institute of Mental Health he served for nearly three decades as director of the Office of Scientific Information. He is the author of six books, including *Sleep, Insomnia: The Guide for Troubled Sleepers, A Child's Journey, Growing Up Smart and Happy,* and, with Jerome Kagan, a leading textbook, *Psychology: An Introduction.* With his wife, Zelda, he writes a monthly column for *Parents* magazine, to which he is a contributing editor. He writes on mental health and human development for professional journals and major national magazines. Dr. Segal is the winner of the science writer's award of the American Psychological Association and of the American Medical Writers Association. He served on President Carter's Mental Health Commission and was awarded the Superior Service Award of the U.S. government.

Judith S. Wallerstein is executive director of the Center for the Family in Transition, Corte Madera, California, and is a senior lecturer at the School of Social

Welfare, University of California at Berkeley. She is the principal investigator of the California Children of Divorce Project and the results of her investigations have been widely published in scientific journals and lay publications. She is on the editorial boards of *Behavioral Sciences and the Law Journal, International Journal of Psychoanalytic Psychotherapy,* and *Journal of Psychotherapy and the Family.* Dr. Wallerstein has been a Fellow at the Center for Advanced Study in the Behavioral Sciences, Stanford, California, and has received the Distinguished Teaching Award of the University of California, the Koshland Award in Social Welfare of the San Francisco Foundation, and the Citation for Extraordinary Contributions to the Practice of Family Law of the Northern California Chapter of the American Academy of Matrimonial Lawyers.

ACKNOWLEDGMENTS

Roland Ciaranello

The author gratefully acknowledges the help of Norma Varon in typing and editing the manuscript. The studies described in this chapter that were conducted in the author's laboratory were funded by grants from the National Institute of Mental Health (MH-25998); from the National Science Foundation (PCM 78-14183, PCM 79-10793, and PCM 80-11525) and from the Scottish Rite Schizophrenia Research Foundation. The author is the recipient of a Research Career Development Award (Type II), MH-00219 from the NIMH.

Norman Garmezy

Preparation of this chapter was facilitated by grants from the National Institute of Mental Health (MH-33222), the William T. Grant Foundation, a Research Career Award (MH-14914), and the Spencer Foundation. Appreciation is expressed to past and present members of Project Competence, a program of research that has been underway in the Department of Psychology at the University of Minnesota for a decade. The chapter was developed while the author was a Fellow at the Center for Advanced Study in the Behavioral Sciences.

Jerome Kagan

Preparation of this chapter was supported, in part, by research grant HD-10094 from the National Institute of Child Health and Human Development, United States Public Health Service and grants from the Spencer Foundation and the Foundation for Child Development.

P. Herbert Leiderman

This chapter was completed while a member of The Stanford Center for the Study of Youth Development, Stanford University, and derived from participation in the Seminar on Stress and Coping at the Center for Advanced Study in the Behavioral Sciences, 1979–80. I want to thank Erica Leiderman for her judicious editorial comments and Deborah Lewis for coping with several drafts and the final manuscript.

Seymour Levine

The research described in this chapter that was conducted in the author's laboratory was supported by grants from the National Institute of Mental Health (MH-23645), the National Institute of Child Health and Human Development (HD-02881) and a National Institute of Mental Health Research Scientist Award (MH-19936).

Lewis Lipsitt

The author is indebted to the James McKeen Cattell Fund and Brown University for support of his sabbatical year at the Center for Advanced Study in the Behavioral Sciences, Stanford, California, and to the Harris Foundation, the William T. Grant Foundation, and the March of Dimes Birth Defects Foundation, for several years of research support relating to problems of stress in early development. While at the Center, support of the Spencer Foundation facilitated work on this chapter.

Eleanor E. Maccoby

The author gratefully aknowledges helpful comments and contributions of references by Stanford colleagues: John Flavell, Nathan Maccoby, Ellen Markman, Margaret Ellis Snow, and Richard Thompson. The research reported herein was supported by the Stanford Center for the Study of Youth Development at Stanford University.

Gerald R. Patterson

The manuscript was the outcome of a year's seminar at the Center for Advanced Study in the Behavioral Sciences. The effort was supported by stipends provided by the W. T. Grant Foundation, National Institute of Mental Health Section for Crime and Delinquency, and the Center for Advanced Study in the Behavioral Sciences. The ideas presented here reflect a general orientation that emerged during the year of study and discourse at the Center. This was brought into further focus as a result of extended discussions with my colleagues at the Oregon Social Learning Center: John Reid and Rolf Loeber.

Lee N. Robins

The research described in this chapter was supported in part by Public Health Service, National Institute of Mental Health research grants (MH-33883, MH-00334, and MH-31302).

Michael Rutter

The ideas expressed in this paper owe a great deal to the many stimulating discussions with colleagues at the Center for Advanced Study in the Behavioral Sciences during the 1979–80 year; the author thanks the Grant Foundation, the Foundation for Child Development, the Spencer Foundation, and the National Science Foundation (BNS 78-24671) for financial support. A slightly modified version of this chapter appeared in Volume 22 (1981) of the *Journal of Child Psychology and Psychiatry*.

Julius Segal

This chapter is an outgrowth of work begun while the author was a Fellow at the Center for Advanced Study in the Behavioral Sciences, Stanford, California 1979–80. Grateful acknowledgement is made of the assistance provided by Mr. Robert Isquith, of the National Institute of Mental Health (NIMH). Ms. Vivian Bauer, Ms. Lenore Gelb, Ms. Harriet Schnapper, and Mr. Phil Sharman, also of NIMH, participated as well in the preparation of this manuscript.

Judith S. Wallerstein

This paper was written during a Fellowship year at the Center for Advanced Study in the Behavioral Sciences, Stanford, California, 1979–80. Support was provided by the Spencer Foundation, the Rockefeller Foundation, and the National Institute of Mental Health. Support for the research on which this paper is based was provided by the Zellerbach Family Fund, 1971–77.

A final conference during which the work was reviewed in relation to other contributions to this volume was sponsored by the Grant Foundation at the Center for Advanced Study in the Behavioral Sciences in March of 1980.

Dr. Wallerstein is Executive Director for the Center for the Family in Transition, Corte Madera, California, which is supported by a grant from the San Francisco Foundation.

INDEX